Transnasal Systemic Medications

Transnasal Systemic Medications

Fundamentals, Developmental Concepts and Biomedical Assessments

edited by

Yie W. Chien

Controlled Drug Delivery Research Center, Rutgers University, College of Pharmacy, Busch Campus, Piscataway, New Jersey, U.S.A.

ELSEVIER
Amsterdam — Oxford — New York — Tokyo 1985

ELSEVIER SCIENCE PUBLISHERS B.V.
Molenwerf 1,
P.O. Box 211, 1000 AE Amsterdam, The Netherlands

Distributors for the United States and Canada:

ELSEVIER SCIENCE PUBLISHING COMPANY INC.
52, Vanderbilt Avenue
New York, N.Y. 10017

ISBN 0-444-42460-1

Printed in The Netherlands

Table of Contents

PREFACE

The theme for the 1984 Industrial Pharmaceutical R & D Symposium at Rutgers University, College of Pharmacy, is devoted to another new frontier: Intranasal Drug Administration for Systemic Medications. This symposium was organized with the objective of providing scientific information and technical knowhow to those interested in the fundamentals of intranasal drug administration and/or in the development of novel nasal drug delivery systems for effective administration of systemically active drugs, which are either macromolecules, such as proteins, or small molecules, such as progesterone. These drugs are either easily inactivated when taken orally, due to the extensive hepatic first-pass elimination, or too large to be absorbed efficiently via transdermal absorption. Hopefully, at the completion of this symposium, most of the participants will recognize this potential non-parenteral method of drug delivery as a viable alternative for a number of drugs that have traditionally been administered by the parenteral route.

To organize the 1984 conference with a theme as timely as Transdermal Controlled Release Medication (1982 symposium) and Oral Controlled Drug Administration (1983 symposium), a number of excellent ideas were proposed and discussed. After several brainstorming sessions over a time-span of 6 months, the merits of using the intranasal drug administration for systemic medications as the theme for 1984 symposium were increasingly recognized.

With the help of invaluable suggestions from Dr. Kenneth S. E. Su of Eli Lilly and Dr. Norman L. Henderson of Hoechst-Roussel, the list of lectures and proposed speakers was drawn up.

This 1½-day symposium consisted of 8 lectures organized in a logical format of 3 sessions. These 8 lectures were delivered by 4 academicians and 4 industrial scientists with a fine reputation in the science and the technology of intranasal drug administration for systemic medications.

Professor Donald F. Proctor of Johns Hopkins Medical Institutions, Professor John L. Colaizzi of Rutgers University and Professor Anwar A. Hussain of the University of Kentucky accepted our invitation to review the fundamentals of intranasal drug administration from the physiological, pharmacokinetic and physicochemical aspects. Dr. Kenneth S. E. Su of Eli Lilly outlined the concepts behind the development of nasal drug delivery systems. Dr. Walter Petri and Dr. Juergen Sandow of Hoechst AG in Germany, Dr. Brian H. Vickery of Syntex Research and Professor Jeffrey S. Flier of

Harvard Medical School took time out from their busy schedule to discuss their experience in the development, animal testing and clinical evaluation of nasal delivery systems. We at Controlled Drug Delivery Research Center believe we have again provided you with a valuable scientific program.

As the organizer, I wish to express my sincere thanks for the encouragement, input and support from Dean J. L. Colaizzi, Professor N. G. Lordi, Dr. N. L. Henderson and Dr. K. S. E. Su. We greatly appreciated the speakers taking the time, and in some cases coming so far, to share their scientific knowledge and technical expertise with us. We were happy to be able to welcome participants in this annual event from both the U.S.A. and other parts of the world. The able assistance of Ms. M. Boslet, Dr. D. S. T. Hsieh, Dr. Y. C. Huang, Dr. J. C. Liu, Ms. E. Skurkay, and Dr. K. Tojo is also commendable. Without their invaluable input and support, the symposium could not have been such a success.

With the cooperation of all the speakers and the able assistance of Ms. Marline Boslet, we have now completed the proceedings of the symposium. This volume contains not only the valuable scientific information presented at the conference by all the speakers, but also an up-to-date literature review on the historic development of transnasal systemic medications prepared by Dr. S. F. Chang and myself. We believe that this symposium proceedings offers a wealth of scientific documentation organized in a logical sequence, which will be useful to everyone who is interested in or working in the research and development of intranasal drug administration for systemic medications.

To provide a better definition of the objective and scope of this multidisciplinary area of R & D, we give this proceedings volume the title: Transnasal Systemic Medications.

Yie W. Chien
Controlled Drug Delivery Research Center
Rutgers - The State University of New Jersey
College of Pharmacy

WELCOMING ADDRESS

On behalf of Rutgers University, welcome to the third annual Industrial Pharmaceutical Symposium on Specialized Drug Administration. The first two symposia in this series on transdermal and oral administration of drugs were very successful and useful to all involved. Similarly, we hope and expect this third symposium on intranasal drug administration will also be valuable. We are very pleased that you are here and welcome you to New Brunswick and to this fine Hyatt Regency Hotel, and if you have an opportunity we invite you to visit our New Brunswick campuses and the College of Pharmacy in Busch Campus.

I see from the program that an exciting symposium has been assembled bringing together many of the world's experts in intranasal drug administration both from the theoretical and the practical application aspects. This is an exciting and important field where major advances are being made and an ideal area for collaborative research programs between universities and industry.

It has been my pleasure these past two years to chair the Rutgers University Committee on University-Business Cooperation. Over the past decade, Rutgers has been giving major priority to and making important progress in improving its interaction and service to industry. But in the past two years, we have planned and are establishing new interdisciplinary university-industrial research centers in biotechnology, ceramics and materials science, food technology, computer aids for industrial productivity, and hazardous and toxic substance management. Some of these ventures are being made jointly with other colleges and universities in the State but each is being designed with major input from industries including the pharmaceutical industry which is so important to New Jersey. Most importantly, the State of New Jersey through the Governor's Commission on Science and Technology is providing major support for the creation of these centers through proposal for an $80 million dollar bond issue that will be before the New Jersey voters in November, and through the proposal for the creation of a free-standing permanent commission to be operated out of the New Jersey Department of Commerce and Economic Development, which will be charged to support and oversee the operation of these centers. In addition, the University through this new program is putting major emphasis on increased service to industry in many areas, including the encouragement of more workshops and symposia such as this one, which bring researchers from universities and the various industries together to discuss and learn the latest advances in their fields.

Therefore, we are very pleased that so many distinguished pharmaceutical scientists from industry are participating in this conference today, and that so many distinguished speakers have agreed to come.

We are especially grateful to Professor Yie W. Chien and Dean John L. Colaizzi whose leadership and support have made this conference possible. We hope you enjoy the services of the Hyatt-Regency Hotel without which this conference would surely have been less enjoyable and less successful, and we offer you whatever assistance by way of travel arrangements or other help you may need to make this symposium more enjoyable.

I do hope that while you are here you will take the opportunity to visit the College of Pharmacy. The College, under Dean Colaizzi, has experienced spectacular increases in the quality of its graduate and under-graduate programs, students, and faculty. In particular, it has developed strong Ph.D. programs in the areas of pharmaceutics, pharmaceutical technology, pharmaceutical analysis, and pharmacology/toxicology. The College has splendid facilities even though it has been packed to the limit with its recent successes and expansion.

Again, I extend to you a most cordial welcome on behalf of the faculty and the administration and hope your stay will be most stimulating and productive.

Paul L. Leath
Office of Provosts at New Brunswick
Rutgers - The State University of New Jersey
June 21, 1984

INTRODUCTORY REMARKS

Welcome to the segment of the Rutgers Symposium on Intranasal Drug Administration dealing with the development and assessment of nasal drug delivery systems. The first Rutgers Industrial Pharmaceutical R & D Symposium on drug administration was held in 1982. The topic was transdermal controlled release medication. At that time, in 1982, transdermal drug delivery was in its infancy. In a short time, however, by the end of 1983, sales of transdermal devices had reached 106 million dollars. The market is continuing to grow at a rapid pace, which indicates wide acceptance of this new technology. In 1984 intranasal administration of drugs is also in its infancy. It will be interesting to see what type of market success these types of systems will achieve in the next few years.

The term "drug delivery systems" is certainly the "in" topic today. It is a term that has become an umbrella for many different topics, disciplines and activities. Unfortunately, the various disciplines under the umbrella seem to be on different wavelengths. When asked about drug delivery systems, a chemist will think of prodrugs, a biologist will think of liposomes or monoclonal antibodies, and a pharmaceutical scientist may think of some type of formulation or device. Hopefully, conferences such as this one will help to get everyone in the field of drug delivery systems on the same wavelength.

In the pharmaceutical industry the term "drug delivery systems" was first used in the late 1950's when it was recognized that the "inert" ingredients in a formulation could have an effect upon the degree and duration of drug activity. At that time, the term "drug delivery system" was probably borrowed from the vernacular of space age weapons technology to promote the idea that a formulation was a carrier which delivered a drug to the body. In that sense, drug delivery systems could be considered to be a type of systems hardware. They could also be considered "magic guns" for "magic bullets." Now, as our technology improves, drug delivery systems will be forthcoming that are a combination of hardware and software; that is, they will pull the trigger of the magic guns at the right time and place.

Drug delivery system technology certainly promoted the search for new orifices or cavities in the body. During the past few years there have been numerous publications on the use of rectal or vaginal drug delivery systems to evade first-pass metabolism effects or to avoid the gastro-intestinal inactivation of drugs. There is even a recent publication by Professor Chien on a navel delivery system. Perhaps the next Rutgers Symposium will be on implant systems, ophthalmic systems or even otic systems.

Norman L. Henderson
Hoechst-Roussel Pharmaceuticals Inc.
Somerville, New Jersey
June 21, 1984

Transnasal Systemic Medications, edited by Y.W. Chien
Elsevier Science Publishers B.V., Amsterdam, 1985 — Printed in The Netherlands

HISTORIC DEVELOPMENT OF TRANSNASAL SYSTEMIC MEDICATIONS

Y. W. CHIEN and S. F. CHANG
Controlled Drug Delivery Research Center
Rutgers University, College of Pharmacy
Piscataway, New Jersey 08854

A) Introduction

B) Cardiovascular Drugs
   1. Propranolol
   2. Nitroglycerin
   3. Hydralazine
   4. Clofilium tosylate

C) Antimicrobial Biologicals
   1. Interferon
   2. Vaccines

D) The Anterior Pituitary Hormones
   1. Growth hormone
   2. Adrenal corticotropic hormone

E) Gonadotropin-releasing Hormone
   1. Natural and synthetic LHRH
   2. Buserelin-LHRH agonist for contraception
   3. HOE471 - synthetic LHRH analog for cryptorchism
   4. Synthetic GnRH for ovulation induction
   5. Synthetic GnRH for delayed puberty
   6. Combined LHRH/clomiphene treatment for ovulation induction
   7. Nafarelin - LHRH agonist for contraception

F) The Posterior Pituitary Hormones
   1. Oxytocin
   2. Vasopressin

G) Adrenal Hormones

H) Sex Hormones

I) Pancreatic Hormone - Insulin

J) Autonomic Drugs
   1. Sympathomimetics
   2. Parasympathomimetics
   3. Parasympatholytics

K) CNS Stimulants - Cocaine

L) Prostaglandins

M) Miscellaneous Therapeutic Agents
   1. Antimicrobial & antiviral agents
   2. Histamine & antihistamines
   3. Diagnostic drugs
   4. Inorganic salts

A) INTRODUCTION

For systemic medications, drugs are administered routinely by oral and parenteral (i.v., i.m., or s.c.) routes. Recently, it was discovered that systemically active drugs can also be administered topically by transdermal administration through the intact skin to achieve a systemic effect. There are situations in which a systemic medication is required, but the parenteral administration may be either undesirable or impractical, whereas the oral administration may not be suitable, due to some potential systemic bioavailability problems associated with gastrointestinal stability and/or hepatic first-pass metabolism. In view of the vascularity underlining the nasal mucosa, possibility of bypassing the hepato-gastro-intestinal first-pass elimination, and the ease of administration, the nasal route would seem to be an ideal alternate for daily administration of some drugs.

The use of nasal route for the administration of drugs has engaged the attention of mankind since ancient times. Nasal therapy (Nasaya Karma) is a recognized form of treatment in the Ayurvedic system of Indian medicine. Psychotropic drugs and hallucinogens have been used as snuffs by the Indians in South America. In more recent years, many drugs have been demonstrated to achieve a better systemic bioavailability by self-medication through the nasal route. Nasal absorption could achieve therapeutic levels for certain drugs which require only a very small dose for biological activities. Several factors, however, need to be resolved before the intranasal route of drug administration can be considered for wider application. This chapter intends to review various classes of drugs which have been evaluated for the potential of intranasal administration, to compare the methods of application, to study its effectiveness and side effects in comparison with other routes of drug administration, i.e., i.v., i.m., s.c., oral or sublingual. Hopefully, this extensive review will be beneficial to those who are interested in the research and development of intranasal systemic medications with improved bioavailability and ease of self-medication.

B) CARDIOVASCULAR DRUGS

1. Propranolol

Propranolol, the adrenergic β-receptor blocking drug, is capable of suppressing the heart rate, contractibility, and bronchodilation as well as increasing the vasoconstriction in those vascular beds (ref. 1). It is, thus, widely used for the management of hypertension and the treatment of angina pectoris. It is usually given by mouth, but in the treatment of arrhythmias it may be given intravenously (ref. 2).

In 1970, Shand et al. (ref. 3) reported that the oral administration of propranolol in 5 human subjects yields a considerable variation in plasma drug levels. Peak plasma levels among the subjects could vary as wide as sevenfold, while the dose given intravenously to the same subjects was observed to vary only twofold. This indicated a considerable variability among individuals in the amount of drug reaching the systemic circulation by oral administration. However, the plasma levels of propranolol were seen to remain relatively constant in the subjects given the single doses repeatedly. Furthermore, the systemic bioavailability of propranolol from an oral dose (80 mg) varied from 16 to 60% of that of an i.v. dose (10 mg). The observed variability in blood levels as well as the resultant low bioavailability from the oral intake may be attributed to an extensive drug metabolism during absorption and first passage through the liver.

In order to enhance the bioavailability of propranolol and to minimize the variation in blood levels from the nonparenteral route, Hussain et al. (ref. 4) investigated the feasibility of intranasal administration of propranolol. Drug was administered in 0.1 ml of pH 7.2 isotonic buffer to the nasal cavity of Sprague-Dawley male rats (anesthetized with pentobarbital sodium), using a micropipet. They found that the blood propranolol levels following intranasal administration are identical to those by i.v. injection, whereas the oral administration resulted in considerably lower blood levels. The results also indicated that:

1) propranolol is rapidly absorbed from the nasal mucosa, the peak plasma level is attained within 5 minutes of nose drop instillation.
2) the nasal route appears to be superior than the oral route and is as effective as the intravenous route.
3) the area under the blood level curve is directly proportional to the dose administered nasally.

In 1980, Hussain et al. (ref. 5) studied the nasal absorption of propranolol from different dosage forms (solution and sustained-release formulations) in the rats, by _in situ_ nasal perfusion technique (See the chapters by Hussain et al. and by Su and Campanale in this volume), and in the dogs, by micropipet technique, respectively. The results confirmed that:

1) intranasal administration of the drug solution in both rats and dogs results in plasma drug levels similar to those of i.v. administration, whereas oral administration yields a considerably lower blood level.
2) intranasal administration of propranolol in the sustained-release formulations produces a low initial, but a prolonged blood level with the bioavailability identical to that of the intravenous administration.

3) intranasal administration of propranolol is superior to the oral route and as effective as the intravenous route.

The nasal absorption of propranolol was also evaluated in humans in comparison with intravenous and oral administrations (ref. 6). A 10 mg of propranolol HCl in 0.5 ml of 2% methylcellulose gel was administered into the nasal cavity while the subjects were in a sitting position. The results demonstrated that the serum drug level after the intranasal administration is identical to that by intravenous infusion of 10 ml propranolol HCl solution at a rate of 0.73 mg/ml, whereas the oral bioavailability of propranolol HCl in tablets, as calculated from the AUC ratio, is only 25%. The results also suggested that propranolol HCl is absorbed rapidly from the nasal mucosa. Once again, the clinical bioavailability studies confirmed the earlier observations in laboratory animals that for propranolol administration the nasal route appears to be superior than the oral route and is as effective as the intravenous route.

The nasal ciliary epithelium is known to affect the removal of dust, allergens, and microorganisms that are deposited during inhalation (See the chapter by Proctor). As propranolol is used in the chronic medication, the effects of long-term intranasal administration of propanolol on the ciliary beat frequency may be important, which was investigated recently by van de Donk and Merkus (ref. 7) in chicken embryo tracheas and human adenoid tissue. They found that 1% or 0.1% of propranolol in nose drops inversibly arrested the ciliary movement of chicken and human cilia, respectively, within 20 minutes.

2. Nitroglycerin

Nitroglycerin is the most widely used vasodilator for angina pectoris, its primary action is to induce the relaxation of both peripheral and coronary vascular smooth muscles, which thus results in a reduction of the central venous pressure, the lowering of cardiac output, a fall in the systemic arterial pressure, the decrease in both left ventricular size and cardiac stroke volume. The net effect of nitroglycerin is a reduction of myocardial oxygen consumption (ref. 8). It has been suggested that organic nitrates are inactive by oral administration, because of its almost complete destruction during a single passage through the liver (ref. 9). Alternatively, nitroglycerin (NTG) may be administered orally as sublingual tablets, topically as ointments or as transdermal patches to bypass the hepatic first-pass elimination. Intravenous NTG is useful for its rapid action, but the preparation, standardization and stabilization of such a solution have potential problems and can be rather costly.

Hill et al. (ref. 10) initiated a study to determine the time course, vascular distribution, and dose-related uptake of intranasal nitroglycerin solution. All the patients studied were scheduled for coronary artery by-pass surgery. NTG solution (0.8 mg/ml in saline) was instilled intranasally. Two experiments were performed with the first group of 5 patients receiving one ml of NTG solution, while the second group of 13 patients received, on a random basis, ½, 1, or 1½ ml of NTG solution. Plasma NTG levels were determined, using gas-liquid chromatography with electron capture detector, after extraction with n-pentane.

The highest NTG concentrations were detected in the central venous blood, followed by the arterial and peripheral venous blood. The NTG levels in the central venous blood was observed to peak at 1 minute and remained above the therapeutic level for 8 minutes. The arterial NTG levels peaked at 1-2 minutes, while the peripheral venous levels peaked at 2 minutes. In all the patients, the desired clinical effects, as indicated by the lowering of pulmonary artery pressure and/or the improvement in the S-T segment changes, were observed within 2 minutes. The results of this study, therefore, suggest that intranasal administration of NTG in solution is a rapid and convenient alternative to intranvenous injection.

The clinical effects and pharmacokinetics of nitroglycerin following intranasal administration were further studied by Hill et al. (ref. 11). The NTG solution was prepared and one ml (0.8 mg/ml) was instilled intranasally through a Teflon i.v. catheter into five patients undergoing elective coronary artery bypass surgery.

As observed earlier (ref. 10), the desired clinical effects were detected in all five patients within two minutes of administration. NTG levels were found to be at highest in the central venous blood, reaching a peak within 1-2 minutes after administration. On the other hand, the arterial and peripheral venous levels were found to be progressively lower, peaking at 1-2 and 2 min., respectively. Apparently, NTG is rapidly absorbed into the vascular space following an intranasal instillation and its time course of absorption is rather similar to a bolus intravenous injection. Blood levels were noted to decline rapidly, after the peak concentration was reached, as a monoexponential function and became barely detectable at 16 min. The apparent volume of distribution (123.5-312.5 l) was large, indicating that NTG is either stored, pooled or bound to a specific biological substance. The rates of clearance (15.8-37.2 l/min) were high and the plasma half-live (5.41-5.82 min) of NTG were similar as determined from all three sites of blood sampling.

Infrarenal aortic cross-clamp during the abdominal aortic aneurysmectomy or the aortofemoral bypass procedure has been known to increase systolic blood pressure (SBP) and pulmonary capillary wedge pressure (PCWP), to produce a little change in heart rate and a decrease in cardiac output. All these reponses are the result of a sudden increase in the after-load. The maximum rate of these hemodynamic changes was observed to occur within 1 to 3 min. after clamp. Moon et al. (ref. 12) recently used the intranasal administration of NTG to relieve the cardiovascular stress associated with the aortic cross-clamp by decreasing the arterial BP and PCWP, since intranasal NTG acts rapidly within only 2 min. Usually, 0.4 mg NTG (i.e., in 0.5 ml of the solution) was squirted into the nostril without a nasogastric tube. The results indicated that systolic BP was lowered to a near preclamp level, with only a little change in the heart rate. If the blood pressure was still high after 2 to 3 min., as compared to the preclamp level, another 0.5 ml was given and the effect seemed to last for 10 to 15 min. Intranasal NTG can also be used in many other situations during anesthesia, such as at the end of a coronary bypass operation. If the patient's BP happens to rise just before or during the transfer from the operating room to the special care unit, a small squirt in the nose could solve the problem.

3. Hydralazine

Hydralazine, 1-hydrazinophthalazine, is a vasodilator, which has been used virtually always in conjunction with other antihypertensive drugs for the treatment of essential, early malignant hypertension and hypertensive emergencies. Although hydralazine is known to be quickly and almost completely absorbed after oral administration (ref. 13, 14), its oral bioavailability is always relatively low as a result of the extensive hepatic first-pass metabolism. In order to improve the systemic bioavailability of hydralazine, Kaneo recently studied the nasal absorption of hydralazine in Sprague-Dawley male rats and the effect of surfactant and solution pH (ref. 15) using the in situ nasal perfusion technique and in vivo nasal absorption studies developed by Hirai et al. (ref. 16). As the control, hydralazine was also administered intravenously and intraduodenally for comparison.

In the in situ nasal perfusion experiments, the results indicated that hydralazine disappears from the perfusate at a first-order kinetics and the disappearance of the drug is due to the absorption through the nasal mucosa. No dependence of the nasal absorption on the initial concentration was noted at either pH 5.0 or pH 9.0. Although a good linear relationship between the absorption rate constant of hydralazine and the fraction of its undissociated species as calculated from the pka value, the classical partition theory could not be applied to the pH dependency of the drug absorption. An asymptotic minimum absorption was obtained at a solution pH that was much lower than the pka of this basic drug, suggesting that the aqueous channel could be one of the important pathways for the transport of hydralazine across the nasal mucosa (ref. 17). The absorption of hydralazine was also noted to be markedly enhanced by the surfactants, such as 0.5% polyoxyethylene-9-lauryl ether or 1.5% (30 mM) sodium glycocholate, at pH 5.0 and 9.0. These findings also suggested that the nasal absorption of hydralazine is by passive diffusion process.

The in vivo nasal absorption experiments in rats also showed that hydralazine is well absorbed through the nasal mucosa from the saline solution (pH 3.0). However, the peak plasma level was attained in 30 min., indicating that the nasal absorption is at a relatively slow rate. By increasing the pH of the drug solution to pH 6.5 or by addition of a surfactant, like 0.5% polyoxyethylene-9-lauryl ether, the nasal absorption was found to be facilitated and the plasma peak level was obtained within 10 min. after the administration.

Hydralazine was also found to be rapidly absorbed following a direct administration into the duodenum, but the plasma concentration was observed to be lower than that of the intranasal administration and its systemic bioavailability was found to be 78% of the level achieved by the intravenous administration.

The nasal bioavailability of hydralazine in pH 3.0 saline solution, pH 6.5 phosphate buffer solution, and pH 3.0 saline solution with surfactant, as calculated from the AUC ratio, was found to be 127%, 83% and 113%, respectively, of the intravenous injection.

4. Clofilium Tosylate

Clofilium tosylate, [4-(p-chlorophenyl) butyl] diethyl heptylammonium tosylate, is a newly synthesized quaternary ammonium compound with antifibrillatory activity (ref. 18, 19). The oral absorption of clofilium tosylate in rats was found to be poor (ref. 20). To improve the systemic bioavailability, Su et al. recently studied the feasibility of intranasal administration of clofilium tosylate in rats (ref. 21). Oral and intravenous administrations were also conducted for comparison.

A substantial variation in the blood levels and a low absorption rate were noted following the oral administration of [^{14}C] clofilium tosylate. The blood level of the radiolabelled clofilium tosylate after oral administration was only 1% of the level obtained from the i.v. dose, whereas the intranasal administration achieved a level which was 70% of the systemic bioavailability by intravenous injection at the same dose. However, the difference in the blood levels between the intranasal and intravenous administrations was found to be statistically insignificant ($p > 0.05$). At the nasal dose of 0.3-0.6 mg/Kg, the amount of drug absorbed was observed to be directly proportional to the dose administered in accordance with the law of diffusion. This observation is in agreement with the absorption of quaternary ammomium compound by a diffusion mechanism (ref. 22).

At the dose of 0.3 mg/Kg, the nasal bioavailability was found to be 21 folds greater than the oral absorption. The peak blood level, after the intranasal administration, was attained within 10 minutes. The results indicated that clofilium tosylate is rapidly absorbed from the nasal mucosa and the intranasal administration appears to be superior to oral administration.

Typical lesions were noted in some specimens of the nasal mucosa exposed to the low concentrations of clofilium tosylate, while only occasional epithelial cells were found necrotic with large areas of the mucosa were unaffected. There was no histological difference between the nasal mucosa exposed to the dose of 0.3 or 0.6 mg/Kg. However, necrosis of a larger area of mucosa was found to occur after exposure to a higher concentration.

One hour after the intranasal administration of clofilium tosylate, high levels of radioactivity (relative to the blood) were detected in the heart, lung, liver and kidney tissues. There was a gradual accumulation of the drug in the heart, with the peak level attained within 4-6 hours; and after 6 hours, the total activity in the heart appeared to be about 18 times greater than that in the blood. The data suggested that the [^{14}C] clofilium ion and/or its metabolite(s) tend to concentrate in the heart tissues and that the blood levels of radioactivity may not be an accurate index of the cardiac levels or biological responses (see the chapter by Su and Campanale).

C) ANTIMICROBIAL BIOLOGICALS

1. Interferon

Interferon is a proteinaceous molecule, which is produced in the body in response to the exposure to an active or inactivated virus or even certain bacteria, which enables the cells to become refractory to the infection by other viruses (ref. 23). It is species - specific and is a relatively nontoxic substance with a broad antiviral spectrum and a high therapeutic index (ref. 24). The prospects of interferon as an antiviral agent have been actively investigated since its discovery in 1957 (ref. 25). The Soviets conducted the first and only field trials of interferon in 1967 and 1969 (ref. 26, 27). During an influenza A2 epidemic involving 14,000 people, interferon was given by intranasal administration for 3-7 days. Out of the 3,129 control subjects given placebo, 551 (17.6%) became ill; On the other hand, out of the 2,994 subject treated with interferon, only 231 (7.7%) were not protected. In 1970, a small double-blind controlled trial was conducted, which was aimed for the prophylaxis of rhinovirus infections, in volunteers, using human leucocyte interferon given intranasally (ref. 28). This study failed to show any protective effect, although 180,000 units of interferon were given to each volunteer. In 1973, Merigan et al. (ref. 29) studied the inhibition of respiratory virus infection by intranasal administration of human leucocyte interferon. They applied interferon locally, so that they could take advantage of the nasal epithelial barrier to minimize the systemic availability of interferon and also avoid the possibility that the interferon might disappear rapidly from the circulation and not reach the nasal mucosa in adequate concentrations. From this study, they found that 800,000 units of human leucocyte interferon, which were given as 16 doses by nasal spray on the day before influenza challenge, could only slightly delay the onset of the influenza B infection and did not prevent the occurrence of the illness or reduce its severity. However, by using a high daily dose (14,000,000 units) and combining one day of prophylaxis with 3 days of treatment, a statistically significant decrease in the severity of symptoms and in the frequency of virus-shedding were achieved after challenging 16 volunteers with rhinovirus 4. Even with these high doses, however, interferon titers in the nasal washings never exceeded the level of 300 units/ml, which suggests the possibility of either an extensive dilution occurs or the rapid upake or destruction of interferon in the nose and/or nasopharynx. Johnson et al. (1976) reported that the intranasally applied human leucocyte interferon, at a dose of 10,000 units by a Pasteur pipette, could be recovered locally in 9 of 10 chimpanzees and 3 of 3 human volunteers tested at a rate ranging from 200 to 1,000 units (ref. 30). The amount of interferon recovered at 5 to 60 minutes after the intranasal application was only 5 to 50 folds less than the reference sample. Harmon et al. (ref. 31) reported that the human nasal epithelial cells responded equally to both leucocyte and fibroblast interferons, with development of a resistance to the virus replication that was time- and dose-dependent. In 1978, Greenberg et al. (ref. 32) compared the activity of interferon applied intranasally either in nasal drops or in a saturated cotton pledget. The nasal drops were instilled once every 5 minutes for 1 hour by a Pasteur pipette, while the saturated cotton pledget (an absorbent cotton saturated with 0.5 ml of phosphate-buffered saline containing interferon) was placed on one inferior turbinate for 1 hour. No significant reduction in the mean value of virus yield was found in the volunteers, who received 80,000 U. by nose drops. However, a significant reduction ($p<0.025$) in the mean value of virus yield was found in the cells obtained 4 hours after intranasal administration of 80,000, 50,000 or 20,000 U. of interferon by cotton pledget as well as in the volunteers taking oral antihistamines prior to receiving 80,000 U. by nose drops. These investigations suggested that nasal epithelial cells can be made antiviral *in vivo* by the intranasal administration of human leucocyte interferon and a significant antiviral activity could be achieved, depending on the method of delivery of interferon to the nasal mucosa and the extent of interferon contact with the nasal epithelial cells.

The prophylactic effect of human leucocyte interferon (HuIFN-α) at low doses against the rhinovirus infection was evaluated in human volunteers, who were given an antihistamine (chlorpheniramine) before the intranasal administration of either a single or multiple doses of HuIFN-α by saturated cotton pledget or by aerosol (ref. 33). Volunteers were then challenged with rhinovirus. The cotton pledgets were saturated with 0.5 ml of phosphate-buffered saline (PBS) containing 5×10^5 units of HuIFN-α and were then placed between the inferior and middle turbinates of each nasal cavity. For aerosol administration, a nebulizer, which sprays the aerosol at a mean particle diameter of 2 μm, was used. Totally, 1×10^6 units or 3×10^6 units of HuIFN-α was delivered in PBS (15 ml) over 1 hour. The untreated (control) volunteers inhaled a placebo aerosol, which consists of 0.3 mg of human serum albumin in each ml of PBS to make it comparable to the HuIFN-α preparation, for 1 hour. A significant improvement in the mean symptom scores was obtained only in the volunteers who received HuIFN-α by cotton pledget. No significant side effects were noted in the HuIFN-α-treated volunteers. The investigators proposed two approaches that can increase the fraction of the HuIFN-α dose in contact with the epithelial cell surfaces: administration of a highly concentrated HuIFN-α formulation, at intermittent manner, to the nasal mucosa or prolongation of the contact of nasal mucosa with a less concentrated preparation.

Recently, Scott et al. (1982) initiated a double-blind placebo-controlled study (ref. 34) and reported that repeated nasal sprays, using the Pisdon spray gun, of a purified human leucocyte interferon (2 x 10^6 U) have reduced the incidence and the severity of colds in the volunteers under the challenge with human rhinovirus 9. Interferon activity was still detectable in the nasal washings, for as long as 26 hours after the last dose, in about one half of the volunteers under active treatment.

The prophylactic effect of recombinant leucocyte A interferon (γIFN-αA) by intranasal spraying (10 x 10^6 units/day for four days) against the infection by rhinovirus Type 13 was measured in 26 volunteers in a double-blind, placebo-controlled study by Samo et al. (ref. 35) in 1983. Significant reduction was observed in the illness frequency, mean sympton scores, nasal secretion weights, and frequency of virus isolation. However, there was no significant difference in the rates of infection between γIFN-αA- and placebo-treated volunteers. In the two double-blind, placebo-controlled tolerance studies with γIFN-αA, 26% of the volunteers treated with γIFN-αA for more than five days reported some local nasal irritation with mild epistaxis and erosions of the nasal mucosae.

Recently, Hayden et al., (ref. 36) reported the human tolerance and histopathologic effects of long-term intranasal administration of interferon-α2. Using a metered-pump sprayer, 52 volunteers self-administered daily a dose of 8.4×10^6 IU HuIFN-α 2 for four weeks. HuIFN-α 2 was found to be associated with the signs of mucosal irritation (e.g. dry mucous membranes, crusts, and friability) and/or symptoms (blood-tinged mucus) in 23% of the recipients; and a moderate or marked acute epithelial inflammation with ulceration in 19% of the recipients. Additionally, pronounced submucosal lymphocytic and mononuclear cell infiltrates were found to develop in 58% of the HuIFN-α 2 recipients. Their results indicated that long-term or indefinite intranasal administration of HuIFN-α 2 at the daily dose of 8.4×10^6 I.U. is not a feasible strategy for the prophylaxis of respiratory viral infections.

Interferon therapy can also be instituted by administering an inducer rather than the interferon itself. Most inducers are complex macromolecules with formidable toxic properties (ref. 24). Poly I · Poly C (polyriboinosinic-polyribocytidylic acid), a double-stranded RNA-type synthetic interferon inducer, is an example (ref. 37). It was reported (ref. 38) to have a protective effect against the in vitro infection by respiratory viruses. Intranasal application and aerosolization of poly I. poly C in mice was found to afford a protection against pneumonia and influenza viruses (ref. 39). In the same year, Heberling et al. (1970) reported that the baboons treated with a combined intravenous and intranasal administration of polyI.poly C are protected against influenza A2/Hong Kong virus (ref. 40). Hill et al. (ref. 37) conducted a well-controlled study on the effect of intranasal polyI.polyC on upper respiratory virus. The polyI.polyC was administered intranasally to volunteers for a 7-day period, beginning one day prior to the inoculation, with 100 TCD_{50} units of rhinovirus Type 13 or 10^5 TCD_{50} units of Type A2 influenza virus/Hong Kong/68. The results indicated that:

1) no detectable toxic effect was noted
2) low-to-undetectable levels of nasal interferon were found
3) the symptoms of rhinovirus Type 13 and Type A2 influenza virus infection were reduced
4) the reduction of rhinovirus Type 13 shedding occurred in only one of the two trials, while no reduction of Type A2 influenza virus shedding was observed
5) no effect on the antibody production was detected.

However, their results were rather encouraging, since they demonstrated that the low levels of interferon induced by the intranasal administration of poly I.poly C is associated with some degree of protection against the infection by respiratory tract virus.

In 1972 Todd et al. (ref. 41) undertook the investigation to study the factors involved in the early onset of protection against the infectious bovine rhinotracheitis virus (IBR) following the intranasal administration of an avirulent strain of IBR (AV-IBR). A high level of interferon was found to develop in the nasal secretions after the nasal AV-IBR administration. The time of first appearance was noted to coincide with the time at which resistance to the virulent IBR virus challenge became evident.

Later, Gatmaitan et al. measured the nasal interferon level and activity caused by the infection with rhinovirus and assessed the effect of a chemical interferon inducer, CP-20961 [N, N- dioctadecyl- N'-N'-bis (2-hydroxylethyl)-propanediamine] by Pfizer, on the time course of viral shedding in a double-blind test (ref. 42). In six of the 11 subjects challenged with $10^{0.5}$ TCD_{50} units of rhinovirus 21, nasal interferon was produced to a level which was sufficient to inhibit the replication of rhinovirus 21 in a tissue culture. In eight of the 14 subjects, who were similarly challenged after a 24-hr treatment with CP-20961 in a nasal spray emulsion, the nasal interferon was observed to be produced 24 hours earlier with a slightly higher level. This alkyl-substituted propanediamine-type interferon inducer, if applied intranasally alone, was also found to induce interferon production in four out of 8 subject. Apparently, intranasal administration of this alkyl-substituted propanediamine can induce nasal interferon production and also enhance the production of virus-induced interferon. However, the results suggested that there is no difference in the rates of infection or the incidences of illness between the drug- and placebo-treated groups, except that the severity of the symptoms is reduced. Similar conclusions were also reached by Douglas and Betts in their investigation on the intranasal administration of CP-20,961, suspended in a vehicle consisting of equal parts of glycerin and polysorbate 80, in 29 volunteers infected with rhinovirus 13 (ref. 43).

One year later, Panusara et al. (ref. 44) followed the same treatment protocol as above, but used a modified interferon inducer preparation, in which the size of the particles in the suspension was less than 2 μm. The results showed that the treated group has produced a significantly higher level of interferon, a decrease in the virus shedding, and a marked reduction in the symptoms of the illness, as compared to the control group.

2. <u>Vaccines</u>

Vaccine is a term originally developed to designate the biological substance used in the immunization against the smallpox. It is a glycerinated suspension of the lymph tissue obtained from the vesicle of the calves following the inoculation with vaccinia or cowpox. Later, the meaning of vaccine was extended to include all the antigenic materials generated from viruses, and, in later years, to those produced by bacteria and rickettsiae as well.

1) Influenza virus vaccine

Influenza is a disease resulting from infection of the respiratory epithelium. Therefore, antibody in the respiratory tract may be important in the prevention of infection. The use of nasal route for vaccination against epidemic influenza offers several theoretical advantages as well as some disadvantages (ref. 45). Among the advantages are that the intranasal administration is both ease and comfort, low incidence of side reactions, and short duration of illness. One of the most obvious objection to the nasal vaccination is the possibility of establishing an infection, which could then be transmitted from one individual to another. It was reported that among the 11 human subjects inoculated intranasally with PR8 strain of the virus of epidemic influenza, only one shows a rise in antibody level following the intranasal administration, while none of the remaining 10 subjects exhibits any significant signs or symptoms of infection. Burnet (ref. 46) also observed that 68 to 80% of the subjects he studies do not show any significant changes in the antibody titer, following the inhalation of an "attenuated" influenza virus preparation. However, Mawson and Swan (ref. 47) demonstrated that inhalation of an active influenza virus can yield a modified form of the disease and result in a good antibody response. By using the serologically determined antibody response as a basis for comparing the effectiveness between the intranasal and subcutaneous administrations, Henle et al. (ref. 48) concluded that inhalation of an active or inactive virus, which is mostly unconcentrated, is not as effective as the vaccine by subcutaneous injection. Ouilligan and Francis (ref. 49) conducted a study in 80 children to determine the antigenic effect of inactive virus, in concentrated form, given intranasally by a single or multiple sprays. The effect was compared with subcutaneous vaccination. Each individual was sprayed with a solution of 5x dilution in each nostril for 1 minute. For subcutaneous administration, one ml solution of 40x dilution was given. The data indicated that a single intranasal inhalation of the inactivated influenza virus preparation produces a rather good antibody response and that the use of 5 daily sprays yields a slightly higher level of antibody. Comparison of the effect of 2 different doses on the sera taken 5 months after the intranasal vaccination suggested that the higher dose results in a more persistent elevation in the antibody titer. It was also found that subcutaneous vaccination produces a higher and also a more persistent level of antibody responses with a smaller dose, while only a minimal reaction is obtained following the intranasal inhalation of the combined inactivated virus. On the other hand, Beare et al. (ref. 50) discovered that the live, attenuated influenza vaccine administered intranasally yields a better protection than the intramuscular administration. Waldman and his associates (ref. 51) undertook a study to evaluate the effectiveness of a vaccine aerosol by determining the rates of infection by influenza during the epidemic in the 1967-68 winter by giving either (i) the aerosolized vaccine of inactivated influenza virus in 386 volunteers, (ii) the same vaccine given subcutaneously in 269 volunteers, or (iii) saline solution administered to 1,490 volunteers. When compared to the control, the group receiving aerosolized vaccine had a 79% fewer illness as compared to 27% in the subcutaneously immunized volunteers. In addition to its superiority in its ability to protect the volunteers against the infection by the naturally occurring influenza, the aerosolized vaccine also led to a significantly fewer incidence of side effects and to a significantly shorter duration of illness in those few who became ill.

2) Para-influenza virus vaccine

Para-influenza viruses have been known as a major cause for respiratory infections, especially in children, in whom the life-threatening infections occur in the lower respiratory tract. Wigley and his colleagues (ref. 52) initiated a study in 56 volunteers to compare the antibody responses in the serum and the respiratory secretions following the intranasal aerosol spray or subcutaneous injection of an inactivated para-influenza Type 2 vaccine. The results indicated that the neutralizing antibody levels in the nasal secretions and sputum are risen at a rate which is greater in the group of of men receiving the vaccine by nasal aerosol than in the group vaccinated by subcutaneous injection ($p<0.01$ for sputum and $p<0.05$ for nasal secretions). Both intranasal and subcutaneous groups showed a significant rise in serum antibody levels as measured by both neutralizing and hemagglutination inhibiting tests. The greater rise observed in the subcutaneous group was not statistically significantly different from the intranasal group.

3) Measles vaccine

Measles has been a serious, uncontrolled public health problem in many parts of the world. The subcutaneous or intramuscular route is generally employed for the inoculation of live measles vaccine. By these routes of inoculation, measles virus is known to uniformly induce an effective immunity in the susceptible children. Black and Sheridan (ref. 53) conducted a study to compare the effectiveness of vaccination by subcutaneous injection and other routes that might be involved in the natural transmission of the disease. A dose of 0.15 ml vaccine A (containing ~50 $TCID_{50}$ of virus) was given by subcutaneous injection to 9 seronegative subjects. Another dose of 0.2 ml vaccine A seed pool, which had a titer of 3,000 $TCID_{50}$/0.1 ml, was also given to 10 seronegative subjects. The conjunctival instillation of attenuated measles virus was carried out in two groups of 5 seronegative children each. The first group of 5 received 1 drop of vaccine A seed pool (~1,500 $TCID_{50}$) in the left conjunctival sac, while another group of 5 were inoculated with 2 drops of the vaccine B seed pool in each conjunction sac (a total of 6,000 $TCID_{50}$). The attenuated measles virus was also administered intranasally by swabbing of the anterior nares in two groups of children. The first group of 5 children was each receiving a nasal dose of 0.2 ml vaccine A seed pool (containing about 5,000 $TCID_{50}$), whereas the second group of 6 children each received about 10,000 $TCID_{50}$ of vaccine B seed pool. The results suggested that immunization by the nasal route is apparently successful in 4 out of 11 subjects (a successful rate of 36%), but as compared to the 100% successful rate by subcutaneous injection, this intranasal immunization cannot be recommended for routine use. In contrast to the shortened incubation period observed with subcutaneous injection, the subjects receiving vaccine intranasally showed an incubation period comparable to those resulted from the natural infection.

Intranasal inoculation of children with the first generation of chorioallantoic passage measles virus was reported to result in the occurrence of "vaccination measles" in about ¼ of the subjects and also produce a marked rise in the antibody titer in these children (ref. 54). With virus of the second or later genertions, the "vaccination measles" was not observed, but a rise in the antibody titer was observed in some subjects, who became immune against the natural infection. The monkeys vaccinated with the second generation of chorioallantoic passage virus by inhalation and injection methods were observed to yield a remarkable rise in the antibody titer without any clinical manifestation. McCrumb et al. (ref. 55) studied the clinical and immunologic reactions in 71 children, who had been exposed to measles vaccine propagated in canine renal cell culture. The results indicated that administration of attenuated virus intranasally in an aerosol formulation is associated with a milder response and a lower incidence of high fever as compared to the intramuscular injection or the instillation to conjunctival sacs. The observations led to the conclusion that man can be rendered immune to measles by the use of the vaccine from a live attenuated measles virus.

A group of 121 susceptible children were successfully immunized with the live attenuated measles virus vaccine by several methods (ref. 56). It was concluded that vaccination by intranasal route has the disadvantages of high reaction rate and unpredictable take-rate. Administration of a pooled human γ-globulin following the parenteral inoculation of attenuated measles virus vaccine was found to produce a marked modification of the clinically overt reaction.

The Toyoshima strain of measles virus can be serially cultivated over many generations in the amniotic cavity of a developing chick embryo (ref. 57). This long-term egg-amniotic passaged virus was employed for vaccination by inhalation method. When a definite dose (10 $TCID_{50}$ per person) or more of virus was given by nasal spray to children, mild measles-like symptoms, the so-called "vaccination measles", appeared in nearly all the children at approximately 8 to 9 days after the vaccination, and a satisfactory antibody response was observed in every subject.

The clinical and antibody responses following the inhalation of live attenuated measles virus, Sugiyama, were studied in 51 home-dwelling seronegative children (ref. 58). The seroconversion rate obtained was found to be 79% in the 19 children by inhalation, whereas 100% in the 32 children by subcutaneous injection, which are statistically significant. However, the mean CF antibody titer at one month after the vaccination was not significantly different between these two methods of vaccination. The onset of fever and rash was much delayed and scattered in a wider range in the case of inhalation as compared with that for subcutaneous injection. The mean value of maximal temperature was noticed to be somewhat higher by subcutaneous injection than by inhalation. The duration of fever and rash was not significantly different between these two groups of children.

An attempt was made by Okuno et al. (ref. 59) to develop a practical method for the use of live vaccine, which would maintain a high antibody titer following the inoculation with killed virus and would also evoke a sufficiently large antibody response. The feasibility of using inhalation method to deliver the combined vaccine of killed and live (K & L) viruses was evaluated. The results indicated that the use of combined K & L viruses causes a less clinical reaction than the live virus vaccine alone, though it does produce a fever of more than 39°C in some children. It was suggested that in practice, following two injections of killed virus vaccine, live virus vaccine should be inhaled, by which most children will be expected to gain a sufficient immunity without developing the clinical symptoms.

Russian investigators (ref. 60) reported an effective immunization of 1- to 8-year old children by exposing them, in a large tent or chamber, to the aerosol of attenuated measles vaccines. Recently, Sabin et al. (ref. 61) carried out a study to determine whether the inhalation of an aerosolized measles vaccine might provide a practical new approach to the elimination of measles in the countries, in which the measles is a serious problem during the first year of life. Inhalation of an undiluted, aerosolized measles vaccine was reportedly immunogenic in 100% of the 4-6 months old children or older with and without residual maternal antibody, when the human diploid cell (HDC) vaccine, which contains the Ikic (Edmonston-Zagreb) strain and 1% human albumin, was used. On the other hand, a smaller percentage of infants became immunogenic when receiving the chick embryo fibroblast (CEF) vaccine.

Prevaccination with the residual placentally transmitted plaque-neutralizing antibody was reported to prevent the immune responses by the subcutaneous injection of measles vaccine, but did not inhibit the immune responses by the inhalation of aerosolized vaccine. No immediate clinical reactions were observed in the 160 children who had inhaled the aerosolized vaccines, and no significant subsequent reactions were noted among the 96 children who were successfully immunized.

4) Poliovaccine

Poliovirus antibody activity has been found in the γA class of immunoglobulin in the nasal and duodenal secretions. Ogra and Karzon (ref. 62) investigated the secretory antibody responses in nasal secretions following the intranasal inoculation of large doses of inactivated poliovaccine. Six of the 8 children manifested antibody responses of varying degrees. In 7 of the eight children, no significant rise in γG level could be demonstrated. Secretory γA antibody appeared in the nasal secretions as early as 5 days after the first dose of a primary series of 3 nasal vaccine doses, and the antibody activity disappeared by 77-100 days. The responses to a secondary intranasal inoculation with an inactivated vaccine at 3 to 4 months later, although short-lived, was found to be generally similar to the primary responses.

5) Rhinovirus Type 13 vaccine

Perkins et al. (ref. 63) studied the antigenicity and protective action of the inactivated rhinovirus Type 13 vaccine, by intranasal administration, in adult male volunteers. After intranasal vaccination, fourteen of the 17 vaccinees developed a more than 4-fold increase in the antibody levels in the nasal secretions and/or serum. A significant protective effect was achieved, when the men were challenged with $10^{1.7}$-$10^{2.5}$ $TCID_{50}$ of Type 13 virus. Whereas 11 of the 13 seronegative controls became ill, only 4 of the 12 vaccinees developed illness. The difference in the rate of illness between these 2 groups was statistically significant ($p<0.05$).

6) Respiratory Syncytial virus vaccine

Respiratory syncytial (RS) virus is the most common viral agent implicated in bronchiolitis and Pneumonia in the infants and young children. Considerable efforts have been extended toward the development of a safe and effective vaccine for the prevention of clinical illness due to RS virus. Wright et al. (ref. 64) initiated a clinical evaluation, following a controlled, double-blind protocol, to assess the intercurrent illness and to detect the resistance of respiratory syncytial virus ts-1, which is a live attenuated experimental vaccine. The respiratory syncytical virus ts-1 was administered intranasally to 25 infants with 11 to 19 months of age. At the low dose (100 $TCID_{50}$), 8 of the 25 recipients were successfully infected, as determined by the virus shedding or antibody response. On the other hand, the transmission of the virus to the 9 control subjects given the placebo did not occur. However, the incidence of illness observed in the vaccinees during the trials was found to be comparable to that in the control subjects. The vaccinated children were further followed up through the subsequent natural RS virus epidemics. The results indicated that re-infection has occurred in both vaccinated and control subjects; however, there was no evidence of potentiation of the natural illness by the live attenuated RS virus vaccine. This study suggested the feasibility of using live attenuated virus vaccines by intranasal administration for prophylaxis against the viral respiratory illness.

D) THE ANTERIOR PITUITARY HORMONES

The pituitary body is known as the "master gland", because it has so many important actions in the body and it also regulates the functions of several other glands. The anterior lobe of the pituitary body is capable of producing at least six different hormones which control the functions of sex, growth, adrenal cortex, thyroid and parathyroids.

1) Growth Hormone

The growth hormone (GH) can induce growth, which results in the increase in the weight and the height of the body, affect the metabolism of protein, carbohydrates, fats and electrolytes and also exert a prominent effect on the kidney's function. Human pancreatic tumor GH-releasing factor-40 (hpGRF-40), when administered intravenously, was found to selectively stimulate the secretion of GH in the normal subjects (ref. 65) and in some of the adult patients with GH deficiency (ref. 66). HpGRF-40, if used for therapeutic purposes, may require a repeated administration of multiple doses during the day. Thus, the intranasal route of administration will obviously be more acceptable than the injection. The feasibility of intranasal administration was evaluated recently by Evans et al. by studying the effects of intranasal hpGRF-40 on GH release in six normal subjects (ref. 67). Following the intranasal administration of hpGRF-40 (30 μg/kg), serum GH levels increased significantly with the peak concentration reached within 30 minutes. Their results demonstrated that hpGRF-40 can be effectively absorbed intranasally and can significantly stimulate the release of GH from the anterior lobe of the pituitary body.

2) Adrenal Corticotropic Hormone

Adrenal corticotropic hormone (Adrenocorticotropin, Corticotropin, ACTH) is a polypeptide, which contains 39 amino acid residues and has a molecular weight of about 4,500. It maintains and controls the functions of the adrenal cortex and, thus, indirectly affects the metabolism of carbohydrates, proteins, and minerals (ref. 23). ACTH is widely used in the clinical practices for the diagnosis of various adrenal disorders and to differentiate the primary and the secondary adrenal insufficiency. It is also used in the symptomatic treatment of a variety of conditions, such as rheumatoid arthritis and asthma (ref. 68).

The nasal insufflation was applied as a method of administering ACTH, by R. W. Smith et al. (ref. 69), to observe the blood eosinopenic responses in 20 normal volunteers. In this study, lyophilized ACTH powder (Armour), at the dose of 10 or 20 mg, was delivered to the nasal membrane using a posterior pituitary powder insufflator. The eosinopenic responses to the 20 mg dose, which was administered as two divided dosages at thirty minutes apart, were found to be significant at the second hour and at maximum by the fourth hour. Local effect on the nasal membranes was characterized by only a transient mild irritatiion and a slightly burning sensation.

The clinical uses of ACTH has been limited by the fact that it could be administered only by either intramuscular or intravenous injection. Oral administration of ACTH has proved unsuccessful, because it is extensively denatured by the proteolytic enzymes in the intestinal tract (ref. 70).

As early as in 1952, Gelfand and Shearn already studied the effect of ACTH, by intranasal administration, upon the circulating eosinophils in 6 normal individuals (ref. 71). ACTH was dissolved in water or propylene glycol and dispensed by a hand nebulizer (De Vilbis No. 40) or the Vaponefrin nebulizer for nasal absorption. They observed no significant drop in the circulating eosinophils level, which suggested that ACTH is not absorbed effectively by the nasal route. On the other hand, Paulson and Nordstrom demonstrated that ACTH can be absorbed through the nasal mucosa provided a suitable preparation is used (ref. 72). A lowering of the circulating eosinophils level was achieved by daily intranasal administration with a higher dose of 30 to 50 units, which induced the remission of rheumatoid arthritis. Two years later, Mckendry et al. (ref. 73) also observed that a suitably prepared ACTH preparation, when given at 40 I.U. to the normal individuals, can be absorbed from the nasal mucosa to sufficient concentration to lower the circulating eosinophils by more than 50% and to produce a considerable increase in the urinary 17- ketosteroids.

Tetracosactrin (β^{1-24} - corticotropin) is a synthetic polypeptide, which stimulates the synthesis and release of certain adrenal steroids in man (ref.

68). Its parenteral administration has yielded an increase in the plasma cortisol levels, a rise in the excretion of 17- ketosteroids and 17-hydroxysteroids, as well as a fall in the eosinophil count and urinary sodium/potassium ratio.

Tetracosactrin has been administered to six healthy dexamethasone-suppressed subjects by nasal insufflation using a Marvic inhaler (ref. 74). A pronounced increase in the plasma level of fluorogenic corticosteroids was observed within 60 minutes following the insufflation of tetracosactrin, which suggested that this peptide is well absorbed by nasal route.

α^{1-18}-ACTH (D-Ser^{1}, Lys$^{17,\ 18}$ -α^{1-18}ACTH) is a long-acting ACTH, which has a prolonged activity, presumably due to its delayed degradation in the circulation (ref. 75). In 1969, Felber et al. studied the corticotropic action of α^{1-18}-ACTH in humans by nasal spray (ref. 76). This polypeptide was administered as a liquid suspension via a nebulizing flask and the results indicated that the rise in the plasma levels of corticosteroid occurs at all dose levels tested (0.1 mg, 0.3 mg, and 1.0 mg) and the duration of action appears to be dose-dependent. It was thus concluded that the intranasal administration of α^{1-18}-ACTH appears to be a viable means to circumvent the difficulties associated with the repeated administration by injection.

The potency and duration of adrenocorticotrophic actions of α^{1-18}-ACTH after intranasal administration were compared with intramuscular, subcutaneous and sublingual administrations in normal subjects by Keenan et al. in 1971 (ref. 75). Powdered α^{1-18}-ACTH was given in three doses. After the intranasal administration by a pressurized insufflator, the α^{1-18}-ACTH was found to be well absorbed and the mean plasma level of corticosteroids rose rapidly, reaching a peak level of 37 ± 3.7 μg/100 ml within four hours, and remained at the elevated level for about 24 hours. On the other hand, following the intramuscular injection of 1 mg α^{1-18}-ACTH, the mean plasma concentration of fluorgenic corticosteroid rose to a level of 45 ± 4.7 μg/100 ml within six hours and then returned to the baseline level after 30 hours. After the subcutaneous injection of 0.5 mg α^{1-18}-ACTH, the mean plasma corticosteroids concentration rose to a peak level of 30 ± 1.9 μg/100 ml within two hours and dropped down to the baseline values between 16 and 20 hours. However, the sublingual administration of α^{1-18}-ACTH did not produce any rise in the plasma level of corticosteroids. Side effects were not encountered during the administration of α^{1-18}-ACTH by either intranasal or intramuscular route. The results confirmed that α^{1-18}-ACTH is rapidly and effectively absorbed when administered intranasally, intramuscularly and subcutaneously, but not from the buccal mucosa. The corticotropic action of α^{1-18}-ACTH after intranasal applications by aerosol was evaluated in 14 normal volunteers by Baumann et al. in 1976 (ref. 77). In this investigation, α^{1-18}-ACTH was prepared as a suspension in the oil and administered intranasally as an aerosol by an automatic dose-controlled nebulizer. The results indicated that the plasma cortisol concentrations and the urinary levels of 17-ketogenic steroids and 17-ketosteroids rose substantially in all subjects ($p<0.001$). It becomes apparent that the intranasal administration of α^{1-18}-ACTH may provide a simple, painless and effective way to stimulate the secretion of the endogenous corticosteroids.

E) GONADOTROPIN RELEASING HORMONE

The secretion of an anterior pituitary hormone is not constant, but rather undergoes intrinsic cyclical variations. For each anterior pituitary hormone, there is one hypothalamic releasing hormone from the hypothalamus to control the intrinsic cycles by negative feedback loops. For example, the hypothalamus controls the release of luteinizing hormone (LH) and follicle-stimulating hormone (FSH) by releasing the gonadotropin-releasing hormone (GnRH), such as luteinizing hormone-releasing hormone (LHRH), to stimulate the gonadotrophs of the anterior pituitary to secrete both LH and FSH (ref. 78, 79). The exact nature and number of steps involved in the process between the interaction of LHRH with its receptors on the external membrane of the pituitary cells and ultimate release of LH and FSH into the circulation are not known (ref. 78).

1. Natural and Synthetic LHRH

The structure of LHRH, as determined from the porcine (ref. 80) and the ovine (ref. 81) hypothalamic tissues, is a decapeptide: <Glu-His-Trp-Ser-Tyr-Gly-Leu-Arg-Pro-Gly-NH_2. This structure is common to all mammalian species. The natural and synthetic LHRH was proved to share the same biological properties (ref. 82-86). The development of automatic instruments, for solid-phase peptide synthesis, and of rapid methods, for peptide purification, has led to the synthesis of several potent agonist and antagonist analogs of LHRH (ref. 78). These synthetic LHRH analogs are valuable in the diagnostic investigations of the hypothalamic-pituitary gonadal axis and have therapeutic potentials in the treatment of hypogonadotropic hypogonadism, cryptorchidism, amenorrhea, hypospermia and retarded puberty (ref. 78). The therapy calls for the administration of LHRH analogs by intravenous, intramuscular, or subcutaneous injections (ref. 78, 87). However, many studies have begun to utilize the nasal spray as the mode of drug delivery, thus providing a simple and practical means for the administration of LHRH and analogs (ref. 78). Such synthetic LHRH peptides were found effective when administered intranasally, although a much higher dose is required than the parenteral administration (ref. 78).

In 1973, London and his associates studied the hormonal responses to the intranasal administration of synthetic LHRH in five healthy male subjects (ref. 88). The LHRH (5 mg) was dissolved in 0.5 ml of either normal saline or distilled water and then placed, dropwise, into each nostril alternately over a period of 3 mins. The results indicated that the intranasal administration of LHRH produces a rise of serum gonadotrophin concentrations in a pattern similar to that following the i.v. administration of 100 μg LHRH. The maximum effect on LH was observed at a nasal dose of 2.5 mg LHRH, whereas the FSH responses were much smaller and did not display the same dose dependency as the LH.

Another study in five young healthy males with a nasal dose of 2 mg LHRH (dissolved in 0.5 ml of distilled water) by single instillation into both nostrils was reported to yield a clear increase in the LH levels in all subjects within 30 minutes. The elevated LH concentrations were observed to last for up to 180 minutes (ref. 89). A definite release of FSH was also noted in 2 subjects.

In 1973, Jeppson et al. compared the effects of LH/FSH-RH (Hoechst) by intravenous (100 μg), intranasal (2 mg) and sublingual (4 mg) in 10 amenorrhoeic women (ref. 90). All the women responded to the intranasal administration at a level similar to the intravenous injection; and the rise in the plasma levels of LH and FSH after administration by both routes was statistically significant ($0.05 > p > 0.01$). However, the sublingual administration produced no response at the 4 mg dose level.

Ten healthy volunteers, 5 males and 5 females, were administered a dose of 0.1, 0.5, 1.0 or 2.0 mg LHRH in saline, using a nasal spray (Hoechst AG) designed to deliver a quantity of 100 μl per application (ref. 91). In the male subjects, the intranasal application of 0.5 mg, 1.0 mg and 2.0 mg LHRH led to an apparent increase in the LH release in all subjects with the mean (±SEM) LH values of 13.9 (±7.4) mIU/ml, 18.4 (±6.9) mIU/ml and 30.2 (±7.3) mIU/ml, respectively. A linear dose-dependency was observed over the dose range of 0.5-2.0 mg when the net values of LH increase were calculated. However, the FSH release was not apparent in all cases. In the female subjects, the results showed only a limited success.

Mortimer et al. (ref. 87) compared the duration of action of LH/FSH-RH (Hoechst) following the intranasal, intravenous, intramuscular and subcutaneous administrations in three healthy male subjects. The results showed that 100 μg of the synthetic LH/FSH-RH given by i.v., i.m. or s.c. injection produce virtually the same amounts of LH and FSH release with identical time courses, irrespective of the routes of administration. However, the results suggested that the intranasal administration is a less reliable route than the others and is less effective in promoting the release of gonadotrophin, despite the use of a higher dose. Unfortunately, their suggestion was based on the results obtained in only two subjects and the method of intranasal application they used appeared to be both time-consuming and inconvenient (ref. 92).

Fink et al. (ref. 93) initiated a study in 5 healthy male volunteers to compare the intranasal with the intravenous administrations of LH-RH with respect to the pituitary responses and the plasma levels of releasing hormone obtained. The volunteers were administered intranasally with LHRH in 0.2 ml of saline solution (pH adjusted to 3.8-4.2), through a small graded plastic nasal catheter (Rhinyle, Ferring), 100 µg LHRH at the start of the test, 500 µg after 2 hours and 1000 µg after 4 hours. Four of them were given LHRH as a rapid intravenous injection at a weekly dose of 1, 10, or 100 µg. The results indicated that the intranasal administration of LHRH yields an increase in the plasma LH concentrations, which are dose-dependent with the peak levels reached 1 hour after the adminstration. The intravenous route was found to be approximately 100 times more effective than the intranasal route in terms of the LHRH dose necessary to achieve an LH response of similar magnitude. The investigators were convinced that the intranasal administration is a safe, rapid and convenient means for the administration of LHRH to man and seems to be an attractive alternative for long-term therapy.

The optimal dosage and the method of application of LHRH was studied by Happ et al. in 1975 (ref. 94). Nine males with idiopathic hypogonadotrophic hypogonadism were treated with synthetic GnRH (Hoechst) for 6 months. Seven of them received 200 µg by nasal spray every 2 hours, 8 times daily; the remaining 2 received 500 µg by subcutaneous injection, 3 times daily. GnRH tests (25 µg i.v.) were conducted before and during the treatment. The best result was achieved in the patient treated with intranasal GnRH, which showed a rapid increase in the basal levels of LH and FSH. The responses of LH and FSH decreased on the 2nd day and returned to the original level for FSH after 4 days and for LH after 2 weeks. The LH and FSH responses were observed to decrease with the rise in the basal Testosterone level. The researchers presumed that the success of GnRH therapy depends on the special features of gonadotrophin deficiency, rather than on the dose of GnRH.

2. Buserelin - LHRH Agonist for Contraception

Buserelin (D-Ser(TBu)^{6}-LH-RH-EA^{10}, HOE-766) is a synthetic analogue of LHRH and is a nonapeptide with the following amino acid sequence: Pyr-His-Trp-Ser-Tyr-D-Ser(t-Bu)-Leu-Arg-Pro-NH-C_2H_5 (ref. 95). It contains a t-butyl-D-serine residue, instead of a glycine at position 6, and the terminal amino group has been added an ethyl group. The biological activities of this synthetic analogue is, qualitatively, the same as the natural LHRH, but, quantitatively, it is 50-70 times more potent (ref. 95). It was originally used in the veterinary practice in stock animals to increase the rate of ovulation. Recently, this analogue was also tested for its ability to terminate the pregnancies (ref. 95).

The intravenous injection of buserelin in 4 normal male volunteers at 4-day intervals with 1.0, 2.5, 5.0, and 10.0 µg showed that a significant LH release, but no FSH release, is observed after the dose of 1.0 and 2.5 µg, while a dose-dependent increase of LH and an imposed elevation of FSH are obtained after 5.0 and 10.0 µg (ref. 96). The peak levels of LH were achieved after 30 minutes, while FSH were reached after 2 hours. This analogue produced a prolonged effect on the release of LH and FSH, which lasted for a duration of up to 8-10 hours. Following the release of LH and FSH after the doses of 5.0 and 10.0 µg buserelin, there was a late stimulating effect on the secretion of testosterone and estradiol.

The subcutaneous injection of buserelin in 16 normal cyclic women (ref. 97) yielded the results that it is approximately 40 times as effective as LHRH in stimulating the release of LH and FSH, with the serum levels reaching their maxima 4 hours after the injection of Buserelin as compared to 30-45 minutes after the administration of LHRH.

Following the 4-wk subcutaneous administration (50 ng/day) in the intact Sprague-Dawley male rats, buserelin was reported to induce "paradoxical" antifertility effects (ref. 98), whereas in the castrated male rats, the same dose of buserelin produced a direct inhibitory effect on gonadotropin secretion in the absence of gonads.

The result of subcutaneous administration of buserelin at a daily dose of 5 µg to 5 postmenopausal women for a period of 10 days demonstrated that buserelin produces a significant decrease in both the basal levels of LH and FSH and the gonadotropin responses to this LHRH agonist, while the serum estrogen level remains unchanged during the study period (ref. 99). The results suggested that buserelin could have a direct inhibitory effect at the pituitary level.

In another clinical trial, 2 groups (5 each) of normal males were received either 1.25 or 2.5 µg buserelin subcutaneously every morning at 8 a.m. over a period of 12 days, while a third group was administered 5 µg at 2-day intervals (ref. 100). After the daily administration of 1.25 or 2.5 µg, a regular increase in LH and FSH release was observed with a marked reduction of this stimulation seen in the second week. On the other hand, the administration of 5 µg in a 2-day interval produced a clear LH and FSH release.

In 1977, Wiegelman et al. (ref. 101) studied the effect of buserelin in normal men by intravenous injection (1.0, 2.5, 5, 10, and 20 µg) and intranasal administration (200, 400, and 800 µg). After the intravenous administration, the increase in LH release, with a peak level reached at 30 min., was obtained with all the dose levels administered, while the FSH release, with a peak level observed at 2 hour, was measurable only after 5, 10, and 20 µg. A dose-response relationship was established for LH release after 5 and 10 µg. The releasing effect of gonadotropin was found to last for 8 to 10 hours. After the intranasal application of buserelin in ointment formulation, the LH response was observed with a peak value being reached between 2 and 6 hour, and this stimulating effect was seen to continue for 10 hours. The FSH and testosterone responses following the intranasal application of 800 µg buserelin were similar to those after the intravenous injection of 5 µg.

The contraceptive efficacy of buserelin by intranasal administration was studied in 27 women, using a nasal spray, for 3-6 months (ref. 102), in which 13 women received a daily dose of 400 µg and other 14 women received a daily dose of 600 µg. Ovulation was successfully inhibited for all, but 2, of the 89 cycles during the treatment. Among the 27 women, 21 had shown a slight menstrual-like anovulatory bleeding during the 3-6 month trial, while the remaining 6 women were rapidly returned to amenorrhoeic ovulatory menstrual cycles after discontinuation of the treatment. This treatment was found well tolerated and capable of inhibiting the ovulation without producing any side effects. The majority of the women found that the nasal spray is very convenient and practical to use.

Bergquist et al. (1979) investigated the effects of intranasal administration of various buserelin doses on the ovulation in 39 normally ovulating women over a duration of 26-35 days (ref. 103). The nasal spray bottle can deliver a dose of 87 µg per spray application. Eight women (Group I), who were treated with a daily nasal dose of 87 or 174 µg, showed signs of follicular growth during the treatment and 6 of them were detected with a raised serum level of premenstrual progesterone. Three out of the 5 women in Group II, who were treated with a daily dose of 348 µg, had anovulatory cycles and the other two yielded a very low progesterone value. Anovulation was achieved in all but 2 of the 26 women in Group III, who received a daily nasal dose of 400 or 600 µg. All of the 39 women ovulated within 4 weeks after discontinuation of the treatment and none of them had any dysfunctional uterine bleeding. The results suggested that it might be possible to use the intranasal administration of buserelin at a daily dose of 400 µg or more to control the fertility in humans.

At almost the same time, Lemay (1979) studied the effect of buserelin after the intranasal administration of 2 doses, 500 µg each, at 8 a.m. and 5 p.m. on one day between Days 4 and 9 after the LH peak, in 6 normal women for two consecutive menstrual cycles (ref. 104). The results indicated that the luteal phase is shortened from 13.6 (±0.3) days to 10.9 (±0.3) days, while the plasma progesterone level is reduced to 61.3 (±9.2)% of the control. The data implied that the intranasal administration of buserelin can induce luteolysis and control the time for the occurrence of menses in the normal women (see the chaper by Sandow and Petri).

3. HOE471 - Synthetic LHRH Analog for Cryptorchism

Another synthetic LHRH analog, D-Leu^{6}-des-Gly^{10}-LHRH-EA^{10} (HOE471) showed a slightly less potent than the buserelin (HOE766). The intravenous injection of HOE471 was shown to be slightly more effective than the subcutaneous administration. The gonadotropin release after the intranasal administration of 50 μg HOE471 was found to be comparatively small and was approximately as effective as the subcutaneous dose of 5 μg, but lasted for about the same duration as i.v. injection with 5 μg, i.e. 7-9 hours (ref. 105). The net increase in the serum LH level produced by the intranasal administration of 50 μg HOE471 matched that by 25 μg LHRH administered intravenously. By a constant i.v. infusion of 1 μg HOE471 for 15 hours, a continuous increase of serum gonadotropins was observed with the serum LH levels reaching a plateau after 7 hours and serum FSH after 9 hours (ref. 105).

Illig et al. (1977) investigated the effect of nasal HOE471 in 84 boys with unilateral or bilateral cryptorchidism in a controlled double-blind study (ref. 106). The results of the 4-wk therapy with intranasal HOE471 in six doses daily (1.2 mg/day) indicated that the success rate does not depend upon the patient's age, but is related to the initial testicular position and is also inversely related to the percentage of testes initially not palpable. On the other hand, by intranasal administration of HOE471 (1 mg/ml) sprayed into both nostrils, 6 times daily with a total dose of 1.2 mg, to 55 boys for 4-5 weeks (ref. 107). The results suggested that the intranasal LHRH agonist is suitable for the initial treatment of cryptorchidism, since 24 of the 67 patients have achieved their testicular descent and this treatment is simple, non-invasive, painless, no adverse side effects, and does not require hospitalization.

Another trial was also conducted to evaluate the effect of intranasal administration of HOE471 (1 mg/ml, 6 times daily over a period of 4 weeks) on the plasma gonadotropins levels in the treatment of uni- or bilateral cryptorchidism (ref. 108). After 4-wk treatment with the synthetic LHRH analog, a significant increase in the basal and peak LH values was observed with a remarkable fall in the peak FSH level. This opposite effect on LH and FSH suggests the possibility of a separate regulation of the two gonadotropins. No significant increase in plasma testosterone concentration was noted after the 4-week therapy.

Happ et al. (1975) reported the effect of nasal GnRH on the maldescended testes (ref. 109). Aqueous solution of 10 μg synthetic LHRH analog (HOE471) was sprayed into each nostril, six times a day. Descensus of the testicles occurred in 16 out of 17 boys with uni- and bi-lateral cryptorchidism. No adverse side effect was observed. The researchers concluded that the LHRH analog is effective in the treatment of cryptorchidism and the administration of LHRH analog by nasal spray is of great advantage for therapy in the children. A similar study was also carried out by Illig et al. in 1977 (ref. 110). The results are outlined as follows:

			Position of testes after 4-wk therapy		
Therapy	Patients	Undescended testes before therapy	in scrotum	improved	no change
LHRH	27	38	16	14	8
placebo	26	36	1	10	25

Twenty-five boys (1-10 years old) with unilateral or bilateral cryptorchidism were treated with 200 μg of synthetic LHRH analog (Hoechst), by intranasal administration, six times a day (ref. 111). Of the 11 patients with bilateral cryptorchidism, treatment yielded a complete descent of both testes in 6 patients. Of the 14 patients with unilateral cryptorchidism, treatment was completely successful in 10 patients, partially successful in 2 patients, and unsuccessful in 2 patients. The rate of success seemed to be greater in the unilateral than in the bilateral cryptorchidism and was directly related to the stage of testicular descent before treatment, regardless of age. Before the treatment, the basal serum LH concentration in the patients was 6.6 (±1.9) mU/ml, and the patients' LH response (LH) to the synthetic LHRH analog was 7.9 (±5.0) mU/ml. The basal FSH level was 3.3 (±1.4) mU/ml and the FSH response (FSH) was 5.1 (±3.4) mU/ml. Based upon the results, Happ et al. (ref. 111) concluded that the intranasal application of the synthetic LHRH agonist, at a dosing schedule of 200 μg and six times a day, represents a harmless, convenient, and very effective

Twenty-two prepubertal children with unilateral cryptorchidism were treated with nasal spray of synthetic LHRH agonist (Hoechst AG) for 7 days (ref. 112). Nine boys insufflated 100 μg LHRH in each nostril 6 times a day (equivalent to 1200 μg/day), and the remaining 13 boys insufflated 500 μg every 12 hours (equivalent to 1000 μg/day). The intranasal treatment of these 22 cryptorchidism cases resulted in 32% of the patients achieving the descent of the testis into the scrotum. The basal levels of LH and FSH in the circulation and pituitary body were not altered after the therapy and did not differ from those of the control group. However, no correlation was found between the responses to the treatment and the bone age, basal plasma testosterone level, basal values of LH and FSH, or pituitary reserves of LH and FSH. No side effects were reported during or after the LHRH nasal spray treatment.

Recently, Zabransky reported the LHRH nasal spray treatment of 188 boys with 232 retained testes (ref. 113). A complete descension was obtained in 52% of the patients after a 4-wk therapy with LHRH nasal spray (1.2 mg/day). In another 21% of the cases, the position of the testes was improved. Only 27% of the patients showed no success. It was also reported that no side effect is detected. It was concluded that this intranasal application can be considered as the method of first choice in the hormonal treatment of undescended testes.

4. <u>Synthetic GnRH for Ovulation Induction</u>

In 1977, Potashnik et al. assessed the pituitary responses to the intranasal and intramuscular administrations of a synthetic gonadotropin-releasing hormone (GnRH) in 3 oligospermic and 2 azoospermic men (ref. 114). A 100 μg of GnRH preparation (Ayerst Laboratories) was administered intramuscularly to each patient or 3 mg of GnRH in nasal drops (500 μg/drop) were administered (three alternating drops in each nostril), using a standard nasal dropper, over a period of 2 minutes. A second nasal preparation (Ayerst Laboratories), which contains 3 mg of GnRH in a solution of natural plant gum (which, when in contact with human mucosa, becomes gel that remains in place and does not run down the throat), was administered to the two patients who had received earlier the aqueous solution. Thirty to sixty minutes following the IM injection, the peak LH values of 8.8-120 mIU/ml, which were 3 to 10 times higher than the mean basal values, were obtained. On the other hand, intranasal application of 3 mg of GnRH in the aqueous solution produced the peak LH levels of 13-31 mIU/ml, which were 5 to 8 times higher than the mean basal values, within 30 to 90 mins. The intranasal administration of 3 mg of GnRH in the natural plant gum solution produced the peak LH levels ranging from 11 to 18 mIU/ml, which were 2 to 5 times above the mean basal values at 30 min. A broader LH peak, which lasts for at least 90 min., was obtained as might be due to the gelling properties of this solution when in contact with human nasal mucosa, which produces a gradual absorption of GnRH. In three patients, the peak plasma FSH values, which ranged from 9.6 to 11.5 mIU/ml and were 2 to 3 times higher than the mean basal values, were found within 30-120 minutes after the IM injection. The peak FSH values of 7.1 - 7.4 mIU/ml, which were 2 to 3 times higher than the mean basal values, were reached within 90-120 minutes following intranasal application of GnRH in nose drops. Intranasal administration of 3 mg GnRH in natural plant gum solution produced a peak FSH level of 13 mIU/ml at 180 minutes in one patient, which remains at the peak level for at least another 120 minutes, but no response in two patients who did not respond to the IM injection. The results demonstrated that with the intranasal administration of 3 mg GnRH in either aqueous or plant gum solutions, one can obtain the pituitary LH and FSH responses similar to those achieved by IM administration. These findings, therefore, suggested that intranasal administration may have a practical application in those cases, where long-term therapy with GnRH is indicated.

The synthetic GnRH nose drops (Ayerst Laboratories) was also administered to 5 amenorrheic patients in an attempt to assess its therapeutic value in anovulatory infertility (ref. 115, 116). After the induction of follicular maturation with human menopausal gonadotropins (HMG), a total daily dose of 7.5 mg of GnRH in nose drops was self-administered at 2-hr intervals for 6 hours on 3 consecutive days. The plasma LH levels were significantly elevated in four patients over a period of at least 8 hours. After the first nasal application of GnRH, the plasma progesterone concentration increased to 9.5 ng/ml within 48 hours and continued to increase to 13.5 ng/ml on the 5th day. In three of these patients, there was a definite upward shift in the basal body temperature (BBT) curve, and uterine bleeding occurred within 6-9 days after the first dosing of GnRH. In the fourth patient, ovulation was induced as indicated by the appearance of biphasic BBT curve, the achievement of a plasma progesterone level of 13 ng/ml, and the observation of a 15-day luteal phase. On the other hand, only a borderline LH response was observed in the remaining patients. The results indicated that the nasal administration of GnRH in the form of a nose drop preparation is effective in eliciting and maintaining an elevated plasma LH level in the patients, whose follicular maturation has been induced with HMG and that this regimen can lead to the ovulation. In addition, the results also suggested that intranasal self-administration of GnRH is convenient and may provide a viable alternative for the long-term therapy with GnRH.

5. Synthetic GnRH for Delayed Puberty

Recently, Happ et al. (1980) studied the treatment of delayed puberty by intranasal administration of GnRH in 7 male patients (ref. 117). Each of the patients received a nasal dose of 200 μg GnRH, 6-8 times a day, for a period of 3-6 months. Before treatment, the serum testosterone in all patients was found to be low and at prepubertal levels, while the basal serum gonadotropins and the gonadotropin responsiveness in the GnRH tests were found to be within the adult range in most of the patients. In the two patients who are anosmic, a decreasing gonadotropin responsiveness was observed after 2-4 weeks of treatment, and no, or only transitory increase in the serum testosterone level was found. In another patient, in spite of a sustained gonadotropin responsiveness to GnRH tests throughout the treatment, no increase in the serum testosterone level was seen. In the remaining 4 patients, an increase of serum testosterone level was observed which, however, did not reach the middle of the normal adult range; and no significant effect on the clinical parameters was noticed with this GnRH therapy. The findings may be the result of the short duration of therapy as well as the change in the serum testosterone levels during the treatment.

6. Combined LHRH/Clomiphene Treatment for Ovulation Induction

LHRH has also been used in the attempt to induce ovulation in the infertile patients with persistent anovulation. Zarate et al. (ref. 118) have been able to induce the ovulation by parenteral administration of LHRH. In their study, two of the three patients treated with intravenous infusion with LHRH ovulated, and five of the ten patients treated by daily intramuscular injections showed the evidence of ovulation. Intranasal LHRH therapy with other fertility drugs, such as clomiphen, was reported to induce follicular development prior to LHRH administration (ref. 119). Successful induction of ovulation was reported in 12 of the 21 clomiphene-failed patients by LHRH infusion for 5 to 8 days after clomiphene therapy. Similar success was also obtained by using the intramuscular injections of LHRH after clomiphene therapy. Studies were also undertaken by the same investigators to evaluate the efficacy of the intranasal administration of LHRH, following the clomiphene therapy, in inducing the ovulation in 8 chronically anovulatory patients (ref. 119). Each patient received 100 mg of clomiphene citrate from Day 5 to Day 9 of a spontaneous or provera-induced cycle. Synthetic LHRH was administered intranasally (3 μg/ul in saline solution), from Day 11 to Day 14, in an attempt to induce the late follicular development and ovulation. Five of the 8 patients treated with the combination of clomiphene and nasal LHRH were ovulated, and three of them became pregnant. Of the 3 patients who remained anovulatory, two had spontaneous menses 7 to 14 days after the therapy. These patients had not had a spontaneous menstrual period for several years already. A small increase in LH level at 30 min. and a maximal response at 150 min. were observed in three patients who showed evidence of ovulation. The LH response was inadequate in the two patients who failed to ovulate. The plasma estradiol levels in three patients who ovulated were in the midfollicular phase range, while the plasma estradiol levels in those who failed to ovulate were comparable to early follicular phase levels. The study apparently demonstrated that the intranasal administration of LHRH, following clomiphene medication, can be effectively used for the induction of ovulation in chronically anovulatory patients. Besides, the ease of self-administration and the lack of side effects suggest an important role for this mode of therapy in some selected cases of infertility.

7. Nafarelin - LHRH Agonist for Contraception

Many laboratories have made attempts to synthesize analogs of LHRH with the intention to derive a more potent agonist. There was particularly noticeable for the successful development of nafarelin acetate, [6-D-(2-naphthyl)-alanine]-LHRH or [D-NaI(2)^{6}]-LHRH, which shows a biological activity of approximately 200 times the potency of LHRH (ref. 120, 121). The nasal absorption of nafarelin acetate was recently studied in 6 adult female rhesus monkeys, aiming to evaluate the effects of dose and concentration on the systemic bioavailability of nafarelin acetate by intranasal administration and to establish the nasal dose equivalent to a therapeutic subcutaneous dose (ref. 122). Approximately 100 µl of a buffered aqueous nafarelin acetate solution was sprayed into each nostril while the rhesus monkeys was held with the head in a vertical position and the body in a supine position for 5 minutes after dosing. Nasal absorption of this polypeptide was found to be rapid and very reproducible, with peak levels occurring within 15 minutes. In comparing the plasma level profiles following nasal delivery with that obtained after the subcutaneous injection, the plasma level for the 270-µg nasal dose was almost superimposable with that for the 5-µg subcutaneous dose, which gives a nasal bioavailability of about 2% relative to the subcutaneous dose. The result also agreed fairly well with the bioassay data, which indicated the minimum effective dose for the inhibition of ovulation in the female rhesus monkeys was 250 and 5 µg, respectively, for nasal spray and subcutaneous injection (ref. 120). The reason for the relatively low bioavailability of this polypeptide may be possibly due to its enzymatic degradation in the nasal membrane by, for example, the leucine amino peptidase, or some loss of the solution via postnasal drip. In these studies, a pronounced nonlinearity was observed between the doses administered and the drug levels achieved in the plasma; and this nonlinearity was noted to be associated with the changes in the absorption phase. The nonlinearity observed also appeared to be related to the concomitant increase in drug concentration in the solution administered. These observations can be explained by the increase in the flux across the nasal membrane due to the use of a higher drug concentration or the saturation of the binding sites and/or the enzyme systems in the nasal membrane (see the chapter by Vickery and his associates).

F. THE POSTERIOR PITUITARY HORMONE

1. Oxytocin

Oxytocin is synthesized in neurons in the hypothalamus. Purified oxytocin contains 500 to 600 USP units/mg (ref. 123). Oxytocin is known to stimulate the contraction of smooth muscle in the uterus and can also induce the contraction of the myoepithelial cells around the breast alveoli, thus, squeezing milk into the larger ducts and also increasing the flow through the nipple. Therefore, oxytocin is the drug of choice for the maintenance of labor once the pregnancy is at term, used to assist an ongoing abortion, utilized in the treatment of breast engorgement, or to increase milk flow to the infant.

Following the introduction of oxytocin (Extracts of posterior pituitary) in obstetrics, different concentrations and methods of administration have been used to induce and augment labor or lactation for a variety of obstetric indications. Since the oxytocin is easily destroyed in the digestive tract, it was routinely administered by parenteral route in the form of subcutaneous, intramuscular or intravenous injection or by intravenous drip.

1) Induction of labor

Uses of pituitary extracts, which contain oxytocin, were begun as early as 1911 by Hofbauer as a powerful stimulant for uterine contractions during labor, which represents an important development in modern obstetrics (ref. 124). Hofbauer discovered that the most convenient method of administering oxytocin is by subcutaneous injection. In 1920, B. T. Watson attempted to induce the labor by supplementing the well-known combination of quinine and castor oil with the hypodermatic administration of 0.5 cc pituitary extracts at 30-min. intervals until labor set in or until six doses had been given. He claimed that this technique has a successful rate of 90% in his application and yields no maternal deaths. However, it had a fetal mortality of just over 6%. In 1927, Hofbauer and Hoerner inserted a cotton pledget, which had been soaked in a solution of posterior pituitary extracts, into the nasal cavity of 80 patients (ref. 124). At the end of 1-2 hours, the pledget was withdrawn and a fresh one was applied to the opposite nostril for an identical duration. They found no marked changes in the nasal mucous membrane following the repeated applications of pituitary extracts and claimed that this intranasal administration of pituitary extracts is a safe and efficient procedure for accelerating a labor already in progress.

Morton (ref. 125) employed a combination of castor oil and quinine, intranasal administration of pituitrin (oxytocin), and artificial rupture of the membranes in an attempt to induce labor in 150 obstetric cases, whose pregnancies had progressed beyond the period of viability. The efficiency of this method was reported to be 98.7 per cent. The average duration from the rupture of the membranes to the onset of good pains was 1.81 hours for primiparas or 1.93 hours for multiparas. The average duration of labor was 9.65 hours for primiparas or 3.93 hours for multiparas, which is considerably below the averages for the labor with spontaneous onset over the same two-year period.

Bartholomerv (ref. 126) reported a method to induce labor or to combat uterine inertia using the nasal drops of pituitary extracts. He suggested the physician to instill 3 or 4 drops of the pituitary extracts into each nostril, turn the patient's head, alternately, to either sides and to compress the nostrils to improve the spreading of the solution all over the mucous membrane. A definite increase in the frequency and the strength of contractions was noticed within 5-10 minutes and persisted for 30 minutes or more.

Hendricks and Gabel (1960) evaluated the effect of a nasal synthetic oxytocin product, called syntocinon (Sandoz, Inc.) by intranasal administration in a group of 23 pregnant women (ref. 127). Among these women, 16 were at or beyond term, the remainder had pregnancy for 12 to 38 weeks. The oxytocin was administered, either by a small bottle of solution (8 I.U. oxytocin/ml) with a curved nasal dropper or a small plastic squeeze bottle (40 I.U. oxytocin/ml), into both nostrils on each application. It was found that one nasal application of 1,000 mU of oxytocin is roughly equivalent to the intramuscular administration of 50 mU. of oxytocin, which, in turn, is comparable to the intravenous infusion of 2 mU. of oxytocin per minute continuously for 5 minutes. The results indicated that only a minute fraction of the oxytocin dose administered intranasally is actually absorbed, whereas the bulk of the drug dose simply passes through the nasopharynx and is eventually swallowed by the patient. Following the intranasal administration of oxytocin, the uterine activity was usually detected to increase within 5 to 7 minutes and the peak activity was normally attained within 10 to 20 minutes, after which there usually began a slow decline toward the level of spontaneous activity. The results also indicated that the contractions stimulated by the nasal oxytocin are indistinguishable in all characteristics from the spontaneously-occurring contractions and the level of response is primarily dependent upon the sensitivity of the uterus to oxytocin.

Hendricks (ref. 128) continued the evaluations of the clinical applicability of momentary nasal exposure to the oxytocin solution, which was administered either as nasal spray or nose drops. It was found that the extent of increase in the uterine activity and the progress of actual labor are primarily dependent upon the "readiness to labor" of the uterus at the time when the labor induction is started. The results suggested that the intranasal administration of oxytocin has a high degree of safety, without the risks of excessive uterine activities or excessive tonus, and may have a great usefulness in some selected cases, where a weak stimulus to uterine contractibility is indicated.

Baumgarten and Hofhansl (ref. 129) investigated the feasibility of replacing the intravenous drip of oxytocin for labor induction by nasal spray.

The syntocinon was applied to each nostril for a duration of only a quarter of a second. Contractions were soon observed and 2-4 applications were frequently found to be sufficient to establish labor, but, in some cases, the treatment had to be repeated during the first stage of labor, and, occasionally, even until the second stage. The investigators also noted that the nasal spray method is also useful in the cases of primary and secondary inertia, even in the third stage of labor.

Baumgarten and Hofhansl (ref. 130) also used a nasal spray containing a solution of syntocinon (40 IU/ml) to determine the sensitivity of the uterus at or past term prior to the induction of labor. The test was regarded as a positive if a painful uterine contraction was felt within 5 minutes of nasal application. A single dose from the nasal spray was found to produce a uterine activity which is corresponded to 0.01 and 0.02 IU by intravenously injection. In 90 per cent of the 190 women with a positive nasal oxytocin sensitivity test, only two occasions with labor commenced within 24 hours of rupturing the forewaters. It was concluded that the nasal oxytocin sensitivity test provides a safe and reasonably accurate guide to the prospects of a patient beginning her labor.

Intranasal administration of syntocinon was also carried out in 74 cases of induced labor, 138 cases for the enhancement of labor, 39 cases for oxytocin sensitivity tests, and 15 cases for the enhancement of prelabor (ref. 131). The oxytocin was administered as a nasal spray from a small plastic squeeze bottle by a quick squeeze to both nostrils. Applications of the placebo nasal spray formulation from an otherwise identical bottle produced no alteration in uterine activity, whereas each application of oxytocin nasal spray brought about an increase in uterine activity above the previously existing level. Following the first nasal application, a rise in the uterine activity was observed at approximately 7 minutes thereafter. Following a second application 15 minutes later, the uterine activity was raised to a higher level. A small additional increment in the uterine activity was brought about after the third application 15 minutes later. Approximately at 15 minutes after the last application, the uterine activity reached the peak level, after which the uterine activity showed a gradual subsidence toward the usual baseline level and was dropped back to the original pretreatment level 30 minutes after the final dose. The oxytocin administered by nasal route was observed to be an extremely weak stimulus, the fraction of applied dose absorbed appeared to be not much more than 1-2%. However, the investigators (ref. 131) felt that the very low dose actually delivered systemically is the greatest strength of this method of administration. This method of intranasal administration can be especially useful in enhancing the uterine activity during the inertial periods in labor, in inducing labor when combined with anmiotomy, as well as in the oxytocin sensitivity test.

A study on the safety and effectiveness of nasal oxytocin was conducted in 1000 patients by Clement et al. in 1962 (ref. 132). The oxytocin solution was instilled directly into each nostril using a standard tuberculin syringe and a 25G needle. An initial dose of 0.5 minim was delivered, followed by a one minim dose in each nostril at 15 to 20 minute intervals for as long as necessary to maintain a satisfactory uterine contraction, unless contraindications to its use arose. The effectiveness for the elective induction of labor with nasal oxytocin was 91.5% in 47 primiparas and 79.4% in 184 multiparas. Induction for medical reasons was successful in 85.6% of the 14 primiparas and in 94.4% of 36 multiparas. From the data presented, the intranasal administration of oxytocin appears to offer a satisfactory method for the induction of labor and/or the stimulation of uterine contractions. Besides, the margin of safety for the intranasal oxytocin administration was noted to be considerably greater than the intravenous route of oxytocin delivery. In approximately the same time, Borglin (ref. 133) also made comparative studies on the effectiveness of oxytocin in the induction and stimulation of labor by intranasal and intravenous drip administrations. Oxytocin drip was given in 5.5% glucose solution (1 IU/100 ml) through the cubital or forearm vein, while nasal oxytocin solution (100 IU/ml) was given to 96 women at a dose of 5-40 IU through a polyethylene tube. The patients were instructed to blow the entire nasal dose into one of the nasal cavities and this intranasal administration was usually terminated before the child was delivered. The data indicated that the intranasal administration of oxytocin produces a rapid and reliable effect in inducing or stimulating labor with a successful rate of 88.5%, which is as good as that obtained by intravenous drip (90.9%). In this series of studies, complications were found equally common in both routes, but were less severe in the group that received the hormone by intravenous drip, whereas no fetal deaths occurred in the group that received oxytocin intranasally. The investigator thus concluded that the intranasal application of oxytocin is a simple, practical and convenient method to patients.

The efficacy of oxytocin delivered by nasal spray or intravenous injection in the induction or stimulation of labor, as measured by uterine contractility, was compared in 15 pregnant women at or near term (ref. 134). One nasal spray delivered 500 to 800 mU of oxytocin to each nostril, which produced uterine responses within 6 minutes with magnitude equivalent to the intravenous infusion of 0.7 mU/min. of oxytocin continuously for 15 minutes. Application of second spray achieved a response which is approximately equal to the response resulted from the intravenous infusion of 1.5 mU/min. of oxytocin continuously for 15 minutes.

Hinde (ref. 135) reported the results and clinical impression on the intranasal administration of oxytocin in 109 obstetrics cases. The oxytocin was administered from a 5 ml plastic bottle, which delivered a spray of 2.5 IU of oxytocin by directly squeezing the container. The investigator described his clinical impression as that the intranasal administration is as efficacious as the intramuscular injection, but is much safer. He also suggested that oxytocin nasal spray should replace the intramuscular injection for the induction of labor and it is useful in the case of inertia labor, as an adjuvant to the artificial rupture of the membranes during the induction of labor, or as a form of medical induction of labor in the case when the cervical conditions are not favorable.

Intranasal administration of oxytocin by an aerosol-activated spray was studied to evaluate its efficacy and safety using the technique of continuous recordings of the amniotic fluid pressure (ref. 136). The aerosol-activated spray was calibrated to release 1 IU (±10%) of syntocinon with each depression of the triggering device. A nasal dose of 2 (±0.2) IU was applied to each nostril on each emission. Each patient received 1-8 emissions at intervals varying from 15 minutes to 1 hour. The level of uterine activity achieved with the intranasal oxytocin of 2 IU was most often found to be approximated to the intravenous infusion of 2 mU/min of oxytocin over a 10-min. period, or a total dose of 20 mU. The data, therefore, suggested that approximately 1 per cent of the nasal oxytocin dose administered by the aerosol spray is actually absorbed. This weak stimulus to uterine contractility, due to the limited absorption by the nasal mucous membrane, was often desirable in the obstetric condition, which require only a minimal enhancement of the uterine contractility. Repeated applications of the nasal oxytocin aerosol spray were noted to produce, in some patients, an increase in lacrimation and rhinorrhea. A considerable variation in the responses to intranasal administration of oxytocin was detected in the individual patient and some undesirable stimulation of the uterine activity was also noted.

Talledo et al. (ref. 137) designed a study to evaluate the uterine responses, as measured by the changes in the intra-amniotic pressure, to the intranasal administration of oxytocin in 15 pregnant women at term. None of the subjects was in labor and all had intact membranes. The oxytocin was given intranasally, using a tuberculin syringe and a 26G needle, at an applied dose of 0.5 to 2.0 minim in each nostril (which was equivalent to 666 to 2,664 mU). After intranasal application, the initial uterine response appeared, generally, in 5-7 min. and the duration of this response varied from 15 minutes to one hour. The levels of uterine response were found to be comparable to that achieved by an intravenous infusion of oxytocin at a rate of 2 mU/min. The investigators concluded that the unpredicability of the amount absorbed and the uterine response makes this intranasal route of application relatively unsafe. Thus, they did not recommend the routine uses of oxytocin by intranasal administration in the management of pregnant patient.

The safety of an oxytocin-nasal spray was evaluated in 102 patients by Bradfield in 1965 (ref. 138). The oxytocin was applied from a "squeeze bottle", each contains 5 ml. of solution (40 IU/ml), and a single sharp spray of the solution delivered 1.9-3.8 IU. The efficacy of the spray in labor induction was confirmed, but the investigator commented that the nasal spray in its present form lacks the precision needed; and, in the complicated pregnancy, the intravenous infusion of oxytocin at controlled rate is preferable. The clinical effectiveness of oxytocin nasal spray was further evaluated in a group of 39 pregnant women for the induction and enhancement of labor (ref. 139). It was found that this method of oxytocin administration is particularly successful in the induction of labor in those women whose membranes have already been ruptured, but it is also worth using in the cases with an unruptured membrane, since it may bring about the ripening of the cervix.

In 1967, Gent et al. (ref. 140) used another nasal oxytocin product, called Partocon (Ferring AB), in 22 pregnant patients to induce labor while measuring the intra-uterine pressure through a saline-filled vinyl catheter introduced transabdominally. Partocon is a 2-ml bottle, which contains oxytocin solution (100 IU/ml), supplied with a rhinyle, which is a plastic application tube with a graduation of 0.05, 0.1, and 0.2 ml. The patient was asked to blow the content in the rhinyle into the nose. An enhanced uterine activity became visible within 5-6 min. after dosing. The duration of uterine activity after the first dose lasted about 20 minutes; after which the level of activity following an additional dose generally remained higher than the level achieved with the first dose.

A comparative study was conducted to evaluate the effectiveness, safety and convenience of oxytocin administration by the intravenous, intranasal and transbuccal routes (ref. 141). The study involved 300 consecutive cases of attempted labor induction, with 100 cases for each route of administration. Intravenous injection was done as a drip infusion of 5 IU of oxytocin (syntocinon®). Intranasal administration was carried out by a spray arrangement, which deposits 100 IU/ml of oxytocin (partocon®) in the nasal cavity. Transbuccal oxytocin was given in tablets, which contains 100 IU of oxytocin (Syntocinon®). The tablet was placed in the buccal sulcus, alternatively, on either the right or left side at an interval of every 30 min. until, at most, all 8 doses had been administered. The results indicated that no substantial difference in the degree of safety is found among the three methods of administration. Neither maternal death nor rupture of the uterus was reported. The rates of success for the intravenous and transbuccal administrations were practically the same, whereas the rate for intranasal route was somewhat lower. Among these 3 routes of administration, the transbuccal method was considered to be most convenient to the patient and the medical staff.

DeVoe et al. (1967) studied the safety and the effect of nasal oxytocin on the pregnant uterus using a continuous recording of amniotic fluid pressure (ref. 142). Twenty-six patients received intranasal administration of synthetic oxytocin by nasal spray from a plastic squeeze bottle. Eleven of these patients were given one nasal application and then an intravenous infusion of oxytocin at a later time for comparison of the responses. The remaining 15 patients received one nasal application at 20-min interval. Another 15 patients with spontaneous labor were also recorded as the control. After the application of nasal oxytocin, there was an increase in the uterine activity, which occurred at an average rate of 9 minutes. This increased activity was noted in both the intensity and the frequency of contractions, and was associated with a better coordination of the contractions. In most instances, the maximum effect was attained within 10-15 minutes. One spray of nasal oxytocin into each nostril every 20 minutes gave essentially the same level of responses as an intravenous infusion of 1-2 mU/min of oxytocin. The observations led to the conclusion that intranasal administration of oxytocin can be safely used as a gentle stimulus to the antepartum uterus.

Bergsjo and Jenssen (1969) reported the results of a controlled clinical trial comparing a nasal and a buccal oxytocin preparations in the induction of labor (ref. 143). The subjects comprised of 110 primiparae and 12 multiparae. The nasal oxytocin (Partocon/Ferring) was administered through a graded polyethylene tube at a dosing interval of 5 IU/15 min. The buccal oxytocin (Pitocin/Park Davis) was given in buccal tablet at a dosing interval of 100 IU/30 min. The total dose of oxytocin administered nasally and buccally was 260 and 4,200 IU, respectively. The data revealed no significant difference in the rates of success between nasal and buccal routes in the induction of labor. However, the nasal oxytocin was observed to produce an immediate response and trigger off the labor at a rate faster than the buccal oxytocin, whereas the buccal oxytocin initiated a higher proportion of labor in the later hour.

The effect of intranasal and transbuccal administrations of oxytocin on the induction of labor was also compared in 468 women without a ruptured membrane (ref. 144). For comparison, 128 intranasal and 123 transbuccal inductions were studied in parallel. In the transbuccal group, 39 patients received a dose of 50 IU oxytocin [Syntocinon/Sandoz] and 84 patients were given 100 IU of oxytocin. (Another 217 women were also induced by the transbuccal administration of 100 IU of oxytocin.) In the intranasal group, oxytocin was administered as a solution (100 IU/ml of oxytocin, Partocon/Ferring). With the dose levels used, the results were found to be in agreement with the data by Muller and Osler (ref. 141). Overall, 54-64% were successfully delivered by transbuccal administration as compared with 43% in the intranasal group. It was concluded that the administration of oxytocin by intranasal and transbuccal routes is simple and produces, at most, some minor discomfort. And, there was no obvious difference between intranasal and transbuccal administrations.

Laine reviewed in 1970 a clinical trial comparing the intranasal, transbuccal and intravenous administrations of oxytocin in 445 cases of labor induction (ref. 145). The average oxytocin doses for P.I.N. (Partocon IN® solution/Ferring), S.B. (Syntocinon Buccal® tablets/Sandoz), and S.I.V. (Syntocinon® i.v. infusion/Sandoz) were 175, 1916 and 3.8 IU, respectively, for the total series. A fairly satisfactory result was achieved with all these three methods of administration. The percentage of successful induction in the P.I.N. group, S.B. group and S.I.V. group was 79%, 75% and 67%, respectively. The intranasal preparation (Partocon IN®) appeared to be a little more effective than the other preparations. It was concluded that the intranasal, transbuccal and intravenous oxytocin are all good tools for the obstetrician provided that the indications for induction are carefully considered, the patient's readiness for induction is observed cautiously, the timing is correct, and the procedure is closely supervised.

Hoover (1971) reported a study on the safety of intranasal oxytocin in 1,806 patients (ref. 146). Of these patients, 75% received intranasal oxytocin for elective stimulation of labor or stimulation of prolonged labor. The remaining 25% of the patients elected for induction of labor. Oxytocin solution (10 IU/ml) was administered by a glass or plastic dropper with each drop containing 0.4 to 0.8 IU of oxytocin. Initially, 1-2 drops were applied as the test dose and then 2-4 drops were administered at 15-20 minute intervals for a total of 8 to 9 doses. Among the 449 cases of labor induction, 366 received intranasal oxytocin only, 60 received a combination of intranasal and intramuscular oxytocin, and 23 received a combination of intranasal and intravenous oxytocin. A total successful rate of 88 per cent was obtained with an overall cesarean rate of only 1.5 percent; and no major maternal complications was noted.

2) Stimulation of lactation

Oxytocin induces not only the contraction of myometrium, but also the contraction of myoepithelial cells in the breast. The contraction results in an increase in the intramammary pressure [IMP], which is followed by "milk ejection" (ref. 147). The smooth course of breast feeding is dependent upon adequate function of the let-down reflex (ref. 148). Stimulation of the nipple in the lactating woman results in the release of an oxytocic factor into the blood stream through the mediation of the central nervous system and the posterior lobe of the pituitary gland. This factor then acts on the myoepithelial elements surrounding the alveoli of the breast, causing them to contract and force milk into the larger ducts, where it becomes readily available to the baby. As early as in 1958, Newton and Egli already demonstrated the artificial production of the let-down (ejection) reflex by intranasal administration of oxytocin during early lactation (ref. 148). Their results indicated that application of 0.5-1.0c.c. of oxytocin produces a significant increase in the flow of milk, suggesting that let-down has occurred and oxytocin has been absorbed from the nasal mucosa. It was recommended that intranasal application of 0.5 to 1.0 c.c. of oxytocin, given about 5 minutes before a breast feeding, may help the mother overcome the inhibition of let-down reflex.

Wenner (1959) also reported a good galactokinetic (milk let-down) effect by the nasal spray of synthetic oxytocin (Syntocinone®) (ref. 149). Generally, 3-4 IU of oxytocin were found sufficient and should be administered 5 minutes before a breast feeding.

The efficacy of oxytocin nasal spray (Syntocinon®) in stimulating milk ejection from the parturient engorged breast was reported by Stewart and Nelson (ref. 150). The results on the milk-letdown phenomenon in the nursing or nonnursing mothers demonstrated that the intranasal administration of oxytocin is of value in the stimulation of breast secretion, although it is perhaps not quite as efficient as the intramuscular route.

Hollenbach (1960) investigated the effects of nasal spray of synthetic oxytocin (Syntocinon®) in 351 patients and found that it is as effective as parenteral administration (ref. 151). It was estimated that about 4-5 units of oxytocin are delivered when the vaporizer is compressed for 1 second. Whenever a patient required this "milk ejection hormone", a unilateral nasal spray was applied just before a feeding was due. Hollenbach noted that oxytocin helps to relieve the painful tension due to engorgement of the breast and also diminish the trauma on the nipple by reducing the duration of the feeding.

Berde and Cerletti (1960) studied the effect of variation in the applied dose of synthetic oxytocin (Syntocinon®) on the lactating mammary gland of the rabbits (ref. 152). Oxytocin was given by intranasal administration, intramuscular injection or intravenous infusion. It was found that it needs approximately 1.5 to 8.0 times as much by intramuscular injection and approximately 10 to 100 times as much by intranasal administration to elicit the responses with intensity and character approximately identical to those produced by intravenous infusion.

A series of double-blind, controlled and randomized studies were conducted by Friedman and Sachtleben (1961) to determine the effect of synthetic oxytocin, administered in nasal spray or sublingual tablet, on the initiation, enhancement, and maintenance of the early phase of lactation (ref. 153). The nasal preparation was applied by self-administration as a short, firm spray (0.3-0.6 ml, or 12-24 IU) just before the feeding (usually about 5 minutes). The sublingual tablet was allowed to dissolve sublingually, usually beginning within 20 minutes before the feeding. The nasal spray produced a very rapid, high intensity and short-lived milk-ejection response. Major response was seen in about 2 minutes, reached an extremely high peak of pressure, and lasted for a variable length of time (which usually does not exceed 2 minutes). Following this intensive reaction, no further activity could be elicited again by any means, indicating the existence of an inhibitory effect, which perhaps accounts for the clinical ineffectiveness of this intranasal administration. On the other hand, the oxytocin, administered as a sublingual (10 IU) tablet prior to a feeding, was found to produce a prompt initiation of lactation, as demonstrated by a significantly greater amount of milk delivered to the newborn. However, this effect was not increased by a ten-fold increase in the dosage (100 IU), nor by the addition of hyaluronidase to aid sublingual absorption. It was thus concluded that the nasal spray give only a short-acting, quickly-dispelled actuation, whereas the sublingual tablet produces a prolonged, low-dosage stimulation.

In a group of 24 patients to whom oxytocin (Syntocinon®) was administered using a nasal spray was compared with another group of 24 patients who received a placebo only (ref. 154). By depressing the nozzle, the patient inhaled 4-5 IU of synthetic oxytocin. The nasal spray was noted to produce an early establishment of breast-feeding and also an improvement of milk production. No significant difference was detected in the incidence of early breast engorgement between the treated and control groups. No serious side-effects were noted.

Heckmann (1961) reported his clinical experiences with intranasal administration of oxytocin in 125 women, who were treated with the nasal spray of oxytocin between the second and eleventh day of the puerperium (ref.

155). Another 106 untreated women were used as the controls. It was found that the spray causes a moderate increase in the milk yield in 86% of the subjects, a great rise in the output in 13% and no effect in 1%. Measurement of the total milk output between the fourth and eighth day of the puerperium showed that in 80% of the patients, the oxytocin nasal spray produces an increase in the yield which exceeds the yield in the normal controls for up to a maximum of 26 percent. It was also noted that under the influence of oxytocin, an apparently empty breast can still produce 30-80% of the previous milk output.

Sandholm (1968) recorded the intramammary pressure (IMP) in 18 lactating women on the fourth day of the puerperium (ref. 147). Three patients were given oxytocin intranasally in Partocon® (Ferring AB) at doses of 2.5, 1.25 and 0.625 IU in order to establish the smallest dose required to produce an increase in the IMP. In another 15 patients, the IMP was first measured for a few minutes and then oxytocin was infused intravenously at a rate of 5 mU/min. After the intranasal administration of oxytocin, the IMP showed an increase within 1-1.5 minutes, which persisted for 10-20 minutes. The minimal nasal oxytocin dose needed to produce an effect on the IMP was determined to be 1-2 IU. The effect of oxytocin at a nasal dose of 5 IU was found to last for about 10 minutes, while 10-20 IU persisted for up to 20 minutes. It was also noticed that the nasal dose of oxytocin required is about 100 times greater than the dose needed by intravenous infusion to produce a comparable effect.

3) Secretion of insulin and glucagon

The effectiveness of oxytocin to evoke the secretions of insulin and glucagon by the nasal route of administration was recently studied by Altszuler and Hampshire in 1981 (ref. 156). Oxytocin (1.5-2.0 IU/kg) was given intranasally to 8 normal, conscious dogs by dropper from a stock solution of 180 IU/ml. The same volume (0.2 ml) of saline solution was administered to the control animals. 50 and 500 μU/kg/min of oxytocin was also infused intravenously to another group of 8 dogs. Intranasal instillation of oxytocin was observed to produce a prompt and striking increase in all the measurements of glucose, insulin and glucagon in the plasma, whereas similar instillation of saline yielded no effects. Intravenous infusion of oxytocin also produced a prompt, modest rise in the plasma glucose level and a significant rise in the plasma concentrations of insulin and glucagon. Following the intranasal instillation of 1.5-2.0 IU/kg of oxytocin, the effects on the plasma levels of glucose, insulin and glucagon were somewhat greater than those observed with the intravenous infusion of oxytocin at 500 μU/kg/min. No unwanted side effects of oxytocin were evident with the administration by either routes.

2. Vasopressin

Vasopressin is synthesized in neurons in the hypothalamus (ref. 157). Human and most mammalian vasopressin, called arginine vasopressin, is a polypeptide with peptide chain of:

Cys-Tyr-Phe-Glu (NH_2)-Asp (NH_2)-Cys-Pro-Arg-Gly (NH_2)

It is usually named antidiuretic hormone (ADH). Lysine vasopressin is another naturally-occurring antidiuretic peptide, which is presented in the pig and related species.

Vasopressin promotes water retention, but also increases the excretion of sodium and chloride. When there is a defect in the hypothalamicopituitary secretion of ADH, diabetes insipidus develops. Polyuria and polydipsia are the major symptoms. The long-term treatment of diabetes insipidus has been either the intramuscular injection of Pitressin® tannate in peanut oil (Parke-Davis) or the nasal insufflation of crude posterior pituitary powder (5-20 USP units, 3 or more times a day)(ref. 158). The use of Pitressin tannate has been reported to yield a water retention and allergic reactions to the oil and the peptide (ref. 158), whereas the posterior pituitary snuff has the disadvantages of requiring frequent administration as well as uncertain action, and in some patients it even produces nasal irritation (ref. 158), asthma (ref. 159) or pulmonary fibrosis (ref. 160).

Recently, Blumgart (1982) reported the use of posterior pituitary extract powder sprayed intranasally in the treatment of polyuria and polydipsia and found that intranasal administration is as effective as parenteral administration (ref. 161).

1) Lypressin - A synthetic vasopressin analogue

The possibility of vasopressin synthesis has led to the commercialization of a nasal spray containing synthetic lysine-8-vasopressin (Lypressin). Such a preparation proved effective in the patients with diabetes insipidus, who experience a generalized allergic reaction to the natural hormone (ref. 162, 163). As early as in 1963, Barltrop already demonstrated that administration of lypressin by intramuscular or nasal routes can effectively control the insipidus in 9 young child subjects (ref. 164). With a lypressin dose of 14 units t.d.s. given intranasally for over a 6-month period can control the diabetes insipidus, whereas intramuscular administration of lypressin can control the urine output at a dose of 5 units every 8 hours.

Fraser and Scott (1963) evaluated the nasal spray of lypressin (Diapid®/Sandoz) in 8 patients with diabetes insipidus, 6 of them were developed from a complication of pituitary implant for breast carcinoma or diabetic retinopathy (ref. 158). It was found that the optimal dose is two nasal sprayings for each nostril. Since the effect of a single dose lasted anywhere from 3 to 5 hours, mild cases required only 3 intranasal applications a day, while severe cases needed up to 7 applications daily. The results indicated that the nasal spray of lypressin yields a complete control of the diabetes insipidus of moderate severity and partial control of the severe cases.

Sjöberg and Luft (1963) also found lypressin to be effective, following the administration by nasal spray, in 3 female and 5 male patients with verified diabetes insipidus (ref. 165). It was reported that in 7 of the 8 patients, the nasal lypressin spray can replace pitressin tannate, and the patients have been effectively maintained on nasal regimen from one month to more than a year. In all cases, the urine volume became normal after nasal spraying 3 to 7 times a day. Seven of the 8 patients appeared to be satisfied with the nasal spray treatment. Only one of the 8 patients developed a nasal congestion and ulceration of the nasal mucosa, the treatment was thus discontinued (ref. 166). It was concluded that satisfactory control of diabetes insipidus can be obtained by intranasal administration of synthetic lysine-8-vasopressin (lypressin) in nasal spray, and that this form of administration is preferred by many patients.

Additional 13 patients with diabetes insipidus were again satisfactorily and conveniently treated with the nasal spray of lypressin (ref. 167). The nasal spray was applied to the patients 3 to 5 times a day, which yielded a total daily dosage of 35 to 125 units with a mean of 69 units. The vasopressin administered in this way was reportedly effective in reducing the urine volume and increasing the concentration to a normal range. The only adverse effects of the nasal spray were observed to consist of minor nasal irritation in 3 patients. On the other hand, it was reported that lypressin administered subcutaneously is 7.4 times as effective as the nasal spray preparation.

The effectiveness of a nasal spray containing the synthetic lysine-8-vasopressin was also studied in 19 patients with diabetes insipidus by Dashe et al. (ref. 168). Three patients were evaluated in a controlled environment with concurrent plasma vasopressin recovery studies. The lypressin was administered nasally by a squeeze bottle container. Following the administration, there was a slow appearance and peaking of vasopressin concentration in the plasma with detectable vasopressin level for at least 2 hours in 10 patients. Also, a concomitant fall in the urine volume and an elevation of urinary osmolality was observed. Nasal spray of lypressin was found to be remarkably free from any side effects and cleared from the plasma rapidly. The plasma profiles were coincide with the clinical effect, which was only transient (3 to 5 hours). The results suggested that lypressin administered by nasal spray is an effective, rapidly absorbed, apparently nonsensitizing, and nonirritating material, which could be useful in the management of vasopressin-sensitive diabetes insipidus.

Dingman and Hauger-Klevene (1964) reported the usefulness of lypressin nasal solution (8 LVP spray/Sandoz) in the management of 20 patients with vasopressin-deficient diabetes insipidus (ref. 169). Lypressin was delivered as a fine spray into the external nares from a compressible plastic bottle and the patients received 1 or 2 sprays in each nostril every 3-6 hours during the day. The average daily dosage was 1.0 to 1.25 ml of LVP nasal solution of 50 to 62.5 U of lypressin. The antidiuretic action of LVP spray was found to be fairly prompt, with the onset of action within one hour and a duration of activity for 3-8 hours. It produced an average decrease in the urine flow down to 1.5-5.0 L/day, while most patients maintained a urine flow at less than 3 L/day. The lypressin nasal spray was thus recommended for clinical use, since it is ease for administration, no significant water retention, and free from any potential serious allergic reactions.

Chirman and Kinsell (1964) also investigated the intranasal administration of synthetic lysine-8-vasopressin as a nasal spray to three patients with diabetes insipidus and found an excellent control of only one subject (ref. 170). In the other two patients, it was found to be of some value as a therapy supplement to pitressin tannate in oil. It appeared that the intranasal application of lysine-8-vasopressin does provide an adequate control in some patients, but may not be adequate in others, particularly the nocturnal control of thirst and polyuria.

The lypressin was also used, by nasal inhalation, to control the severe diabetes insipidus in six patients (ref. 171). The average dosage requirement was determined to be 10-20 IU per day. Four out of 6 patients with clinically severe diabetes insipidus were well controlled by this treatment, while the other two patients required a higher dose and their symptomatic control was still not satisfactory.

Nasal spray of lypressin was found successful in controlling the manifestations of diabetes insipidus in 3 patients with demonstrable neurohypophyseal insufficiency (ref. 172). Hung (1967) reported his experience in the use of lypressin nasal spray in 5 children with diabetes insipidus (ref. 173). Lypressin was administered from a squeeze-bottle container every 2 to 6 hours during the day and at bedtime. The antidiuretic action of lypressin nasal spray was noted within 1 hour in all patients and the drug was cleared from the plasma in 3-5 hours. The results suggested that lypressin nasal spray is an effective and, apparently, nonirritating agent for the long-term treatment of diabetes insipidus in the children. Based on its ease of administration, its effectiveness in the control of polyuria and polydipsia, and lack of significant adverse effects, the lypressin nasal spray was thus recommended for the treatment of diabetes insipidus.

Mimica et al. (1968) also reported the use of lypressin by nasal spray to achieve a good control of 3 patients with diabetes insipidus, who showed manifested allergic reactions to various antidiuretic hormone preparations of animal origin. Its use did not yield any allergic symptoms or other side effects (ref. 174).

2) PLV-2

A new synthetic posthypophysial hormone-like substance, phenylalanyl-lysyl-vasopressin (PLV-2), was reported to have effects on the blood pressure. It is 5 times more effective, as a vasopressin, than lysine-8-vasopressin, but it shows 10-40 times weaker in diuretic action (ref. 162). It has been used for topical and local vasoconstriction. Topical application to the nasal mucosa by a squeeze bottle, PLV-2 was found as effective as 4% cocaine in providing a nasal decongestion prior to the nasotracheal intubation (ref. 175). It was proposed that PLV-2 may be used as a local vasoconstrictor with a greater degree of safety than epinephrine.

3) D.D.A.V.P.

D.D.A.V.P., [1-β-mercaptopropionic acid, 8-D-arginine]-vasopressin or [1-deamino-8-arginine]-vasopressin, is a synthetic analogue of vasopressin, in which the l-arginine in position 8 has been replaced with d-arginine and the free amino group in position 1 has been removed by replacing the hemicysteine component by β-mercaptopropionic acid.

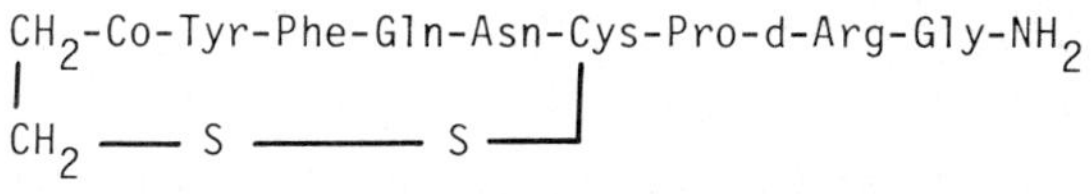

Vávra et al. (1968) reported that in rats, dogs and humans, D.D.A.V.P. has a greater antidiuretic potency than either the natural hormone or any other known synthetic analogues, and that it also produces a prolonged antidiuresis (ref. 176). On the other hand, other activities - pressor, galactogogic, Vagal-like action on the gut - were simultaneously reduced to very low values. D.D.A.V.P. can be administered intranasally as well as by injection.

The effects of D.D.A.V.P. in ten patients with vasopressin-sensitive diabetes insipidus were studied in 1972 by Anderson and Arner (ref. 177). Five patients were given 1 or 2 μg of D.D.A.V.P. intravenously and the effects were observed to last from 5 to more than 12 hours as compared to the 45-90 minutes for lysine-8-vasopressin. D.D.A.V.P. was also administered intranasally at dose of 15 μg, one to three times a day, which reportedly normalized the urine production. During a followup study for 6-12 months by intranasal administration, D.D.A.V.P. proved to be adequately effective and no side effect was observed. It was concluded that D.D.A.V.P. is a safe and effective substance in the treatment of cranial diabetes insipidus.

D.D.A.V.P. was also given, either intranasally or intravenously, to 7 patients with cranial diabetes insipidus and to 2 patients with nephrogenic diabetes insipidus (ref. 178). A marked antidiuresis, without any side effects, was produced in all the 7 patients with cranial diabetes insipidus when treated with 20 μg of D.D.A.V.P. intranasally, twice a day. A similar result was also obtained with 2 μg of D.D.A.V.P. by intravenous injection. On the basis of its slow metabolic clearance, absorption through the nasal mucosa and its lack of side effects, the investigators concluded that D.D.A.V.P. is an ideal drug for the treatment of vasopressin-sensitive diabetes insipidus (ref. 178).

The prolongation of the duration of action of D.D.A.V.P. in diabetes insipidus by clofibrate was reported by Radó and Marosi in 1975 (ref. 179). D.D.A.V.P. was given intravenously in a single dose of either 1 or 2 μg and intranasally in a single dose of 10 μg at 8 a.m.. Clofibrate (500 or 2000 mg) was administered per day. The intravenous and intranasal administrations of D.D.A.V.P. were both found to induce a significant ($p<0.001$) increase ($71 \pm 6.4\%$) in the 24-hr urine osmolality following the intake of clofibrate as compared to the values obtained before clofibrate administration. The results indicated that clofibrate induces an alteration in the time course of D.D.A.V.P. action, indicating a prolongation in the duration of antidiuretic effect as possibly due to a decrease in the metabolic degradation.

Recently, Grossman et al. (1980) administered D.D.A.V.P., either as a nasal spray or as a sublingual lozenge, to two groups of 6 patients with cranial diabetes insipidus, which was compared with the administration of D.D.A.V.P. by rhinyle (ref. 180). In this investigation, a metered-dose nasal spray was used to deliver D.D.A.V.P. intranasally. For sublingual administration, D.D.A.V.P. was formulated in a gelatin-based sublingual lozenge. Two puffs of the nasal spray or one lozenge were taken, which was equivalent to 10 μg of D.D.A.V.P. given by rhinyle. In terms of urine flow or osmolality at any time up to 20 hours,there was no significant difference between the administration by rhinyle and spray or between the applications by rhinyle and lozenges. Each application produced a potent antidiuresis with rapid onset and sustained activity for 10-12 hours, which was followed by a gradual loss in the control of diuresis over the next 12 hours. The investigators concluded that the nasal spray is simple and efficient; it is generally preferred by the patients tested and is better for D.D.A.V.P. administration than the rhinyle (ref. 180).

G) THE ADRENAL HORMONES

The adrenal hormones include both the adrenocorticoids from the adrenal cortex and epinephine and norepinephrine from the adrenal medulla. Adrenal cortical activity is enhanced by the release of adrenal corticotropic hormone (ACTH) from the anterior pituitary, which triggers the secretion of glucocorticoids and mineralocorticoids. These corticosteroids can influence the metabolism of carbohydrate, protein, fat and nucleic acids, the balance of electrolytes and water, and the functional capacities of the cardiovascular system, kidney, skeletal muscle, the nervous system, as well as other organs and tissues.

Corticosteroids have been used since 1950 for the treatment of allergic airway diseases. They can be administered orally, parenterally, or intranasally. Many attempts have been made to apply corticosteroids directly to the mucous membrane, by either spray or injection, in order to obtain a therapeutic activity without the risk of systemic side effects. The intranasal administration of corticosteroids has been reported to produce a great efficacy and a minimum inhibitory effect on the hypothalamus-pituitary-adrenal axis, i.e., without adrenocortical suppression.

Review of the literature suggests that nasal route has been widely utilized by otolaryngologists, since 1952, for the administration of corticosteroids (ref. 181-238). Extensive studies have been initiated and documented for the intranasal administrations of cortisone (ref. 181, 192, 202) and acetate (ref. 193), prednisolone (ref. 202-204) and tebutate (ref. 182-184, 189, 202), methylprednisolone acetate (ref. 187), hydrocortisone (ref. 194-198, 200, 202) and acetate (ref. 195, 196, 201) or hemisuccinate sodium (ref. 199), triamcinolone acetonide (ref. 185-187, 205), dexamethasone phosphate (ref. 206-213), betamethasone valerate (ref. 214, 215), beclomethasone dipropionate (ref. 216-236), fluocinonide (ref. 237), and toxicortol pivalate (ref. 238). However, all of these studies primarily for the relief of nasal obstruction associated with rhinitis, hay fever or nasal polyps as well as the secondary nasal edema from sinusitis or the common colds.

Apparently, the majority of the intranasal drug administrations outlined above have aimed for a localized therapy, not for any systemic medication. To maintain the objective and the scope set for this symposium proceedings, the intranasal administration of adrenal hormones will not be reviewed in great details in this section; however, the literature pertinent to this area of research is still enlisted for those readers who may have a strong interest in this particular mode of medication.

H) SEX HORMONES

The ovarian production of sex hormones is regulated by the gonadotropic hormones from the anterior pituitary. The production of pituitary gonadotropin is, in turn, modulated by the circulatory estrogens and progesterone levels, which, at low plasma concentration appear to stimulate and at high concentration inhibit the production of FSH, LH, and LtH. Thus, a complex positive and negative feedback system subserves the cyclic phenomena of ovulation and menstruation.

Naturally occurring ovarian steroids can block ovulation, but they do so only at a relatively high dose if administered orally or by injection. The undesirable side effects associated with the high dose preclude their use in the conventional methods of hormonal contraception (ref. 239). Synthetic steroids, on the other hand, are effective at low dose, because of their ability to bypass the hepatic first-pass elimination, by which most of the naturally occurring hormones are metabolized; so, the synthetic steroids can reach the target site of action in the brain without the loss of efficacy (ref. 240).

Kumar et al. (ref. 240) conducted a study in rhesus monkeys to determine whether the tritium-labelled estradiol and progesterone, administered intranasally as a spray, could be transferred into the body fluids and then taken up by various tissues. Four groups of two anesthetized monkeys, each of them was either sprayed intranasally (using an atomizer connected to a respiratory pump) or injected intravenously with 0.1 mCi of either ^{3}H-estradiol-17β (0.32 μg) or ^{3}H-progesterone (0.37 μg) dissolved in 0.2 ml of propanediol. Duration of injection or spraying lasted for only one minute.

The results showed that both steroids are able to enter the cerebrospinal fluid (CSF) within one minute after the administration either by intranasal spray or intravenous injection. Considerable amounts of radioactivity was detected in the plasma after spraying with ^{3}H-estradiol, while the amount of radioactivity in the plasma is negligible following the ^{3}H-progesterone spray. A comparison of the plasma: CSF ratio of the two steroids indicated that relatively more steroids enter the CSF after the intranasal administration as compared with the intravenous injection. A salient difference between these two routes of administration is that by nasal spray, the peripheral target tissues, such as the liver, lung, ovary, uterus, vagina and the fallopian tube, show a much lower level of radioactivity than by intravenous injection; on the other hand, the olfactory bulb, olfactory mucosa and respiratory mucosa show a much higher activity following the intranasal administration. The results suggested that steroids can reach the brain preferentially when administered intranasally (ref. 240). There are possibly two pathways by which the steroids can reach the brain: either from the nose, i.e., nasal epithelium, or by way of the olfactory neurons.

Kumar et al. (ref. 241) reported that by intranasal administration progesterone and norethisterone can prevent ovulation in rhesus monkeys. Progesterone or norethisterone was dissolved in a 0.5 ml mixture of ethanol:propylene glycol:water (1:1:3) and sprayed into the monkey's nostril for 10 seconds using a glass atomizer (Brovon Inhaler, Moore Medical Products Ltd), which was regulated by a nitrogen source at a constant pressure. Control animals were sprayed with the solvent alone. The results indicated that intransal administration of steroids can suppress ovulation. Progesterone suppressed ovulation at low dose (2 μg/day), but not in all animals at higher doses (10-30 μg/day). Norethisterone is effective only at the higher doses (9 or 17 μg/day).

Progesterone and norethindrone were given to 15 female rhesus monkeys to determine its systemic absorption through the nasal mucosa and conjunctival sac and to evaluate the existence of a specific pathway from the eye and nose to the cerebrospinal fluid (ref. 241). Suspension of progesterone or norethindrone was prepared in an aqueous opthalmic vehicle consisting of saline and 0.5% methylcellulose and was applied topically into the lower conjunctival sac of each eye, via a polyethylene tubing connected to a microsyringe, or to the nasal mucosa, or was administered intravenously. Measurable plasma levels (0.2-1.6 ng/ml) of norethindrone were obtained within 1 min. after ocular administration. The peak levels (3.6 10.6 ng/ml) were reached after 30 minutes, which stay unchanged for up to 60 minutes. Intranasal administration of norethindrone yielded maximum plasma levels after 30 minutes, whereas the intravenous administration produced its maximum plasma level after 1 minute. On the other hand, ocular administration of progesterone yielded an increase in the plasma levels after one minute and reached a peak plasma level after 3 minutes. The CSF values for norethindrone and progesterone were all much lower than the corresponding plasma levels. The CSF values for progesterone were also very low except the 30-min. point, which was about the same as the serum value. The very rapid absorption of norethindrone and progesterone into the peripheral circulation, after topical administration, and the low steroid levels in the cerebrospinal fluid do not appear to substantiate the concept of a rapid and specific transport of steroids into the CSF as proposed by Kumar (ref. 239). The discrepancy may be due to the difference in the methods of administration. In the present study by Öhman et al. (ref. 242), norethindrone and progesterone were formulated in a suspension form and applied to the nasal cavity as nasal drops, while Kumar used a nasal solution spray instead. The slow and gradual increase in the concentration of norethindrone in the CSF, during the period with high blood levels, make the transport through the blood stream the most likely route for the entry of norethindrone into the central nervous system.

The effects of spraying different doses of progesterone into the nostrils of rhesus monkeys were described by Kumar et al. (ref. 240). Progesterone was dissolved in the combination of ethanol:propylene glycol:water (1:1:3) and sprayed intranasally for 10 days (on Day 5 to Day 14 of the menstrual cycle) to the monkeys. Control animals received only the solvent spray. Blood levels of progesterone did not rise beyond 1.5 ng/ml at any stage of the cycle in all the monkeys treated with 2 μg of the hormone, indicating the suppression of ovulation in all the treated monkeys. On the other hand, ovulation was not suppressed in the monkeys given a higher dose (10-300 μg) of progesterone. This observed pharmacological effect is not surpising, because it is known that progesterone can either inhibit or facilitate the secretion of gonadotropin depending upon its circulatory levels. This study also illustrated that a dosimetric dissection of the facilitatory and inhibitory effects of progesterone can be attained by administering the steroid intranasally.

Kumar et al. (ref. 243) outlined the technique for administering steroids intranasally and the method for monitoring the kinetics of progesterone (P) and norethisterone (NET) in the CSF and blood following the intranasal (i.n.) or intramuscular (i.m.) administrations as well as the effects of steroidal nasal sprays on ovulation in the rhesus monkeys. The steroid solution was prepared by dissolving in the same solvent system as outlined above and was sprayed, using a glass atomizer with its nozzle inserted into one of the nostrils, for 10 seconds at a constant nitrogen pressure. Most of the particles sprayed with this device have a size ranging between 7 and 10 μm. This method of intranasal administration was found to result in the deposit of most sprayed substances in the olfactory region of the nasal mucosa. The investigators believed that the particulate substances thus deposited could transport across the olfactory dendrites, diffuse into the nervous system and uptaken by the submucosal blood vascular system through the supporting cells in the olfactory mucosa.

Serum progesterone concentration was observed to attain its peak level of ca. 600 pg/ml within 10 mins. after nasal spraying (2 μg) to 2 adult ovariectomized monkeys, whereas following i.m. administration of the same dose the peak serum level was reached in 15 minutes with a similar order of magnitude. On the other hand, the peak CSF level of progesterone (ca.

300 pg/ml) was obtained as early as 5 minutes following the i.n. spraying, while the peak CSF level (ca. 100 pg/ml) was reached 30 minutes after i.m. injection. These findings suggest that the intranasal administration of progesterone results in a rapid absorption into the blocd as well as a rapid and higher transfer of progesterone from the blood into the CSF as compared to i.m. injection.

The serum levels of NET following i.n. and i.m. administration of NET (9 µg) to 2 intact adult female rhesus monkeys were found to be almost at a similar order of magnitude, but the peak level was reached within a shorter time following the i.n. administration as compared to i.m. injection (5 vs. 10 min.). The peak NET level in the CSF was found much higher following i.n. spraying as compared to the i.m. route of administration. However, the peak levels of NET in the CSF, unlike those of progesterone, do not precede the peak NET values in the blood.

Progesterone (P) or Norethistrone (NET) was sprayed daily from Day 5 to Day 14 of the monkey's menstrual cycle to determine the efficiency of i.n. spraying of steroids in blocking the ovulation in rhesus monkeys. The most effective dose for inhibiting ovulation was estimated to be 2 µg/day for P and 9 µg/day for NET. Out of the 20 monkeys given 2 µg of P, ovulation was inhibited in 11. Ovulation was not inhibited in all the animals sprayed with the placebo formulation only.

The studies reported above indicate that steroids sprayed intranasally result in a sharp, but shortlived, rise in their concentrations in both serum and CSF as well as a blockade of ovulation in at least 50% of the treated rhesus monkeys with 2 µg of P and 9 µg of NET.

The bioavailability of progesterone, in terms of the area under concentration (AUC) vs. time profiles, and the maximal concentration in the serum and CSF, was evaluated in the adult ovariectomized rhesus monkeys following various routes of administration of 10 µg of progesterone (ref. 244). The maximal serum $AUC \int_0^{60\ min.}$ achieved following the nasal spray (NS) of progesterone, using a precalibrated glass atomizer, was significantly higher ($p<0.01$) than all other routes of administration. The AUC values did not differ significantly among i.v., i.m., nasal drops (ND) and eye drops (ED) routes. The $AUC \int_0^{60\ min.}$ in the CSF was also considerably higher after NS than all other routes of administration, but this difference was not statistically significant. The C_{max} of progesterone in the serum was highest following NS, which was also significantly higher than the i.v., ND and ED administrations ($p<0.05$) and than the i.m. ($p<0.01$). The C_{max} of progesterone in the CSF was apparently higher following NS, but this level was not significantly different from the C_{max} achieved by i.v. However, the C_{max}

value following NS was significantly higher ($p<0.05$) than the i.m., ND and ED administrations.

The aforementioned studies clearly indicated that the bioavailability of progesterone in both the serum and CSF is considerably higher following the intranasal administration by nasal spray and that the enhanced bioavailability is dependent upon the method by which progesterone is administered into the nostrils. This enhanced bioavailability may be the result of a slow rate of entry of the steroid into the body fluids as well as a slow rate of its clearance.

The bioavailability and mean blood levels of progesterone following intranasal, intravenous and intraduodenal administrations were examined by Hussain et al. in Sprague-Dawley male rats (ref. 245). For intranasal administration, three doses (50, 100, and 150 μg) of radiolabelled progesterone was dissolved in 0.1 ml of 1% polysorbate 80-saline solution and administered to the nasal cavity of each rat by a micropipet. For intravenous administration, the same doses were injected through the femoral vein. For intraduodenal administration, the abdomen was opened by a midline incision and a 50-μg dose in 0.1 ml of 1% polysorbate 80-saline solution was injected directly through the duodenum. The blood level of progesterone after the intranasal administration increased rapidly and attained the peak level within 6 minutes, whereas the intraduodenal administration resulted in a considerably lower blood level. The AUC values were found to be directly proportional to the doses administered either intranasally or intravenously. The nasal bioavailability, calculated from the ratio of the AUC values [(nasal/intravenous) x 100], was 100% at all three doses, while the intraduodenal bioavailability achieved only 1.2% of the intravenous bioavailability. The results clearly indicated that the natural steroid, like progesterone, is rapidly absorbed into the systemic blood from the nasal mucosa, without any first-pass metabolism and that intranasal administration is superior to the intraduodenal route of administration for progesterone.

The metabolism of ^{14}C-progesterone by incubation with the nasal mucosa and lung slices from mice and rats was studied by Brittebo (ref. 246). The nasal mucosa (containing both respiratory and olfactory epithelia) was removed from the nasal cavity walls, septum and turbinates. The tissue slices were then incubated with ^{14}C-progesterone (in 1 μl DMSO) in 2 ml of Krebs-Ringer phosphate buffer containing 10 mM glucose (pH 7.0). The incubations were performed at 37°C, under the oxygen atmosphere, for 10 to 180 minutes. At least 3 metabolites were detected after 10-minutes incubation and at least 10-12 metabolites after 30 minutes or longer. The pattern of metabolites appeared to be similar in both mice and rats, but showed a certain difference between the two tissues investigated. The total amount of metabolites formed by incubation with nasal mucosa was observed to increase rapidly; and following 3 hours of incubation, only 8% (mouse) and 20% (rat) of the radioactivity extracted from the incubation medium was identified as the unchanged ^{14}C-progesterone. The ability of the nasal mucosa to metabolize progesterone seems to be significantly greater than the lung, which yielded a considerably lower rate of formation of metabolites. A 60% (mouse) or 50% (rat) of the extracted radioactivity was identified as the unchanged ^{14}C-progesterone after 3 hours of incubation. Addition of metyrapone to the incubation medium containing the nasal mucosa was noticed to produce a marked decrease in the formation of some progesterone metabolites, with a concomitant increase in the formation of other less polar products. The action of metyrapone on steroid hydroxylation is known to be associated with its ability to interact with cytochrome p-450, suggesting the possible involvement of cytochrome p-450-dependent monooxygenase activity in the metabolism of progesterone by the nasal mucosa.

The pharmacokinetics of progesterone in blood and cerebrospinal fluid following the intravenous injection, intravenous infusion, and nasal spray was studied by Kumar et al. in the adult ovariectomized rhesus monkeys (ref. 247). Progesterone was formulated in the solution of ethanol:propylene glycol:water (3:3:4) and administered at the same dose through these three routes. The infusion was carried out at a uniform rate of 1 μg/min. for a total of 10 minutes. Five μg of progesterone was sprayed into each nostril, using a commercially available glass atomizer, over a 10-min. period.

The serum concentrations of progesterone at 3 min. after administration were not significantly different among the three methods of administration. However, in all the samples taken subsequently, the concentrations of progesterone were significantly higher after the i.v. infusion and nasal spray as compared to the i.v. injection; though the serum concentrations of progesterone did not differ significantly between i.v. infusion and nasal spray.

Progesterone concentrations in the CSF after its i.v. injection showed a progressive decline in samples taken at different intervals, whereas after i.v. infusion the progesterone concentrations in the CSF increased in the first 3- and 9-min. samples and, thereafter, the levels declined progressively. When progesterone was sprayed intranasally, its concentrations in the 9- and 15-min. CSF samples were higher than the 3-min. CSF samples and then declined progressively as seen in the 30- and 60-min samples. Progesterone concentrations in the CSF samples taken at 3 min were not significantly different among the three methods of administration. However, in all the subsequent samples, progesterone concentrations were significantly higher after i.v. infusion and nasal spray than after i.v. injection. The CSF concentrations of progesterone were not different significantly between i.v. infusion and nasal spray.

A comparison of the data obtained in the serum for AUC$\int_0^{60}$, AUC$\int_0^{\infty}$, C_{max} and T_{max} among the three methods of administration clearly indicated that the levels obtained after the i.v. infusion are the highest, followed by those values obtained by nasal spray and i.v. injection. However, the slight difference observed in the AUC values between the i.v. infusion and nasal spray was not statistically significant. The C_{max} and T_{max} values for i.v. injection and i.v. infusion were significantly different, whereas the C_{max} values between i.v. injection and nasal spray or between i.v. infusion and nasal spray were not.

The AUC$\int_0^{60}$, C_{max}, and T_{max} values of progesterone obtained in CSF were highest after i.v. infusion, followed by those obtained after nasal spray and i.v. injection. A comparison of these 3 parameters among the three methods of progesterone administration showed that a statistically significant difference is evident between i.v. injection and i.v. infusion as well as between i.v. injection and nasal spray, but is not evident between i.v. infusion and nasal spray.

The concentration of progesterone and its bioavailability in the body fluids after the nasal spray were significantly higher than those observed after the i.v. injection, but were lower than those obtained after the i.v. infusion, though the difference was not statistically significant. In fact, the actual amount of progesterone deposited in the nasal cavity after the nasal spray was much less than that administered by the systemic routes. In conclusion, this study demonstrated the possibility of administering a physiological dose of progesterone as nasal sprays for replacement therapy or contraception purposes.

Estrogen replacement in deficiency states by oral administration of natural estradiol has never adequately achieved the physiological form and amount of estrogen required. The wide use, in recent years, of orally effective synthetic estrogens continues to cause some concerns because of their potential of producing the undesirable endocrine-metabolic effects. In 1977, Rigg et al. (ref. 248) initiated a study in women to determine the serum levels of estradiol-17β (E_2) following intravaginal and intranasal administrations of a micronized estradiol-17β (E_2). The micronized E_2 was suspended in 0.5 ml of normal saline and then placed in the posterior vaginal vault of 16 women, with the assistance of a vaginal speculum, or applied to the nasal mucosa in 11 women, via a nose dropper. Serum concentrations of estrone (E_1), estradiol-17β (E_2), LH and FSH were then measured by radioimmunoassays.

The absorption of E_2, after the intravaginal administration, appeared to be extremely rapid and sustained as reflected by an incremental change in the serum E_2 concentration. A rise in the circulating E_2 level was observed to occur within 5 min and continued to increase linearly as a function of time during the first 30 min, reaching a level (520 ± 90 pg/ml) that is more than 60 times the basal value (8 ± 1 pg/ml). Thereafter, the rate of change in the circulating E_2 seemed to be less rapid, which reached a peak level of more than 110 times the basal level at 2 hours after the administration. The high E_2 level was sustained for 4-5 hours, beyond which it decline slowly. The level at 24 hours was still more than 5 times the basal level. In contrast, the incremental change of serum E_1 level was found to be less rapid and much smaller in magnitude. E_1 attained a mean peak concentration (243 ± 24 pg/ml), which is more than 7 times the basal level (32 ± 4 pg/ml) after 8 hours and then decline more slowly than did the E_2. The E_1 value at 24 hours remained at a level which is more than 3 times the basal level. The biological effectiveness, in terms of gonadotropin suppression, is essentially the same for the 2 E_2 doses (0.5 and 1.0 mg) used. A quantitative decline of LH and FSH levels in response to E_2 administration was found.

Intranasal administration of E_2 at 1 mg dose induced a rapid, but short-lasting increase in the circulating level of E_2. Moreover, a progressive increase in the mean E_1/E_2 ratio was observed, which rose well above unity beginning at 1 hour after intranasal application. This finding may be attributed to the local conversion of E_2 to E_1 in the nasal mucosa, either by an enzyme or a microorganism residing in the nasal cavity.

This study also indicated that the intravaginal, but not intranasal, administration of E_2 can achieve, quantitatively, a much greater level of E_2 and also circumvent the local conversion of E_2 to E_1 normally observed after the oral administration of E_2; and, thus, intravaginal administration represents a practical and highly effective means of delivery E_2 into the systemic circulation.

The absorption of estradiol-17β (E_2) into the blood and CSF following the ocular, intranasal and intravenous administrations was recently studied in women volunteers and rhesus monkeys by Öhman et al. (ref. 249). Estradiol suspension was prepared in an aqueous solution of 0.5% methylcellulose, while estradiol solution was made in a combination of ethanol:propylene glycol:water (1:1:3). An aliquot of suspension was delivered to the nasal cavity or applied to the lower conjunctival sac, using a micro-syringe, in the subjects. The estradiol suspension was also injected into the saphenous vein in two monkeys.

The plasma concentrations of both estradiol and estrone were observed to increase rapidly to reach a rather high plasma level following the ocular administration of 0.5 mg estradiol suspension in the four menstruating women. Following the ocular administration of estradiol suspension in rhesus monkeys, the plasma concentration of estradiol was also seen to increase even at 1 min. After 10 to 30 min., the peak plasma level of estradiol was reached. By ocular administration, on the other hand, the estradiol in a solution form attained a high plasma concentration very rapidly (within 5 minutes after the administration), which was roughly the same plasma level as observed after i.v. injection. When the estradiol suspension was administered to the nasal cavity of rhesus monkeys, a dose-dependent increase in the plasma level of estradiol was observed, which however, was not as high as the ocular instillation. By intranasal administration, estradiol solution induced a great increase in the plasma level of estradiol, which is relatively close to the level reached by i.v. injection. An increase in the estradiol level in CSF was also observed following the ocular, intranasal, and i.v. administration. However, the CSF levels were always lower than the corresponding plasma levels. No great difference in the CSF levels of estradiol was noted between the suspension and solution formulations.

Estrogens administered by parenteral routes are known to suppress spermatogenesis and also to reduce the levels of testosterone in the circulation. Kumar et al. (ref. 250) were interested to determine if testicular function in adult monkeys are also impaired following the intranasal administration of estradiol-17β (E_2), progesterone (P), or norethisterone (NET) at a daily dose of 30 µg, which was sprayed intranasally, using a glass atomizer, over a period of 60 days.

The testes were found to reduce in size after 30 days of steroid administration and the size reduction was more remarkable at the end of 60-day treatment. In the E_2-treated monkeys, the testes were not only reduced in size, but also had retracted into the inguinal canal at the end of 60-day treatment; while the testes of the solvent-treated controls remained unaffected. In the P-treated monkeys, the reduction in the diameter of semininferous tubules was not as marked as that observed in the E_2- or NET-treated monkeys. A progressive decline in the mean values of serum testosterone levels was evident in all the animals treated with various steroids (E, P or NET); and, at the end of the treatment, the reduction in the serum testosterone concentration was statistically significant as compared to the levels at the beginning of the treatment. On the other hand, the serum testosterone levels did not show any change in the solvent-treated controls. The plasma cortisol levels before, during and at the end of treatment with steroids or solvent showed no significant changes at all. Thus, this study demonstrated that there is an impairment of the spermatogenesis and a significant reduction in the levels of circulating testosterone following the intranasal administration of estradiol-17β, progesterone or norethisterone in the adult rhesus monkeys.

The potent natural male sex hormones, testosterone, and its esters are generally administered by intramuscular injection. Although it is readily absorbed orally, it is ineffective due to its extensive metabolism in the GI tract and by the liver before reaching the systemic circulation. In order to enhance testosterone bioavailability from a non-parenteral route, Hussain et al. (ref. 251) investigated the feasibility of nasal absorption of testosterone, in the male Sprague-Dawley rats, and compared it to the intravenous and intraduodenal administrations. Two doses of [^{3}H] testosterone, in 0.1 mL of 1% polysorbate 80-saline solution, were administered to the nasal cavity, using a micropipet, and the nostrils were then sealed with an adhesive. For intravenous administration, the same doses were injected through the femoral vein. For intraduodenal administration, the abdomen was opened by a midline incision and a 25-μg dose in 0.1 mL of 1% polysorbate 80-saline solution was injected directly through the duodenum.

The results showed that the testosterone level in the blood after the intranasal administration increases rapidly and attains the peak level within 2 minute, whereas the intraduodenal administration yields a considerably lower blood level. The blood levels following the nasal absorption were found rather similar to those after the intravenous administration, with the half-life of elimination at 40 minutes. The nasal bioavailability was determined as 99% and 90% for the 25-μg and 50-μg dose, respectively, using the intravenous profile as the reference standard, whereas the intraduodenal bioavailability only achieved 1% of that of the intravenous administration. The results of this study suggested that testosterone is rapidly absorbed from the nasal mucosa into the systemic blood circulation without any first-pass metabolism.

I) PANCREATIC HORMONE - INSULIN

Insulin, an internal secretion produced by the Beta cells in the glandular tissue of the pancreas, is a polypeptide with a molecular weight of around 6,000. It consists of two peptide chains with 21 and 30 amino acids, respectively. These peptide chains are held together by the disulfide linkage of cystines. For diabetes medication, the insulin injection has been the only effective method for many years. It is well known that a polypeptide, like insulin, is subjected to degradation by the proteolytic enzymes during its passage through the mucosa membrane (ref. 252, 253). This reaction has added a limitation to the development of a non-parenteral route of administration for practical application. Numerous efforts have been made to find an effective route for the administration of insulin other than the parenteral injection, such as oral (ref. 254-258), sublingual (ref. 259), rectal (ref. 260), vaginal (ref. 261), aerosol (ref. 262) and subcutaneous implantation (ref. 263). However, the polypeptide nature of insulin has limited the development of a practical nonparenteral application. As early as in 1922, Woodyatt (ref. 264) already initiated experiments to evaluate the efficacy of insulin by intranasal, oral, rectal, vaginal, intravenous and subcutaneous administration. He reported positive effects with subcutaneous and intravenous injections, but a very weak, doubtful or frankly negative results with other routes of administration.

Two years later, Heubner and his associates reported their observation on the lowering of blocd sugar level in diabetics following the inhalation of insulin (ref. 265). In the following year, Gänsslen (ref. 266) confirmed the observation that the blood sugar level in diabetics can be reduced by inhalation of an insulin spray. Collens and Goldzieher (ref. 267), in 1932, studied the absorption of insulin by nasal mucous membrane in human diabetics and the effect of saponin. Insulin solution (100 units) was sprayed directly into the nose by an atomizer and small plegets of cotton were then inserted into the nares to prevent the patient from blowing out the solution. Ninety-six experiments were performed with only 11 failures. It produced the effects similar to those obtained by the subcutaneous injection of insulin. However, this treatment yielded some mild congestion in the nasal membrane and some symptoms of rhinitis.

Major, in 1936, examined the problems of intranasal absorption of insulin and found that insulin in ethylene glycol and trimethylene glycol, when either instilled or sprayed into the nasal mucosa, produces an unquestioned and marked fall in the blood sugar levels in normal rabbits, normal dogs, and also in diabetic patients (ref. 268). However, the dosage employed in this intranasal medication was found to be considerably greater than that required for subcutaneous injection.

No further study was conducted until 1958, in which Hankiss and Hadhazy (ref. 269) investigated the resorption of insulin and adrenaline from the nasal mucosa in both healthy and diabetic patients. It was found that both hormones are resorbed from the nasal mucosa and achieve 53% of the effect as by subcutaneous injection. However, the effect achieved by nasal absorption was unstable and variable, and therefore, the investigators did not recommend the intranasal insulin administration as the means for the treatment of diabetes.

It has been documented that surface-active agents can affect drug absorption and membrane transport. However, the mode of this effect has been shown to be highly variable. Several possible mechanisms have been proposed as follows: (a) Effects on the solubility and dissolution rate of drug, (b) effects on the gastric emptying and intestinal transport, (c) drug-surfactant interactions. The consequence of all the factors listed above have demonstrated in the passage of drugs through the intestinal membrane, as resulted from the direct effects of surfactants on the permeability of biomembranes (ref. 270, 271). A number of reports have concluded that non-ionic, anionic surfactants and bile salts enhance the gastrointestinal absorption of water-soluble, micelle-free drugs, like antibiotics (ref. 272), Vitamin B_{12} (ref. 273), Thiamine disulfide compounds (ref. 274), phenol red (ref. 275, 276), erythritol (ref. 277), electrolytes and monosaccharides (ref. 278), which is the result of enhanced mucosal permeability. Moreover, the rectal absorption of insulin was also reported to be enhanced in the presence of non-ionic surfactants or bile acids (ref. 279, 280).

Yokosuka and his coworkers (ref. 281) studied, in 1977, the nasal absorption of insulin and the effect of several surfactants in 18 healthy adults. The crystalline porcine insulin, at 10, 30 and 50 IU, was dissolved in 0.1 ml of saline solution containing 1% sodium glycocholate at pH 7.6. Following application to nasal mucous membrane, insulin was promptly absorbed with a significant increase in the plasma level of immunoreactive insulin (IRI) and a decrease in glucose concentrations and CPR (C-peptide immunoreactivity) was observed. The peak serum IRI level was noted to increase as increasing the insulin dose, which showed a typical "dose-response" relationship. On the other hand, sublingual administration produced no appreciable change in plasma IRI and glucose levels.

Without the incorporation of sodium glycocholate, intranasal administration of insulin yielded no measurable increase in serum IRI level. Replacement of sodium glycocholate by the surfactants with a larger molecular weight, such as 2% of lysozyme chloride, HCO-60, or Byco-E, nasal absorption of insulin was also negligible. On the other hand, when 1% Na ursodeoxycocholate was added, a decrease in glucose level was not observed in spite of the increase in plasma IRI. Besides, this agent was found to be associated with a marked local irritation of nasal mucosa observed. The results demonstrated that intranasal administration of insulin, which is dissolved in 1% sodium glycocholate solution, yields a relatively prompt increase in plasma IRI level and provides a similar trend of IRI responses as that by intravenous injection, but not to that by subcutaneous administration.

Hirai et al. (ref. 282) investigated the effect of surface active agents on the nasal absorptivity of insulin in dogs. Crystalline pork insulin (25.5 IU/mg) was dissolved or suspended in acetate buffer (0.01M, below pH 6) and in phosphate buffer (0.01M, above pH 6) at a concentration ranging from 2 IU/0.1 ml to 50 IU/0.1 ml. Surfactants, like saponin, sodium glycocholate or polyoxyethylene-9-lauryl ether (BL-9), were added at 1% concentration to insulin solutions. For the parenteral (i.v., i.m., and s.c.) administrations, regular insulin solution (40 IU/ml) was diluted with physiological saline to a concentration range of 0.5-5 IU/ml and used.

After receiving insulin intranasally by a nebulizer spray at a dose of 50 IU/dog (at pH 3.1), the plasma level of immunoreactive insulin (IRI) was noted to increase substantially from 32.8 to 296.7 μU/ml within 30 minutes, while the plasma glucose level decreased by 75.3% from 90.8 to 20.4 mg/100 ml at 2 hours after the administration. In the control dogs, the plasma glucose level was constant throughout the experiment. It was further noticed that the extent and duration of hypoglycemia induced by the nasal absorption of insulin depend on the pH of the preparations. At pH 6.1, which is close to the isoelectric point of insulin, no or only slight hypoglycemia was achieved. But at pH 3.1, the plasma glucose level was decreased by a magnitude of about 45%.

On the other hand, it was observed that incorporation of saponin, sodium glycocholate, or BL-9, at a concentration of 1%, in the insulin preparation at pH 7.4 enhances significantly in either the extent or the duration of hypoglycemia and the plasma glucose level by a magnitude of 25 to 100% at 1-2 hours after the administration. In contrast, the insulin preparation, in the absence of one of the surfactants, produced only a light hypoglycemia. The hypoglycemia effects after the intranasal administration of insulin preparations were noted to be dose-dependent and the dosage required was about 3~4 times the intravenous dose needed to produce hypoglycemia of similar magnitude. This study (ref. 282) suggested that the alteration of nasal mucosa by saponin, sodium glycocholate, or BL-9 appears to increase the permeability of nasal mucosa, which leads to enhancement of the nasal absorption of a macromolecular polypeptide, such as insulin.

Hirai and his associates (ref. 283) continued their investigation in rats to screen other absorption-promoting agents for the nasal absorption of insulin. In the investigation, insulin preparation (0.1 ml/kg, 2-40 IU/0.1 ml) was administered to the nasal cavity by micropipette and the nostril was closed immediately after the administration with an adhesive agent. For the control studies, insulin was administered intravenously, intramuscularly, and subcutaneously to separate groups of rats.

At 10 and 20 IU/kg doses, administration of the pH 3.1 nasal solution resulted in a dose-dependent reduction in the plasma glucose level, which was reduced by 30 and 55%, respectively, of the initial value. On the other hand, the solutions at pH 5.5 and 7.4 produced little or no hypoglycemia.

After the addition of 1% surfactant, the nasal insulin solution (pH 7.4) at 10 IU/kg could produce a reduction in plasma glucose level. This reducing effect was obtained by the surfactants of non-ionic ether type, anionic and amphoteric types, bile salts, saponin and surfactin (a lipopeptide).

On the other hand, the ester type non-ionic surfactants were noted to be less effective than the ether type. Addition of a surfactant with a HLB value of 8-14 was reported to yield a great decrement of the plasma glucose level, whereas the polyoxyethylene butyl ethers and the ester type non-ionic surfactants were exceptions. The degree of reduction in the plasma glucose level was observed to increase gradually as the concentration of the surfactants increased to 0.5% and then plateaued. The absolute bioavailability of insulin, as estimated from the hypoglycemic effect, was 5% by intranasal administration of the pH 3.1 insulin solution without absorption promoter, which was increased to about 30% by the addition of a promoter, such as sodium glycocholate or polyoxyethylene-9-lauryl ether, at 1% level. The results of this study suggested that the surfactants appear to increase the permeability or to reduce the proteolytic enzyme activity of the nasal mucosa, and thereby promote the nasal absorption of insulin.

The mechanism of the promoting effect of surfactants on the nasal absorption of insulin was studied in rats and their effects on the morphology of nasal mucosa was also examined using scanning electron microscope (SEM) (ref. 284). The results indicated that the insulin solution without a surfactant produced only a light hypoglycemia throughout the experiment, whereas the addition of a surfactant significantly decreased the plasma glucose level. The decrement of plasma glucose level showed a maximum of 55.5% with polyoxyethylene-9-lauryl ether (BL-9), which was found to diminish gradually with any increase or decrease in the number of ethylene oxide unit. Both the hemolytic and protein-releasing effects of the surfactants on the biomembrane were also found to reach a maximum with BL-9, which also showed a reduction as the number of ethylene oxide units increased or decreased from 9. A good correlation existed between the effect on the biomembrane and the absorption-promoting properties of the non-ionic surfactants, the anionic surfactants, like sodium lauryl sulfate, and saponin. On the other hand, bile salts, such as taurocholate, cholate and glycocholate, showed a lesser effect on both hemolytic and protein-releasing activities, though their absorption-promoting effects were significant. The addition of BL-9 was noted to yield a slight inhibition of the enzymatic degradation of insulin, whereas the addition of bile salts, especially the sodium glycocholate, resulted in a marked inhibition of the activity of leucine aminopeptidase, which is known to cleave the β-chain of insulin.

By SEM inspection, a morphological change in the microvilli of the nasal mucosa was observed after intranasal administration of the insulin solution containing BL-9, whereas no change was noted with sodium glycocholate. The results of the time course for the nasal absorption of insulin and of SEM studies indicated that the functional and structural changes in the nasal mucosa caused by the surfactants are reversible and they return to normality within a relative short period of time.

Pontiroli et al. recently investigated the efficacy and safety of intranasal insulin administration in normal subjects and in insulin-dependent diabetic patients (ref. 285). The subjects were administered with solutions of regular insulin (40 IU/ml) or a combination of crystalline insulin (110 IU/ml) with sodium glycocholate (1% w/v). In normal subjects, the insulin administered by nasal route was well absorbed and induced hypoglycemia. Serum immunoreactive insulin (IRI) concentration rose sharply after intranasal administration and showed a good correlation with the amount of insulin administered. The fall in blood glucose level occurred at 12.3 ± 1.5 minutes and continued for 51.5 ± 4.7 minutes with a reduction of 41.9 ± 6.4% of the basal blood glucose level. The serum IRI concentrations increased in all subjects with peak values being observed at 13.5 ± 0.7 minutes and an average value of 67.1 ± 16.6 mU/L after insulin administration. Comparison of the hypoglycemia induced by intranasal and intravenous insulin in 3 normal subjects suggested a nasal to i.v. potency ratio of about 1:8. In 4 insulin-dependent diabetic patients, insulin was administered once intranasally and once subcutaneously at a dose ratio of 9:1 and the results indicated that the intranasal insulin is more effective than the subcutaneous insulin in preventing hyperglycemia.

Efficacy and reproducibility of intranasal administration of insulin as an insulin-deoxycholate (1% w/v) aerosol to normal and diabetic subjects were recently studied by Moses et al. (ref. 286) by measuring the blood glucose and serum insulin levels. Insulin (500 IU/ml) was diluted to an appropriate concentration with sodium deoxycholate solution (pH 7.6, with NaCl 0.15M) to give a final insulin solution containing 1% (w/v) of deoxycholate. This insulin-deoxycholate solution was administered intranasally, using a fixed-volume aerosol spray [75 ± 8 μl per spray], into 24 controlled subjects, 4 subjects with Type I diabetes mellitus and 2 subjects with Type II diabetes mellitus.

When insulin alone was administered intranasally in phosphate-buffered saline solution (pH 7.4) at a dose of 0.5 IU/kg, neither a decrease in blood glucose levels, nor an increase in plasma insulin concentration was detected. Following administration of the same insulin dose with sodium deoxycholate by nasal route to 29 fasting volunteers, a peak serum insulin concentration of 103 ± 49 μU/ml, which is 21–222 μU/ml above the baseline, was observed at 10 min. Blood glucose level began to fall by 10 min, reached a 54 ± 14% of the control value by 30 min, and returned to the baseline by 60-80 min. In contrast, following the i.v. administration of one-tenth of the nasal dose (i.e. 0.05 IU/kg), a peak serum insulin level was attained within 2 minutes and returned to baseline within 30-40 min. By comparing the serum insulin levels after i.v. and nasal routes of administration, nasal insulin absorption was approximately 10-20% as efficient as intravenous insulin.

Six normal subjects were further tested with graded doses of insulin by nasal spray, a linear dose-response relationship was observed between the mean peak serum insulin levels and the insulin doses administered. The investigations conducted in the subjects with Type I and Type II diabetes mellitus indicated that serum insulin concentration increases in a manner similar to the pattern in the controlled subjects and a prompt reduction of blood glucose level is accomplished. However, in the Type I and Type II diabetes a prolonged hypoglycemia response was observed, which persisted for as long as 4-6 hour. Both normal volunteers and diabetics tolerated well to the intranasal administration of insulin-deoxycholate combination, with some reports of mild nasal irritation, which last for only approximately 5-10 min. and of minimal nasal congestion, which lasts for 5-15 min. following administration.

This study indicated that insulin, when administered intranasally with an appropriate bile salt, can be absorbed into the bloodstream through the nasal mucosa with reproducible kinetics and good efficiency. It also suggested that the intranasal administration of insulin as a bile salt aerosol may have several advantages over the approaches currently available to parenteral insulin administration, since no injection is required and the absorption is rapid (See the chapter by Flier et al. in this volume).

J) AUTONOMIC DRUGS

1. Sympathomimetics

Ephedrine acts indirectly by activating the release of norepinephrine from adrenergic nerves. At higher doses, it has a direct sympathomimetic action. It penetrates into the brain and, hence, has central nervous activities. Ephedrine has a most important application as a bronchodilator and its weak vasoconstrictor effect also lends itself to the ambulatory management of allergic conditions.

Epinephrine is the predominant sympathomimetic in the adrenal medulla. It possesses all the strong α_1-, β_1-, and β_2 - agonistic activities. Epinephrine is the drug of choice in the management of allergic emergencies, such as anaphylaxis, angioneurotic edema, giant urticaria, and serum sickness, status asthmaticus, topical decongestant and cardiac arrest as well as primary open-angle glaucoma.

As early as in 1931, Childrey and Essex (ref. 287) already undertook a study to determine the absorptive ability of the frontal sinus membranes to ephedrine and epinephrine. Absorption was determined by observations of the blood pressure. When ephedrine was given intravenously, intramuscularly or subcutaneously at doses ranging from 25 to 50 mg., it almost immediately caused a marked rise in the blood pressure, which lasted for as long as 60 minutes; but, administration of 50 mg. ephedrine into the sinus of a dog did not produce any appreciable effect on the blood pressure.

In a cat, intravenous injection of 0.1cc epinephrine in Ringer's solution (0.1%) caused the typical vasopressor response, while a subcutaneous injection of 0.4cc gave negative results as did an injection of 0.5cc into the right frontal sinus. The negative results led the investigators to conclude that ephedrine and epinephrine are incapable of penetrating through the mucosa of frontal sinus in sufficient amount to produce an appreciable systemic effect.

Phenylephrine is a directly acting sympathomimetic drug with a strong α-agonistic, but a negligible β-agonistic and central nervous activities. Phenylephrine can be absorbed orally without being attacked by monoamine oxidase (MAO). It is used in the treatment of paroxysmal atrial tachycardia and wide-angle glaucoma and also used as a nasal decongestant and mydriatric.

An investigation was carried out in 1941 by Alyea and Donnelly (ref. 288) to determine the effects of nasal vasoconstrictors in 11 patients with hypertension, 16 with cardiac disorders, 9 with thyroid disorders and 14 with diabetes. The phenylephrine HCl solution (neo-synephrine HCl/Winthrop), with the strength of 0.25 and 1%, was used. Pulse and blood pressure readings were made at regular intervals for a duration of up to 45 minutes. The results showed that no untoward effects can be detected and the absorption from the nasal membranes is too much retarded to be of consequence in the development of any side effect.

A recent report (ref. 289) concluded that the aqueous solution of ephedrine HCl (0.5%) or phenylephrine (0.25 or 0.5%) is an effective decongestant, when applied intranasally, in the patient with an acute nasal obstruction problem, such as common cold or sinusitis.

Myers and Iazzetta (ref. 290) in 1982 investigated the feasibility of intranasal administration of phenylephrine for the systemic vasoconstriction and for the increase of blood pressure in two groups of high risk patients: 12 patients with chronic nasal congestion, whose blood pressure was normal, and 14 patients with hypertension, who were under the medication of β-blocker (metoprolol). A double-blind study was carried out with the phenylephrine HCl solution or an identical placebo solution administered on separate day in increasing doses at hourly intervals. The results showed no significant increase in blood pressure following the intranasal administration of phenylephrine in either group of patients. Repeated instillation of phenylephrine did not result in a cumulative rise in the mean blood pressure in either group. Alteration in the heart rate after the intranasal administration of phenylephrine or placebo was small.

Lindsay (ref. 291) reported his observations in 93 patients having nasal surgery in the past 12 months, whose bleeding was controlled by diathermy and postoperative application of a nasal aerosol, called Tobispray. Tobispray is a dry, metered-dose nasal aerosol containing a vasoconstrictor (tramazoline), a steroid (dexamethasone isonicotinate), and an antibiotic (neomycin sulfate). In 50 of the 93 patients, the results at the 1- and 2-week follow-up visits were found to be excellent, as evidenced by a clear airway without crusting and mucosal edema. The results were rated as good for another 38 patients, in whom a clear airway with only traces of crusting, mucosa edema or minor adhesions were obtained. This treatment achieved a success rate of 94.6%. No cases of primary or secondary haemorrhage were reported.

The effectiveness and duration of 5 topical nasal decongestants and a placebo solution were evaluated in 21 subjects with nasal congestion (ref. 292). The ability of each decongestant to change the nasal airway resistance was measured at regular intervals for up to a duration of 3 hours. Nasal airway resistance (Rn) is defined in terms of the pressure required for the air to move through the nasal passages at a specific flow rate. The Rn values were determined from the measurements of transnasal pressure and nasal airflow during each breath.

Administration of the placebo solution produced a transient, early increase of Rn. The increase achieved a statistically significant level within 2 minutes ($p=0.023$), after which there was a return toward the control levels. Agent W-37 (0.25% phenylephrine HCl + 1.0% Thonzylamine HCl) was observed to produce a transient, but unimpressive, change in nasal airway resistance. A statistically significant decrease in Rn was seen only 10 and 20 minutes after administration of the decongestant. Agent W-66 (0.25% phenylephrine HCl + 0.25% phenylpropanolamine HCl + 1.0% Thonzylamine HCl) was found to yield a prolonged response, with a statistical difference in Rn values from the controls at 10, 60, 120 and 150 minutes. Agent W-58 (0.25% phenylephrine + 0.25% phenylpropanolamine HCl + 1.0% Thonzylamine HCl + 0.1% volatile oils) produced a slightly more consistent response, but with a shorter duration of effectiveness. Agent 83 (0.25% phenylephrine HCl + 0.12% methapyriline HCl + 0.06% volatile oils) yielded an impressive and prompt decrease in Rn values. Statistically significant decrease in Rn values was seen throughout the period from 2 to 90 minutes, except at 30 minutes, with $p=0.061$. The response to agent W-72 (0.05% metizoline) was not prompt. Analysis of the results demonstrated that (i) the combination of phenylephrine and thonzylamine is least effective as a topical nasal decongestant; (ii) the addition of phenylpropanolamine prolongs the duration of effectiveness for the combination of phenylephrine and thonzylamine (iii) volatile oils provide no effect as the vehicle for the combination; and (iv) methypyrilene has a greater effect than thonzylamine as an antihistamine agent in the combination.

Xylometazoline, 2-(4-t-butyl-2,6-dimethylbenzyl)-2-imidazoline, is a long-acting topical nasal decongestant and used for the relief of congestion due to coryza or allergic rhinitis. Hamilton (ref. 293) in 1981 evaluated the ability of xylometazoline nasal spray in the reduction of nasal congestion in 44 normal subjects with coryza as a result of upper respiratory infection. Rating scales were designed for the subjective response and nasal airway resistance, expressed as nasal conductance (Gn), was measured as the objective response over 6-hr period. The results indicated that the change in Gn values, following the intranasal administration of xylometazoline, is rapid, profound, and persistent. The increase in Gn values was statistically significant ($p<0.05$) at all times from 10 minutes to 4 hours after administration of the decongestant intranasally. A decrease in the congestion was reported for all time periods after the intranasal administration of xylometazoline. No difference was detected in the responses between cigarette smokers and nonsmokers.

The nasal mucosa of 20 healthy subjects were examined before, during and after 6 weeks of regular uses of xylometazoline nose drops (1 mg/ml) at 0.15 ml to each nostril 3 times a day (ref. 294). Mucociliary function was tested and biopsies from the nasal mucosa were taken. The results concluded that the subjects did not suffer any diminish in their mucociliar function during or after the trial. The surface structure of the nasal mucosa was found to have changed when examined with scanning electron microscope (SEM). However, no morphological changes could be detected in the intercellular space, basal membrane or tunica propria examined by transmission electron microscopy. During the test period, 5 of the 20 subjects developed an upper respiratory infection, which was found to temporarily prolong the mucociliar transport time when tested with small saccharin particles. In some of these subjects, the number of ciliated cells was observed to reduce as well as an inflammatory reaction was noted to occur in the region close to the epithelial cells. In the majority of the subjects, one may, therefore, conclude that the intranasal administration of xylometazoline (1 mg/ml) over a 6-week period does not induce any major functional or structural changes in the subjects with a normal nasal mucosa. In the subjects who had common colds, a prolonged mucociliary transport time recovery was observed during the continued use of xylometazoline nose drops.

A synthetic prostaglandin E_2 analog (CL 116,069) was compared with xylometazoline HCl and natural PGE_1, and PGE_2 in the dogs by intranasal administration for their decongestant activity (ref. 295). The drugs were applied to nasal mucosa under in vivo and in vitro conditions. The in vivo technique involved the measurements of the nasal resistance to airflow, i.e., nasal patency. The in vitro technique essentially measured the contraction and relaxation of the smooth muscle of nasal blood vessels isolated from dog's nasal mucosa. The decongestant responses to the CL 116,069 and xylometazoline HCl were found similar in respect to threshold, which showed a near-maximum response to the doses close to the threshold level. The in vitro results also indicated that there is a close similarity between the response characteristics of these two drugs in regard to their threshold and potency.

2. Parasympathomimetics

The action of nicotine in the body is characterized by a primary transient stimulation, followed by a persistent depression of all sympathetic and parasympathetic ganglia. The mechanism of action is related to the depolarization of postsynaptic membrane. The persisting depolarization induced by nicotine produces a block of synaptic transmission. The synaptic stimulatory and depressant effects of nicotine have been known not to be overcomed by atropine. Nicotine is more active on ganglia than on skeletal muscles, and also first stimulates and then paralyzes the central nervous system.

The absorption ability of nicotine by the membranes of the sinus was studied by Childrey and Essex in dogs (ref. 287) and compared to the intravenous and subcutaneous injections. Results indicated that intravenous injection of 1 mg. nicotine is observed to cause an immediate and marked pressor response, which lasts for 2 minutes; subcutaneous injection of 20 mg. nicotine into the same dog yields almost immediately a slight rise in the blood pressure, which lasts 7 minutes, whereas injection of the same amount of nicotine into the left frontal sinus produces no effect during the observation period of 35 minutes. Similar negative results were obtained following the injection of 80 mg of nicotine into the sinus of another dog or 4 mg. into the sinus of a cat.

3. Parasympatholytics

Atopine and scopolamine are antimuscarinic drugs and have been commonly used for the medication of coryza and rhinorrhea caused by allergic rhinitis. Their mode of action is to stop the nasal secretions and to shrink the nasal mucosa by contracting the small blood vessels in the nose.

1) Scopolamine

As early as in 1953, Tonndorf et al. already compared the rapidity and degree of activity of scopolamine administered orally, nasally, or subcutaneously (ref. 296). The drug was administered and salivary secretion was then measured at 15- to 30-min. intervals up to a total period of 2 hours. The control subjects received either no medication, 0.4cc of saline intranasally, or a placebo capsule orally. It was observed that the salivary production in the control group increases slightly, but significantly, during the first hour, after which it remains at a constant level throughout the duration of the experiment. Absorption of scopolamine following subcutaneous injection was found to be rapid and with the peak effect reached after 30 minutes, which was followed by a gradual return towards the normal production. The salivary flow was markedly lower than the control value ($p<<0.01$). Intranasal instillation (0.2 ml) of varying concentrations of scopolamine in saline (pH 5.7-6.0) into each nostril was noted to induce a significant reduction in salivary production to the extent which was below the control level, followed by a gradual return toward the normal level. Neosynephrine was reported to hinder considerably the action of scopolamine when given immediately before the scopolamine nose drops ($p<0.01$), but merely delayed the action when given 15 minutes before the scopolamine nose drop. The subjects treated with scopolamine nasal spray showed a significantly less response than those receiving scopolamine as nose drops, which contained sodium lauryl sulfate to yield a slightly more rapid absorption of scopolamine. With the addition of sodium lauryl sulfate, the nasal spray also demonstrated a striking increase in the degree of scopolamine absorption.

Hyde et al. studied the systemic effect of scopolamine (ref. 297) and observed that sublingual administration of scopolamine is definitely inferior to both the intranasal and subcutaneous routes of administration. Addition of hyaluronidase (1.0 unit/0.4cc) to the scopolamine nose drops was found to yield no significant effect, either in speeding up the initial absorption or in the degree of absorption attained during 90-min. period. To evaluate the difference in the rate and degree of absorption through different parts of the nasal mucous membrane. Scopolamine nose drops were instilled with the head in different positions. The results suggested that at both the 15- and the 30-min. time points, the absorption through the nasal septal mucosa is significantly less than through the mucous membrane on the floor of the nose, the inferior turbinate, and the upper portion of the nose. The thin mucous membrane at the nasopharynx did not absorb scopolamine as rapidly or as completely as did the more vascular mucosa of the inferior turbinates and other portions of the nose. No significant difference in the systemic effect of scopolamine nose drops regardless of whether it was administered to the roof of the nasal cavity, to the floor of the nose, or directly to the inferior turbinate.

2) Atropine

Tonndorf et al. (ref. 296) evaluated the feasibility of using nasal route for the administration of atropine. Trial doses of 0.3 and 0.65 mg of atropine given intranasally to two groups of 5 subjects were found to yield only a slight effect on saliva production. Administration of higher doses of atropine (1.0, 1.5, and 2.0 mg) as nose drops to successive groups of 10 subjects was reported to produce a somewhat more gratifying response, but the only statistically significant difference ($p=0.05$) between the 1.0 mg dose and the 2.0 mg dose was noted to be at the 60- and 120-min. period. Atropine nose drops at 1.5 mg had approximately the same effect as the atropine spray containing a detergent, Duponol (0.01%). Sublingual administration of atropine (1.6 mg/tablet) was noted to be significantly less effective at the 30-minute point than either the spray or the nose drops, but after that the response-time curves ran together. Subcutaneous injection of atropine at a smaller dose (1.0 mg) was found to be definitely more effective than 1.5 mg dose administered sublingually as well as intranasally (at 15-min point). After two hours of observation, there was no significant improvement in the absorption of atropine from the nose drops with either the detergent (0.01% Duponol) or the hyaluronidase (1.0 unit/0.4cc).

Comparison of the intranasal absorption between scopolamine and atropine, it was noted that 0.65 mg of scopolamine produce a systemic effect similar to that resulting from 2.0 mg of atropine. On the other hand, subcutaneous injection of 0.65 mg of scopolamine produced a more rapid and a greater degree of salivary depression than did 1.0 mg of atropine for the 15-, 30-, and 60-minute periods ($p<0.05$). The observed weaker depression of salivary secretion by atropine, after the subcutaneous and intranasal administration, was interpreted as a result of the lower antisialogogic activity of atropine, rather than a slower rate of absorption. More side reactions were noted with the atropine than with the scopolamine.

Atropine sulfate solution (1 mg/ml) was administered intranasally (0.08 mg/nostril), using an atomizer, to 7 patients with rhinorrhea caused by allergic rhinitis and to 24 patients with rhinorrhea caused by viral rhinitis (ref. 298). All, but one, of the 31 patients demonstrated a visible reduction in secretions, and 3 patients showed an obvious vasoconstriction of nasal blood vessels. None of the patients reported the occurrence of dry mouth or visual disturbance. The effects of atropine were noted to last 3-4 hours in the 5 patients who were observed for longer periods.

3) Ipratropium

Ipratropium is a parasympatholytic drug with topical activity and, when supplied in aerosol, has been used as a bronchodilator for the treatment of broncho-constrictive diseases. Borum and Mygind (ref. 299) developed a simple test for the measurement of nasal reactivity in 20 healthy subjects and 10 patients with perennial rhinitis. Each subject was stimulated with increasing concentrations of methacholine, 3 to 48 mg, at intervals of 30 minutes. The dose-response relationship was found to be linear; and the women were noted to produce more secretion than the men ($p<0.001$). The patients produced considerably more secretion than the normal test subjects by a methacholine dose of 6 mg ($p<0.001$). Pretreatment of the normal subjects with ipratropium (40 µg/nostril) at 30 minutes prior to a methacholine provocation resulted in a parallel displacement of the log dose-response curve. Furthermore, a double-blind controlled cross-over trial, with intranasal administration of Ipratropium or placebo at 30 minutes prior to a methacholine provocation, was initiated in 15 healthy experimental subjects. The results showed that ipratropium reduces significantly the methacholine-induced secretion. The maximum effect of ipratropium lasted for up to 4-6 hours, after which it slowly decreased. The investigators suggested that it is possible to effectively block the cholinergic receptors of the glands with 2 puffs (40 µg) of ipratropium in each nostril, 3-4 times a day.

Twenty patients suffering from perennial rhinitis, with hypersecretion as the main symptom, took part in a double-blind, cross-over study. The patients were treated with ipratropium or placebo, in a randomized manner, for two periods, each for 14 days. Of the 20 patients, 14 preferred the active formulation, 3 the placebo, and the remaining 3 had no preference ($p<0.006$). All of the 14 patients, who preferred the active formulation, considered the effect so satisfactory that they were willing to continue the treatment for a longer period.

Borum et al. (ref. 300) recently studied the effect of ipratropium spray on rhinorrhea in 40 adults with naturally occurring common cold. All subjects received a nasal vasoconstrictor (xylometazoline, 0.1%), 5 minutes before intranasal administration of ipratropium or placebo, to ensure adequate mucosal distribution. Treatment with ipratropium as a nasal spray, 4 times a day, for one week resulted in a significant reduction in nasal discharge compared with that of placebo treatment ($p<0.001$). It was noted that ipratropium is especially effective in the first 3 days, when the watery secretion is predominant. Seven subjects in the placebo group and 10 in the ipratropium group showed a slight local reaction. It was concluded that ipratropium nasal spray can be of value in the beginning of a common cold when nasal discharge is a nuisance.

K) CNS STIMULANTS - COCAINE

Cocaine is a stimulant of the central nervous system and also a nonsynthetic local anesthetics. In animals, it was reported to block the re-uptake of endogenous amines by the sympathetic nervous system and to potentiate the effects of exogenous amines (ref. 301). Cocaine has been used in otolaryngology and anesthesiology because of its effectiveness as a local anesthetic and vasoconstrictor. Socially, it has become a major drug of abuse and was reported to produce an intense euphoria 3 to 5 minutes after intranasal application and thereby has gained the reputation of being the "champagne of drugs". Street reports indicate that the "high" is intense, rapid in onset, and brief in duration. The blood concentration pattern of cocaine is rather important since the surgical procedures are often performed immediately after the application of cocaine. The actions of cocaine, if prolonged, may modify physiological responses to the surgical procedures. Cocaine is hydrolyzed and rendered ineffective in the gastrointestinal tract as well as by plasma and hepatic esterases (ref. 301-303).

Byck et al. (ref. 304, 305) measured the plasma concentration of cocaine and evaluated the relationship between plasma concentrations of cocaine and its physiological effect after intranasal administration to 13 surgical patients, among them 9 were undergoing cardiovascular surgery and 4 were dental patients. A 10% cocaine HCl solution was administered topically (1.5 mg/kg) to the nasal mucosa prior to nasal intubation.

Plasma concentration of cocaine were detectable within 3 minutes and observed to increase rapidly for the first 15 to 20 minutes, peaked at 15 to 60 minutes, and then decreased gradually over the next 3 to 5 hours. Maximum plasma concentration of 120-474 ng/ml was obtained with the cardiovascular patients, who appeared to have a significantly greater level than the dental patients. The cocaine was found to be presented on the nasal mucosa for 3 hours following application, suggesting that the prolonged absorption of cocaine, perhaps as a result of its vasoconstrictive action, might explain its persistence in the plasma for as long as 6 hours.

The correlation between blood concentrations and physiological changes after the intranasal administration of cocaine was further studied in 4 normal subjects with a moderately heavy prior use of cocaine (ref. 304). Cocaine was given as a 10% solution by instillation into the nose at doses of 0.19, 0.38, 0.75, and 1.5 mg/kg. All doses used were found failure to produce a discernible effect on the cardiovascular function. Pupillary size was changed at the dose levels of 0.75 or 1.5 mg/kg, but not at the lower dosages. Many subjects fell asleep at approximately 2 to 3 hours after cocaine administration.

Resnick and his associates (ref. 306, 307) undertook a study to assess the physiologic and subjective effects, in 19 volunteers over a 30-min. observation period, by intranasal and intravenous administrations of a single-dose of placebo or 10 mg and 25 mg of cocaine. Another 100 mg of cocaine was also administered by nasal route to five of the subjects. A 0.5 ml of cocaine solution in bacteriostatic water was instilled into the nostrils. The 100-mg nasal dose was given once by drops and once by flakes (mixed with lactose powder). Nasal placebo was 0.5 ml of 1% lidocaine solution or 5 mg of tetracaine powder mixed with lactose powder.

By intranasal administration, 10 mg of cocaine were found to produce no change, 25 mg yielded a minimal change in systolic blood pressure only ($p<0.02$), and 100 mg produced a significant change ($p<0.01$) in the heart rate and also in the systolic and diastolic blood pressures. The magnitude of mean changes after insufflating the cocaine flakes was noted to be greater than after the instillation of cocaine solution. By intravenous injection, all doses (10 & 25 mg) produced a significant ($p<0.01$) change in both the heart rate and the systolic blood pressure. The onset of these effects occurred within 2 minutes and peaked within 5-10 minutes when given intravenously and within 15-20 minutes following intranasal administration. No significant changes in respiratory rate, body temperature, or handgrip strength were detected at any of the doses.

Following the 25 mg nasal dose, a significant change in the subjective effects was observed on the scales of "high" ($p<0.02$), pleasantness ($p<0.05$), and the ARC Inventory ($p<0.02$). The 100 mg nasal dose and both intravenous doses (10 mg and 25 mg) produced a significant ($p<0.01$) dose-related change on all subjective scales, except the strength. By the intranasal route, these subjective effects peaked within 10 min. and 54-68% of the effects were still evident at the end of the 30-min. observation period. By the intravenous route, the onset of these subjective effects occurred within 2 min. and peaked within 10 min. However, no direct relationship between physiologic and subjective effects could be established. A biphasic effect, consisting of an initial euphoria followed by dysphoric effects, was reported by four subjects at 20 to 30 minutes after the 25 mg intranvenous dose and by two subjects at 45 to 60 minutes after the 100 mg intranasal dose.

Dyke et al. (ref. 308) made a comparative study on the efficacy of cocaine by oral and intranasal administrations. In the first study, a 10% cocaine HCl solution was applied topically to the nasal mucosa of 4 human subjects with a total dose ranging from 115 to 246 mg. In the subsequent experiments, the subjects swallowed the same dosage of crystalline cocaine HCl in gelatin capsule. Results indicated that following the intranasal administration, cocaine was detected in the plasma by 15 minutes, reached peak concentrations, which range from 61 to 408 ng/ml, at 60 to 120 minutes, and then decreased gradually over the next 2 to 3 hours. On the other hand, by oral administration, cocaine was not detected in the plasma until 30 minutes, and it then increased rapidly for the next 30 minutes. Peak plasma concentrations, which range from 104 to 424 ng/ml, occurred at 50 to 90 minutes and then decreased gradually over the next 4.5 to 5 hours. There was no significant difference in the peak plasma concentrations between these two routes of administration. Once the peak levels were reached, the concentrations of cocaine decreased in a log-linear fashion with the apparent plasma half-life being 0.9 hour after the oral route and 1.3 hours after the intranasal route.

By intranasal application, measurable effects on the "high" scale were noted within 15 to 30 minutes, peaked at 15 to 60 minutes, lasted for as long as 60 minutes, and then decreased over the next 2 to 3 hours. After the oral administration, measurable effects on the "high" scale occurred within 15 to 75 minutes and peaked at 45 to 90 minutes. Peak effects lasted for as long as 60 minutes and then declined over the next 4 hours. Peak "highs" after oral administration were significantly greater than those reported after intranasal application ($p<0.05$). Despite the common belief that cocaine is not effective when taken orally; however, this study showed that cocaine is well absorbed from the gastrointestinal tract and biologically effective.

In order to investigate the possibility that cocaine is not unique in its psychoactivity, Dyke et al. (ref. 309) recently compared cocaine HCl and lidocaine HCl by intranasal administration at three matched dose levels, i.e., 0.19 mg/kg, 0.38 mg/kg, and 0.75 mg/kg with normal saline as the placebo. The placebo and 0.19 mg/kg dose produced a similar peak "high" rating. The 0.38 and 0.75 mg/kg doses produced a similar mean peak "high" rating that was greater than those of 0.19 mg/kg dose and placebo. The mean peak "high" ratings following three different dosages of lidocaine were very similar to those observed after the same doses of cocaine. Peak "high" ratings were observed to occcur within 5 to 15 minutes for both cocaine and lidocaine, and at 15 minutes for the placebo. The highest dose (0.75 mg/kg) of cocaine and lidocaine was associated with the self-reports of increased pleasantness, but no change in energy or involvement. Following the intranasal administration of 2 lower doses of cocaine and all doses of lidocaine, no change in the pre-post ARCI scores was reported. However, after the 0.75 mg/kg of cocaine there was an increased number of responses on the ARCI. In summary, there was no indication of a unique euphoria or stimulation which differentiated cocaine from lidocaine.

Pharmacokinetics of cocaine following intranasal and oral administrations was assessed in 7 human subjects by Wilkinson et al. (ref. 310). Intranasal doses of 0.19, 0.38, 0.75, 1.5 and 2.0 mg/kg were administered to all subjects as a 10% aqueous solution of cocaine. In another study, 0.38 mg/kg was given nasally to 3 subjects as crystalline cocaine HCl, while four subjects were given cocaine by the oral route in a gelatin capsule (2.0 mg/kg crystalline cocaine HCl). The results indicated that the pharmacokinetics of cocaine following intranasal administration can be described by a one-compartment open model with 2 consecutive first-order input phase and one first-order elimination phase. On the other hand, the disposition of oral cocaine was described by a one-compartment open model with a lag time followed by a single first-order input phase and one first-order elimination phase. The peak plasma levels after the intranasal administration of cocaine in crystalline form were reached slightly sooner than after the same dose of cocaine in a solution formulation (35 ± 13.2 min. vs. 47.1 ± 6.1 min.). The peak plasma levels were found to be dose-dependent. By oral administration, cocaine was not detected in the plasma until 30 minute later and peak level was reached at 64 ± 6.7 min. The mean elimination half-life ($t_{\frac{1}{2}}$) for cocaine following the intranasal and oral administrations was determined to be 75 ± 5 min. and 48 ± 3 min., respectively. The AUCs after the intranasal and oral administrations at the same dose level were not significantly different (23.3 ± 5.0 vs. 22.3 ± 5.4 µg/ml · min). It may be the coincidence that the incomplete absorption of cocaine from the nasal mucosa reduces its systemic bioavailability to the same extent as the hepatic first-pass metabolism after the oral doses. A linear increase in the AUC value was observed as increasing the nasal dose.

Dyke et al. (ref. 311) examined the psychological effects of 3 nasal doses of cocaine HCl in solution (0.2, 0.75, and 1.5 mg/kg) and the plasma cocaine concentrations in four volunteers. Intranasal administration of lidocaine HCl (0.2 mg/kg) was also carried out as a topically active placebo. Results also demonstrated that the mean peak plasma concentrations of cocaine are dose-dependent. For the 0.75 and 1.5 mg/kg doses, plasma levels peaked at 60 minutes and then decreased in a log-linear fashion with an apparent elimination half-life of 1.3 hours. The mean peak "high" ratings were also found to be dose-dependent. The "high" from the administration of cocaine was a pleasant feeling, but was without a distinctive sensation. For the 0.75 and 1.5 mg/kg doses, the increase in the "high" scale occurred within 15 minutes, peaked at 15 to 30 minutes, and then decreased with an apparent half-life of 0.8 hours. On the other hand, all subjects experienced peak "highs" at 30 minutes after lidocaine administration and then this effect decreased until it reached baseline values between the second and fourth hours. The peak "highs" were observed to be related to the dose and the peak plasma concentrations. At a given plasma concentration, "high" ratings were greater when plasma levels were increasing than when they were decreasing. This observation suggested that the acute tolerance by tachyphylaxis occurs after a single dose.

L) PROSTAGLANDINS

In 1935, physiologically active prostaglandins were first isolated from the vesicular glands of sheep. Later, it was found that prostaglandins can be extracted from most animal tissues, but the human seminal fluid contains the highest concentration and the greatest number of prostaglandins. The principal pharmacologic activities of various prostaglandins are numerous, including the stimulation of gastrointestinal and reproductive smooth muscles, relaxation and contraction of respiratory smooth muscle, hypotensive activity, inhibition of lipolysis of fatty acids, secretion of gastric acid and aggregation of blood platelet. Prostaglandins also act on vascular resistance and vasoconstrictor response (ref. 312). Prostaglandins usually depress the effects of sympathetic nerve stimulation and, apparently, inhibit transmitter release from the adrenergic nerve (ref. 313).

Anggard (ref. 314) administered topically PGE_1, PGE_2, and $PGF_{1\alpha}$ (10-15 μg) in 7 subjects and reported the observation of increased nasal patency in 4 subjects taking PGE_1 and PGE_2, but observed no effect for $PGF_{1\alpha}$. The most likely mechanism of action in the increase of nasal patency is a result of the constrictory effect of prostaglandins on nasal blood vessels. Four doses (37, 50, 75 & 100 μg) of prostaglandin E_1 were administered to 15 human subjects as a nasal vasoconstrictor (ref. 315). Good responses were produced in 5 subjects, no response in 3 subjects, and no clear response in the remaining 7 subjects. When a response was observed, it lasted from 3 to 12 hours. The 100 μg PGE_1 dose was noted to induce some degree of nasal irritation, mild burning sensation, lacrimation and nasal throbbing. The effect of PGE_1 and 17-phenyl trinor-PGE_2 on nasal patency was also studied in 6 patients with vasomotor and allergic rhinitis (ref. 316). In 4 out of the 6 subjects, 37.5 μg of PGE_1 were reported to increase nasal patency with some side effects, including nasal irritation, nasal throbbing, lacrimation, severe headache and sore throat, which persisted 15 to 60 minutes.

When administered with the same dose of 17-phenyl trinor PGE_2, all 6 volunteers showed an increase in nasal patency with only one experienced nasal irritation. Further stuides indicated that instillation of 17-phenyl trinor PGE_2 at doses of 12.5, 25, and 50 µg, increases nasal patency in all 14 patients with vasomotor rhinitis (ref. 317). At 50 µg dose, the increase in nasal patency was observed to last for more than 7 hours in 8 of the 14 subjects, whereas 2 patients experienced some mild local irritation and lacrimation.

A synthetic prostaglandin E_2 analogue (CL 116,069) was compared in the dogs with xylometazoline HCl (a nasal decongestant) as well as natural PGE_1 and PGE_2 for nasal decongestant activity (ref. 318). Using both in vivo nasal patency tests and in vitro nasal blood vessel contraction tests, the synthetic prostaglandin E_2 analogue was found to be more effective and very long-acting, with no change in blood pressure, at the effective systemic or topical doses.

Apparently, the natural or synthetic prostaglandins, when given intranasally, result in a good local effect in the treatment of allergic or vasomotor rhinitis as well as nasal congestion.

M) MISCELLANEOUS THERAPEUTIC AGENTS

1. Antimicrobial and Antiviral Agents

A study was carried out by Greenwood et al. (ref. 319) in 1946 to determine the effect of zephiran chloride, tyrothricin, penicillin and streptomycin on ciliary activity of the mucous membrane on upper respiratory tract. The aqueous solution of zephiran chloride (with concentrations of 1:1,000 and 1:2,000) was observed to stop all the ciliary activity of extirpated ciliated mucous membranes in 5-10 minutes. However, the controls, which were treated with plain distilled water, also showed cessation of ciliary action in 5-10 minutes as well. On the other hand, zephiran chloride in isotonic salin solution (at same concentration as above) produced no apparent deleterious effect on the active cilia. Actively beating cilia stopped its beating when treated with aqueous suspensions of tyrothricin (at concentrations of 1:2,000 and 1:5,000) within 5-10 minutes, whereas penicillin (at concentrations of 200 and 500 IU/ml) in isotonic saline solution showed no apparent deleterious effect on the ciliary action of the nasal mucosa from normal healthy rabbits. Streptomycin (at concentrations of 100, 300, 500 and 1,000 units/ml) in isotonic saline solution had no inhibitory or deleterious effect on the ciliary action of either nasal mucosa or tracheal ciliated epithelium from normal healthy rabbits.

It is well known that sulbenicillin, cephacetrile, and cefazolin (ref. 320, 321) are poorly absorbed from the gastrointestinal tract, because of their high water solubility and lack of lipophilic properties. Recently,

Hirai et al. (ref. 322) initiated an in vivo absorption study in the rats to compare the bioavailability of sulbenicillin, cephacetrile and cefazolin following the intranasal, oral and intramuscular administrations. After the oral administration, poor absorption was confirmed for all three drugs, whereas after the intranasal administration, the per cent dose excreted in urine was found to be nearly one-half of that after the intramuscular injection. These results suggested that even the poorly orally absorbed drugs can be easily absorbed following the intranasal administration and the nasal route of administration would be useful as a new route of administration to enhance the systemic bioavailability of poorly orally absorbed drugs.

Absorption of aminoglycoside from the gastrointestinal tract can be enhanced by coadministration with a nonionic surfactant (ref. 323). Rubinstein (ref. 324) recently reported the observations of increased absorption of gentamicin from the nasal passages in healthy human subjects, when the antibiotic (60 mg/ml) was given in a saline solution (0.15M) with sodium glycocholate (1% w/v). The solution was applied to each nostril at a volume of 1 to 2 ml, which were equivalent to a dose of 2 mg/kg. In a control experiment, 3 subjects received an equivalent dose of gentamicin (0.3 mg/kg) in a saline solution, and two others received a saline solution of 1% sodium glycocholate. In addition, 4 subjects received a saline solution of gentamicin (0.3 mg/kg) intramuscularly. Peak concentrations of 2.48 ± 0.42 µg/ml were attained after 30 min in the 4 subjects received intramuscular injection and after 60 min in the 3 subjects received nasal gentamicin dose with 1% sodium glycocholate, beyond which the gentamicin concentrations decreased gradually to 0.94 ± 0.13 µg/ml over 180 minutes. Only a slight local irritation, but no serious side effects, was observed. Amounts of gentamicin in the serum were below the detectable level when 2 mg/kg of gentamicin was given intranasally in the saline solution without sodium glycocholate. Apparently, presence of a surfactant, such as glycocholate, is required to obtain a significant concentration of gentamicin in the circulation.

When antiviral drugs are administered as nasal drops to animals infected with viruses in the upper respiratory tract, the manifestation of antiviral activity is always found to be much less than expected. Bucknall (ref. 325) studied the factors which may be responsible for the reduction of the effectiveness of antiviral drugs taken intranasally. The mice were first infected in the upper respiratory tract with influenza A and then treated with a new antiviral drug, called phenyl-p-guanidino benzoate (PGB). The infection was carried out intranasally by instillation of a 100 $TCID_{50}$ influenza A_0 (DSP) and a good growth of virus in the upper respiratory tract was attained by 30 hours after the infection. If mice were dosed intranasally with repeated doses of PGB solution (4 or 5 times an hour) for 6 hours immediately following infection, there was a reduction in the virus growth. However, there appeared to be a factor or a set of factors which were operating to greatly reduce the effect of the drug when it was given directly into the nose. The most obvious possibility was the mucociliary clearance system which sweeped the drug out of the upper airways after each dose. In an intact mouse, with the mucociliary transport system working normally, the hourly exposure of the upper respiratory tract, with doses given 5 times an hour, was found to be 7½-12½ min, which gave a 9-fold reduction in virus growth, whereas in the in vitro situation a 20- to 40-fold reduction could be obtained with only 1-2 min drug exposure in each hour. Thus, the clearance of drug from the nose by mucociliary transport system must be regarded as only a contributory factor and not the major one, in accounting for the relatively poor performance of the drug given intranasally.

Enviroxime, a substituted benzimidazole derivative, is virustatic for rhinoviruses at concentration of 10 to 40 ng/ml in tissue cultures (ref. 326). Levandowski et al. (ref. 327) recently studied the clinical prophylactic and therapeutic effects of enviroxime given as a nasal spray in a placebo-controlled, double-blind study in 99 volunteers infected with rhinovirus Type 4 (RV4). A metered-dose nasal spray was used to deliver either the enviroxime or a placebo in an alcoholic solution with a Freon propellant. Each spray delivered 284 mcg of enviroxime to each nostril. The concentration of enviroxime in the nasal secretions measured 12 hours after the dosing on Day 3, 4, and 5 was found to range from undetectable to 4,662 ng/ml. In one group of the volunteers, the concentration was 798 ± 310 ng/ml, whereas in the other group the concentration was only 13 ± 5 ng/ml. A level of up to 30 ng/ml was recorded in the volunteers who received only the placebo. Cold symptoms were observed in 27 to 73% of the volunteers in the different test groups. Persons, who were treated with enviroxime before RV4 challenge and had a mean enviroxime concentration of >100 ng/ml in their nasal washes, were observed to experience fewer symptoms during the first 4 days after challenge. Only a slight relief in the symptoms was attained in the volunteers treated with enviroxime after the viral challenge and had an enviroxime level of >100 ng/ml. A total of 20 of the 38 placebo-treated volunteers and 47 of the 61 enviroxime-treated volunteers reported a transient, mild nasal stinging for the first few minutes after intranasal spraying. No abnormalities were observed in the total or differential leukocyte count, hemoglobin concentrations, or the tests of renal and hepatic functions that were attributable to the intranasal administration of enviroxime by nasal spray.

2. Histamine and Antihistamines

Histamine is an important mediator to the development of the symptoms of allergic rhinitis. Its release into the nasal mucosa causes irritation and sneezing, vascular engorgement and congestion, edema of the mucosa and production of excessive nasal secretions. Histamine may also be relevant in the development of the symptoms of vasomotor rhinitis and the common cold.

Antihistamines block the effects of histamine on H_1-receptors. Clinical trials have demonstrated that oral H_1-antihistamines have a greater effect on sneezing and discharge than on blockage in the allergic rhinitis (ref. 328, 329). However, the effect of antihistamines given alone on the symptoms of common cold or vasomotor rhinitis is probably slight and is often unpredictable (ref. 330).

Histamine causes a marked fall in blood pressure when injected intravenously or subcutaneously in the dogs (ref. 331). Injection of 1 mg of histamine, by intravenous and subcutaneous routes, into an etherized dog was found to cause a distinct depressor reponse. The same dose repeatedly injected into the nasal cavity or the sinus produced no effect on the blood pressure. In another dog, injection of histamine, 1 mg first and then 10 mg, into the frontal sinus also yielded no effect on the blood pressure. Apparently, histamine was absorbed so slowly from the mucosa of the sinus that no appreciable changes in the blood pressure were noted.

The effect of antihistaminic drugs in nasal solution on the mucous membranes was investigated in rabbits by Gundrum (ref. 332). Antistine-Privine® (which contains antistine HCl, 0.5% and privine HCl, 0.025%) was found to be most harmful and caused almost a complete necrosis throughout the entire nasal area. Pyribenzamine® (pyribenzamine 0.5%) was the least harmful. Allergan® (pyranisamine maleate, 0.1% and phenylephrine HCl, 0.25%) caused more damage than did Pyribenzamine, but considerably less than Antistine-Privine®.

The potential of intranasal administration of two antihistamines, prophenpyridamine maleate and chlorprophenpyridamine maleate, was evaluated in the patients with allergic rhinitis (ref. 333). In the 83 patients receiving the prophenpyridamine maleate solution (0.5%), 68 patients (82.0%) exhibited a moderate to complete nasal vasoconstriction, which lasted 4-6 hours or longer. In the 61 cases receiving chlorprophenpyridamine maleate solution (0.25%), 48 patients (78.8%) exhibited a moderate to complete vasoconstriction, lasting from 4 to 6 hours on the average. No systemic or latent irritation of the nasal mucosa was reported. Recently, Secher et al. (ref. 334) studied the importance of histamine H_1 and H_2 receptors in the human nose. Twenty-five healthy human subjects were provoked with histamine, after the local pretreatment with a H_1-receptor antagonist, chlorpheniramine maleate, a H_2-receptor antagonist, ranitidine HCl or a combination of these two antihistamines. Results suggested that the histamine-induced increase in the nasal airway resistance is 52% inhibited by the nasal spray containing the combination of these two antihistamines ($p<0.05$), 22% by chlopheniramine maleate alone ($p<0.05$), and 29% by ranitidine. Apparently, the combination was significantly more effective than the H_1-receptor antagonist, chlorpheniramine maleate, alone ($p<0.05$). The observations suggested the equal importance of H_1 and H_2 receptors in nasal blood vessels, and an additive effect of H_1 and H_2 antihistamines.

Sodium cromoglycate is a receptor inhibitor for histamine release. The efficacy of sodium cromoglycate, in powder or solution form, was recently compared with placebo in a group of 39 patients with allergic rhinitis over a period of 4 weeks (ref. 335). A crossover trial was further carried out in 20 patients to compare the efficacy of sodium cromoglycate in powder and solution in those whose main symptoms were nasal obstruction. The data showed that sodium cromoglycate powder and solution are both effective, although the powder formulation appears to be somewhat better than the solution formulation in those patients with rhinorrhoea, which could be related to the fact that the powder is not rapidly washed out by the nasal secretions. However, in those patients in whom blocking was the predominant symptom, the solution appeared to offer some advantages as a result of an effective nasal distribution.

3. Diagnostic Drugs

Phenolsulfonphthalein (phenol red) is a diagnostic aid used for the determination of kidney functions. When injected intramuscularly or intravenously, it begins to be excreted in 5-10 min. in the patients with normal kidneys. In the patients with deficient renal function, the first appearance of its excretion is delayed. In the normal cases, following an intramuscular injection, almost the total amount is excreted within 2 hours. Failure to excrete the full amount within 2 hours may indicate a deficient renal function , and the degree of this functional deficiency may be estimated from the proportionate amount excreted within 2 hours.

The absorptive ability of the sinus membrane on phenol red was studied by Childrey and Essex (ref. 331). As a control, 1cc of phenolsulphonphthalein was injected subcutaneously into a dog, in which the dye first appeared in the urine within 15 minutes, more than 50% was excreted during the first hour, and only traces were present during the third hour. While one cc of phenolsulphonphthalein was injected into the nasal mucosa of another dog, the dye appeared in the urine one hour and fifty minutes after the injection and only faint traces were present at 6 hours and 45 minutes later. If one cc of phenolsulphonphthalein was injected into the right frontal sinus of a normal dog, the first trace of the drug appeared in the urine at one hour and forty-five minutes later and continued to appear for 7½ hours.

Phenolsulphonphthalein was also studied by Hirai et al. in rats (ref. 322) using in situ recirculation method and in vivo nasal absorption technique. From the drug assay data in the in situ recirculation solution, the phenolsulphonphthalein in pH 7.4 buffer appeared to have little nasal absorption within 2 hours.

The urinary recovery data of phenolsulphonphthalein following the in vivo intranasal administration were compared with those by the oral and intramuscular administrations. Results indicated that poor absorption is yielded following the oral administration, while after the intranasal administration, the per cent dose excreted in urine exceeds one-half of that by intramuscular injection. The observed difference in the extent of nasal absorption between the in situ and the in vivo studies is probably due to the difference in the experimental conditions, for example, in the in situ experiments, the volume of the nasal solution (0.2-0.3 ml) is extremely small as compared to the recirculating solution (20 ml).

4. Inorganic salts

Nasal absorption of CsCl, $SrCl_2$, $BaCl_2$ and $CeCl_3$ was studied in Syrian hamsters and compared with G-I absorption (ref. 336). Results indicated that more than 50% of the radioactive cesium (Cs), strontium (Sr), and barium (Ba) deposited on the nasal membrane are absorbed directly into the general circulation, but only less than 4% of the cerium (Ce) is absorbed. For all the isotopes studied, nasal bioavailability was approximately equal to or greater than oral bioavailability in the first 4 hours of post-administration. The data suggested that nasopharynx may be the most important site of absorption for the aerosols with a median mass aerodynamic diameter (MMAD) greater than 5 microns, where nasal deposition greatly exceeds deposition in all other areas of the respiratory tract.

Czerniawska (ref. 337) investigated the possibility of penetration of radioactive colloidal gold (^{198}Au) from the mucous membrane of the olfactory region into the cerebrospinal fluid of the subarachnoid space in the anterior part of the brain. A suspension of colloidal ^{198}Au was injected unilaterally, under the mucous membrane of the roof of the nose, in 2 groups of rabbits (Groups I & III), whereas another group of animals (Group II) received an intravenous injection of radiocolloid ^{198}Au. The results demonstrated that the radioactive isotope, ^{198}Au, penetrates from the mucous membrane of the nasal olfactory region directly into the cerebrospinal fluid of the anterior cranial fossa.

Gopinath et al. (ref. 338) studied the pathways for the transfer of colloidal gold sprayed on the nasal mucosa in rhesus monkeys by electron microscopy. One-fourth ml of the colloidal gold was administered using a glass atomizer with the nozzle directing towards the roof of the nose while spraying. The colloidal gold particles sprayed on the olfactory mucosa were found to enter both the olfactory rods and the supporting cells. The gold particles in the olfactory neurons could be traced to as far as the fila olfactoria. In the supporting cells, the gold particles were observed as either discrete, free-lying particles or aggregated to form larger electron-dense masses in the mitochondria. Gold particles were also detected to be present in the endothelial cells of the blood vessels in the lamina propria, but they could not be detected in the intercellular spaces of the olfactory mucosa. This study revealed that the intranasal route can be used for the administration of drugs directly into the brain as well as into the systemic circulation.

REFERENCES

1) A. Osol; Remington's Pharmaceutical Sciences, Mack Publishing Company, Easton, Pennsylvania (1980), pp. 845.
2) C. T. Dollery, D. S. Davis, and M. E. Conolly; Differences in the metabolism of drugs depending upon their routes of administration, Ann. N. Y. Acad. Sci., 179 108 (1971).
3) D. G. Shand, E. M. Nuckolls and J. A. Oates; Plasma propranolol levels in adults with observations in four children, Clin. Pharmacol. Ther., 11 112 (1970).
4) A. A. Hussain, S. Hirai, and R. Bawarshi; Nasal absorption of propranolol in rats, J. Pharm. Sci., 68 1196 (1979).
5) A. A. Hussain, S. Hirai, and R. Bawarshi; Nasal absorption of propranolol from different dosage forms by rats and dogs, ibid., 69 1411 (1980).
6) A. A. Hussain, T. Foster, S. Hirai, T. Kashihara, R. Batenhorst, and M. Jones; Nasal absorption of propranolol in humans, ibid., 69 1240 (1980).
7) H. J. M. van de Donk and F. W. H. M. Merkus; Decreases in ciliary beat frequency due to intranasal administration of propranolol, ibid., 71 595 (1982).
8) D. D. Mar; New topical nitroglycerin preparations, Am. J. Nurs., 82(3) 462 (1982).
9) B. Heinzow and A. Ziegler; Comparison of the effects of nitroglycerin administered to rats by different routes, J. Cardiovas. Pharmacol., 3(3) 573 (1981).
10) A. B. Hill, C. J. Bowley, M. L. Nahrwold, P. R. Knight, A. R. Tait, M. D. Taylor, M. M. Kirsch, and J. K. Denlinger; Intranasal administration of nitroglycerin, Anesthesiology, 51 S67 (1979).
11) A. B. Hill, C. J. Bowley, M. L. Nahrwold, P. R. Knight, M. M. Kirsh, and J. K. Denlinger; Intranasal administration of nitroglycerin, ibid., 54 346 (1981).
12) G. J. Moon, J. G. Kim, and F. T. Cookinham; Intranasal nitroglycerin (NTG) during infrarenal aortic cross-clamp, ibid., 55 191 (1981).
13) J. M. Lesser, Z. H. Israili, D. C. Davis, and P. G. Dayton; Metabolism and disposition of hydralazine - ^{14}C in man and dog, Drug Metab. Dispos., 2 351 (1974).

14) S. D. Zak, M. F. Bartlett, W. E. Wagner, T. G. Gilleran, and G. Lukes; Disposition of hydralazine in man and a specific method for its determination in biological fluids, J. Pharm. Sci., 63 225 (1974).
15) Y. Kaneo; Absorption from the nasal mucous membrane: I. Nasal absorption of hydralazine in rats, Acta. Pharm. Suec., 20 379 (1983).
16) S. Hirai, T. Yashiki, T. Matsuzawa, and H. Mima; Absorption of drugs from the nasal mucosa of rat, Int. J. Pharm., 7 317 (1981).
17) N. F. H. Ho, W. I. Higuchi, and J. Turi; Theoretical model studies of drug absorption and transport in the GI tract. III, J. Pharm. Sci., 61 192 (1972).
18) M. I. Steinberg and B. B. Molly; Clofilium-A new antifibrillatory agent that selectively increases cellular refractoriness, Life Science, 25 1397 (1979).
19) M. I. Steinberg, M. E. Sullivan, S. A. Wiest, F. W. Rockhold, and B. B. Molly; Cellular electrophysiology of clofilium, a new antifibrillatory agent, in normal and ischemic canine purkinje fibers, J. Cardiovas. Pharmacol., 3 881 (1981).
20) M. I. Steinberg; in "New Drug Annual," Raven Press, New York, N. Y., (1984), p. 103.
21) K. S. E. Su, K. M. Campanale, and C. L. Gries; Nasal drug delivery system of a quaternary ammonium compound:clofilium tosylate, J. Pharm. Sci., 73 1251 (1984).
22) J. A. Hemberger and L. S. Schanker; Mechanism of pulmonary absorption of quaternary ammonium compounds in the rat, Drug Metab. Dispos., II 73 (1983).
23) A. Osol; Remington's Pharmaceutical Sciences, Mack Publishing Company, Easton, Pennsylvania (1980), pp. 1177.
24) M. Ho and J. A. Armstrong; Interferon, Ann. Rev. Microbiol., 29 131 (1975).
25) A. Isaacs and J. Lindenmann; Virus interference. I. The interferon, Proc. Roy. Soc. (Ser. B), 147 258 (1957).
26) V. D. Soloviev, In The Interferons (G. Rita, Ed.); Academic, New York (1968), pp. 233.
27) V. D. Soloviev; The results of controlled observations on the prophylaxis of influenza with interferon, Bull. WHO, 41 683 (1969).
28) Scientific Committee on Interferon; Progress towards trials of human interferon in man, Ann. N. Y. Acad. Sci., 173 770 (1970).
29) T. C. Merigan, S. E. Reed, T. S. Hall, and D. A. J. Tyrrell; Inhibition of respiratory virus infection by locally applied interferon, Lancet, 1 563 (1973).
30) P. E. Johnson, S. B. Greenberg, M. W. Harmon, B. R. Alford, and R. B. Couch; Recovery of applied human leukocyte interferon from the nasal mucosa of chimpanzees and humans, J. Clin. Microbi., 4 106 (1976).
31) M. W. Harmon, S. B. Greenberg, P. E. Johnson, and R. B. Couch; Human nasal epithelial cell culture system: evaulation of response to human interferons, Infect. and Immun., 16 480 (1977).
32) S. B. Greenberg, M. W. Harmon, P. E. Johnson, and R. B. Couch; Antiviral activity of intranasally applied human leukocyte interferon, Antimicrob. Agent and Chemother., 14 596 (1978).
33) S. B. Greenberg, M. W. Harmon, R. B. Couch, P. E. Johnson, S. Z. Wilson C. C. Dacso, K. Bloom, and J. Ouarles; Prophylactic effect of low doses of human leukocyte interferon against infection with rhinovirus, J. Infect. Dis., 145 542 (1982).
34) G. M. Scott, R. J. Phillpotts, J. Wallace, D. S. Secher, K. Cantrell, and D. A. J. Tyrrell; Purified interferon as protection against rhinovirus infection, Br. Med. J., 284 1822 (1982).
35) T. C. Samo, S. B. Greenberg, R. B. Couch, J. Ouarles, P. E. Johnson, S. Hook and M. W. Harmon; Efficacy and tolerance of intranasally applied recombinant leukocyte A interferon in normal volunteers, J. Infect. Dis., 148 535 (1983).

36) F. G. Hayden, S. E. Mills, and M. E. Johns; Human tolerance and histologic effects of long-term administration of intranasal interferon -α 2. ibid., 148 914 (1983).
37) D. A. Hill, S. Baron, J. C. Perkins, M. Worthington, J. E. Van Kirk, J. Mills, A. Z. Kapikian, and R. M. Chanock; Evaluation of an interferon inducer in viral respiratory disease, J. Am. Med. Assoc., 219 1179 (1972).
38) D. A. Hill, S. Baron, and R. M. Chanock; Sensitivity of common respiratory viruses to an interferon inducer in human cells, Lancet, II 187 (1969).
39) M. R. Hilleman; Double-stranded RNAs (poly I: C) in the prevention of viral infections, Arch. Intern. Med., 126 109 (1970).
40) R. L. Heberling and S. S. Kalter; Persistence and spread of influenza virus (A2/Hong Kong) in normal and poly I:C-treated baboons (papio cynocephalus), Proc. Soc. Exp. Biol. Med., 135 717 (1970).
41) J. D. Todd, F. J. Volenec, and I. M. Paton; Interferon in nasal secretions and sera of calves after intranasal administration of avirulent infectious bovine rhinotracheitis virus: Association of interferon in nasal secretions with early resistance to challenge with virulent virus, Infect. Immun., 5 699 (1972).
42) B. G. Gatmaitan, E. D. Stanley, and G. G. Jackson; The limited effect of nasal interferon induced by rhinovirus and a topical chemical inducer on the course of infection, J. Infect. Dis., 127 401 (1973).
43) R. G. Douglas, Jr. and R. F. Betts; Effect of induced interferon in experimental rhinovirus infections in volunteers, Infect. Immun., 9 506 (1974).
44) C. Panusarn, E. D. Stanley, V. Dirda, M. Rubenis, and G. G. Jackson; Prevention of rhinovirus illness by a typical interferon inducer, N. Eng. J. Med., 291 57 (1974).
45) T. Francis, Jr.; Intranasal inoculation of human individuals with the virus of epidemic influenza, Proc. Soc. Exp. Biol. & Med., 43 337 (1940).
46) F. M. Burnet; Immunization against influenza with living attenuated virus, Med. J. Aust., 1 385 (1943).
47) J. Mawson and C. Swan; Intranasal vaccination of humans with living attenuated influenza virus strains, ibid., 1 394 (1943).
48) W. Henle, G. Henle, J. Stokes, Jr., and E. P. Maris; Experimental exposure of human subjects to viruses of influenza, J. Immuno., 52 145 (1946).
49) J. J. Ouilligan, Jr. and T. Francis, Jr.; Serological response to intranasal administration of inactive influenza virus in children, J. Clin. Invest., 26 1079 (1947).
50) A. S. Beare, D. Hobson, S. E. Reed, and D. A. J. Tyrrell; A comparison of live and killed influenza-virus vaccines, Lancet, 2 418 (1968).
51) R. H. Waldman, J. J. Mann, and P. A. Small, Jr.; Immunization against influenza: prevention of illness in man by aerosolized inactivated vaccine, J. Am. Med. Assoc., 207 520 (1969).
52) F. M. Wigley, M. H. Fruchtman, and R. H. Waldman; Aerosol immunization of humans with inactivated para-influenza Type 2 vaccine, New Eng. J. Med., 283 1250 (1970).
53) F. L. Black and S. R. Sheridan; Studies on an attenuated measles-virus vaccine. IV. Administration of vaccine by several routes, ibid., 263 165 (1960).
54) Y. Okuno, M. Takahashi, K. Toyoshima, T. Yamamura, T. Sugai, K. Nakamura, and N. Kunita; Studies on the prophylaxis of measles with attenuated living virus. III. Inoculation tests in man and monkey with chick embryo passage measles virus, Biken J., 3 115 (1960).
55) F. R. McCrumb, Jr., S. Kress, E. Saunders, M. J. Snyder, and A. E. Schluederberg; Studies with live attenuated measles-virus vaccine. I. Clinical and immunologic responses in institutionalized children, Am. J. Dis. Chil., 101 689 (1961).

56) S. Kress, A. E. Schluederberg, R. B. Hornick, L. J. Morse, J. L. Cole, E. A. Slater, and F. R. McCrumb, Jr.; Studies with live attenuated measles-virus vaccine. II. Clinical and immunologic response of children in an open community, ibid., 101 701 (1961).

57) Y. Okuno; Vaccination with egg passage measles virus by inhalation, ibid., 103 381 (1962).

58) M. Minamitani, K. Nakamura, H. Nagahama, R. Fujii, Y. Saburi, and M. Matumoto; Vaccination by respiratory route with live attenuated measles virus sugiyama adapted to bovine renal cells, Jap. J. Exp. Med., 34 81 (1964).

59) Y. Okuno, S. Ueda, H. Hosai, T. Kitawaki, K. Nakamura, T. P. Chiang, S. Okabe, and M. Onaka; Studies on the combined use of killed and live measles vaccine: Advantages of the inhalation method, Biken J., 8 81 (1965).

60) I. I. Terskikh, A. I. Danilov, and G. I. Sheltchkov; Theoretical substantiation and the effectiveness of immunization with aerosols of liquid antimeasles vaccine (Russian), Vestnik Akademii Medicinskikh Nauk SSSR, 26 84 (1971).

61) A. B. Sabin, A. F. Arechiga, J. F. de Castro, J. L. Sever, D. L. Madden, I. Shekarchi, and P. Albrecht; Successful immunization of children with and without maternal antibody by aerosolized measles vaccine I. Different results with undiluted human diploid cell and chick embryo fibroblast vaccines, J. Am. Med. Assoc., 249 2651 (1983).

62) P. L. Ogra and D. T. Karzon; Poliovirus antibody response in serum and nasal secretions following intranasal inoculation with inactivated poliovaccine, J. Immunol., 102 15 (1969).

63) J. C. Perkins, D. N. Tucker, H. L. S. Knopf, R. P. Wenzel, R. B. Hornick, A. Z. Kapikian and R. M. Chanock; Evidence for protective effect of an inactivated rhinovirus vaccine administered by the nasal route, Amer. J. Epidem., 90 319 (1969).

64) P. F. Wright, T. Shinozaki, W. Fleet, S. H. Sell, J. Thompson and D. T. Karzon; Evaluation of a live, attenuated respiratory syncytial virus vaccine in infants, J. of Pediatrics, 88 931 (1976).

65) M. O. Thorner, J. Spiess, M. L. Vance, A. D. Rogol, D. L. Kaiser, J. D. Webster, J. Rivier, J. L. Borges, S. R. Bloom, M. J. Cronin, W. S. Evans, R. M. Macleod and W. Vale; Human pancreatic growth hormone-releasing factor selectively stimulates growth hormone secretion in man, Lancet, 1 24 (1983).

66) J. L. C. Borges, M. C. Gelato, A. D. Rogol, M. L. Vance, R. M. Macleod, D. L. Loriaux, J. Rivier, R. M. Blizzard, R. Furlanetto, W. S. Evans, D. L. Kaiser, G. R. Merriam, J. Spiess, W. Vale and M. O. Thorner; Effects of human pancreatic growth hormone releasing factor on growth hormone and somatomedin C levels in patients with idiopathic growth hormone deficiency, Lancet, 2 119 (1983).

67) W. S. Evans, J. L. C. Borges, D. L. Kaiser, M. L. Vance, R. P. Seller, R. M. Macleod, W. Vale, J. Rivier and M. O. Thorner; Intranasal administration of human pancreatic tumor GH-releasing factor-40 stimulates GH release in normal men, J. Clin. Endocrinol. Metab., 57 1081 (1983).

68) J. Landon, V. H. T. James, R. J. Cryer, V. Wynn and A. W. Frankland; Adrenocorticotropic effects of a synthetic polypeptide-β^{1-24}-corticotropin in man, J. Clinic. Endocri. Metab., 24 1206 (1964).

69) R. W. Smith, Jr., L. C. Dickson, J. B. Bryan and W. D. Lowrie; Nasal administration of ACTH: Observations of effectiveness measured by blood eosinopenic response, J. Clinic. Endocri., 12 958 (1952).

70) E. B. Astwood, M. S. Raben and R. W. Payne; Chemistry of corticotrophin, Recent progress in hormone research, 7 1 (1952).

71) M. L. Gelfand and M. A. Shearn; Absence of eosinopenic response to ACTH administration by the aerosol route in normal subjects, P.S.E.B.M., 80 134 (1952).

72) F. Paulson and S. Nordstrom; Pharmacological and clinical results with ACTH in 112 cases, Swedish Med. J., 49 2998 (1952).
73) J. B. R. McKendry, H. Schwartz and M. Hall; Intranasal corticotropin-its physiological and clinical effects, Can. Med. Assoc. J., 70 244 (1954).
74) J. Keenan and M. A. Chamberlain; Nasal mucosal absorption of tetracosactrin as indicated by rise in plasma fluorogenic corticosteroids, Br. Med. J., 4 407 (1969).
75) J. Keenan, J. B. Thompson, M. A. Chamberlain and G. M. Besser; Prolonged corticotrophic action of a synthetic substituted $^{1-18}$ACTH, Br. Med. J., 3 742 (1971).
76) J. P. Felber, M. L. Aubert and R. Deguillaume; Administration by nasal spray of an 18 amino acid synthetic polypeptide with corticotropic action, Experientia, 25 1195 (1969).
77) G. Baumann, A. Walser, P. A. Desaulles, F. J. A. Paesi and L. Geller; Corticotropic action of an intranasally applied synthetic ACTH derivative, J. Clin. Endocri. Metab., 42 60 (1976).
78) G. I. Zatuchni, J. D. Shelton and J. J. Sciarra, LHRH Peptides as Female and Male Contraceptives, Harper & Row, Publishers, Philadelphia (1976).
79) A. V. Schally, A. Arimura, A. J. Kastin, H. Matsuo, Y. Baba, T. W. Redding, R. M. G. Nair and L. Debeljuk; Gonadotropin-releasing hormone: One polypeptide regulates secretion of luteinizing and follicle-stimulating hormones, Science, 173 1036 (1971).
80) H. Matsuo, Y. Baba, R. M. G. Nair, A. Arimura and A. V. Schally; Structure of the porcine LH- and FSH-releasing hormone. I. The proposed amino acid sequence, Biochem. Biophys. Res. Commun., 43 1334 (1971).
81) R. Burgus, M. Butcher, N. Ling, M. Monahan, J. Rivier, R. Fellows, M. Amoss, R. Blackwells, W. Vale and R. Guillemin; Structure moleculaire du facteur hypothalamique (LRF) d'origine ovine controlant la secretion de l'hormone gondotrope hypophysaire de luteinisation (LH), Compt. rend. Acad. Sci., 273 1611 (1971).
82) A. J. Kastin, A. V. Schally, C. Gual, and A. Arimura; Release of LH and FSH after administration of synthetic LH-releasing hormone, J. Clin. Endocri. Metab., 34 753 (1972).
83) S. S. C. Yen, R. Rebar, G. Vandenberg, F. Naftolin, Y. Ehara, S. Engblom, K. J. Ryan and K. Benirschke; Synthetic luteinizing hormone-releasing factor: A potent stimulator of gonadotropin release in men. ibid., 34 1108 (1972).
84) G. M. Besser, A. S. McNeilly, D. C. Anderson, J. C. Marshall, P. Harsoulis, R. Hall, B. J. Ormston, L. Alexander and W. P. Collins; Hormonal responses to synthetic luteinizing hormone and follicle stimulating hormone-releasing hormone in men, Br. Med. J., 3 267 (1972).
85) D. Gonzalex-Barcena, A. J. Kastin, D. S. Schalch, J. A. Bermuder, D. Lee, A. Arimur, J. Ruelas, I. Zepeda and A. V. Schally; Synthetic LH-releasing hormone (LH-RH) administered to normal men by different routes, J. Clin. Endocri. Metab., 37 481 (1973).
86) A. V. Schally, A. J. Kastin and D. H. Coy; LH-releasing hormone and its analogues: Recent basic and clinical investigations, Int. J. Fertil., 21 1 (1976).
87) C. H. Mortimer, G. M. Besser, J. Hook and A. S. McNeilly; Intravenous, intramuscular, subcutaneous and intranasal administration of LH/FSH-RH: The duration of effect and occurrence of asynchronous pulsatile release of LH and FSH, Clin. Endocri., 3 19 (1974).
88) D. R. London, W. R. Butt, S. S. Lynch, J. C. Marshall, S. Owusu, W. R. Robinson and J. M. Stephenson; Hormonal responses to intranasal luteinizing hormone releasing hormone, J. Clin. Endocri. Metab., 37 829 (1973).
89) H. G. Solbach and W. Wiegelmann; Intranasal application of luteinizing-hormone releasing hormone, Lancet, 1 1259 (1973).
90) S. Jeppson, S. Kullander, G. Rannevik and J. Thorell; Intranasal administration of synthetic gondotrophin-releasing hormone, Br. Med. J., 4 231 (1973).

91) H. G. Dahlén, E. Keller and H. P. G. Schneider; Linear dose dependent LH release following intranasally sprayed LHRH, Horm. Metab. Res., 6 510 (1974).
92) G. Gennser and P. Liedholm; Intranasal administration of luteining-hormone releasing factor, Lancet, 1 865 (1974).
93) G. Fink, G. Gennser, P. Liedholm J. Thorell and J. Mulder; Comparison of plasma levels of luteinizing hormone-releasing hormone in men after intravenous or intranasal administration, J. Endocr., 63 351 (1974).
94) J. Happ, M. Neubauer, A. Egri, K. Demisch, K. Schöffing and J. Beyer; GnRH therapy in males with hypogonadotropic hypogonadism, Horm. Metab. Res., 7 526 (1975).
95) H. Koch; Buserelin: contraception through nasal spray, Pharmacy International, 72 99 (1981).
96) W. Wiegelmann, H. G. Solbach, H. K. Kley, E. Nieschlag, K. H. Rudorff and H. L. Kruskemper; Effect of a new LH-RH analogue [D-Ser(TBU)^{6}-EA^{10}-LHRH] on gonadotrophin and gonadal steroid secretion in men, Hormone Res., 7 1 (1976).
97) J. S. E. Dericks-Tan, E. Hammer and H. D. Taubert; The effect of [D-Ser(TBU)^{6}-EA^{10}-LHRH] upon gonadotropin release in normally cyclic women, J. Clin. Endocr. Metab., 45 597 (1977).
98) J. Sandow, W. V. Rechenberg, G. Jerrabek and W. Stoll; Pituitary gonadotropin inhibition by a highly active analog of luteinizing hormone-releasing hormone, Fertility and Sterility, 30 205 (1978).
99) C. Bergquist, S. J. Nillius and L. Wide; Reduced gonadotropin secretion in postmenopausal women during treatment with a stimulatory LHRH analogue, J. Clin. Endocr. Metab., 49 472 (1979).
100) W. Wiegelmann, H. G. Solbach, H. K. Kley and H. L. Kruskemper; LH and FSH response to long-term application of LH-RH analogue in normal males, Horm. Metab. Res., 9 521 (1977).
101) W. Wiegelmann, H. G. Solbach, H. K. Kley, E. Nieschlag and H. L. Kruskemper; A new LHRH analogue: D-Ser(TBU)^{6}-EA^{10} LHRH effects on gonadotrophin and gonadal steroid secretion in men after intravenous and intranasal application, Acta. Endocr. [Suppl.], 208 37 (1977).
102) C. Bergquist, S. J. Nillius and L. Wide; Intranasal gonadotropin-releasing hormone agonist as a contraceptive agent, Lancet II 215 (1979).
103) C. Bergquist, S. J. Nillius and L. Wide; Inhibition of ovulation in women by intranasal treatment with a luteinizing hormone-releasing hormone agonist, Contraception, 19 497 (1979).
104) A. Lemay, F. Labrie, A. Belanger and J. P. Raynaud; Luteolytic effect of intranasal administration of [D-Ser(TBU)^{6}, des-Gly-NH_2^{10}]-Luteinizing hormone-releasing hormone ethylamide in normal woman, Fertility and Sterility, 32(6) 646 (1979).
105) J. Happ, U. Hartmann, T. Weber, U. Cordes and J. Beyer; Gonadotropin and testosterone secretion in normal human males after stimulation with gonadotropin-releasing hormone (GnRH) or potent GnRH analogue using different modes of application, ibid., 30(6) 666 (1978).
106) R. Illig, F. Kollmann, M. Borkenstein, W. Kuber, G. U. Exner, K. Kellerer, L. Lunglmayr and A. Prader; Treatment of cryptorchidism by intranasal synthetic luteinizing-hormone releasing hormone, Lancet II 518 (1977).
107) R. Illig, H. Bucher and A. Prader; Success, relapse and failure after intranasal LHRH treatment of cryptorchidism in 55 prepubertal boys, Eur. J. Pediatr., 133 147 (1980).
108) R. Illig, T. Torresani, H. Bucher, M. Zachmann and A. Prader; Effect of intranasal LHRH therapy on plasma LH, FSH and testosterone, and relation to clinical results in prepubertal boys with cryptorchidism, Clin. Endocr., 12 91 (1980).
109) J. Happ, F. Kollmann, C. Krawehl, M. Neubauer and J. Beyer; Intranasal GnRH therapy of maldescended testes, Horm. Metab. Res., 7 440 (1975).

110) R. Illig, G. U. Exner, T. Torresani, K. Kellerer, M. Borkenstein, H. Gleispach, F. Kollmann, J. Happ, G. Lunglmayr and J. Spona; Treatment of cryptorchidism by intranasal application of synthetic LH-releasing hormone (LHRH): Results of a collaborative double blind study, Acta. Encocrino. [Suppl.], 212 27 (1977).
111) J. Happ, F. Kollmann, C. Krawehl, M. Neubauer, U. Krause, K. Demisch, J. Sandow, W. V. Rechenberg and J. Beyer; Treatment of cryptorchidism with pernasal gonadotropin-releasing hormone therapy, Fertil. & Steril., 29 546 (1978).
112) D. Pirazzoli, F. Zappulla, F. Bernardi, M. P. Villa, D. Aleksandrowicz, A. Scandola, P. Stancari, A. Cicognani and E. Cacciari; Luteinizing hormone-releasing hormone nasal spray as therapy for undescended testicle, Arch. Dis. in Childhood, 53 235 (1978).
113) S. Zabransky; LHRH nasal spray (Kryptocur), ein neuer aspekt in der hormonellen behandlung des hodenhochstandes, Klin. Pädiat., 193 382 (1981).
114) G. Potashnik, N. Ben-Adereth, B. Lunenfeld, and C. Rofe; Assessment of pituitary response to nasal application of synthetic gonadotropin-releasing hormone in men, Fertil. & Steril., 28 650 (1977).
115) G. Potashnik, R. Homberg, A. Eshkol, V. Insler and B. Lunenfeld; Hormonal and clinical responses in amenorrheic patients treated with gonadotropins and a nasal form of synthetic gonadotropin-releasing hormone. Fertil. & Steril., 29 148 (1978).
116) G. Potashnik, R. Homburg, A. Eshkol, V. Insler, and B. Lunenfeld; Hormonal responses to nasal application of synthetic gonadotrophin-releasing hormone in amenorrheic patients pretreated with gonadotrophins, Int. J. Fertil., 25(3) 234 (1980).
117) J. Happ, V. Schmitr, U. Cordes, U. Krause, W. Atzpodien and J. Beyer; Treatment of delayed puberty by intranasal application of gonadotrophin-releasing hormone (GnRH), ibid., 25(3) 247 (1980).
118) A. Zarate, E. S. Canales, A. V. Schally, L. Ayala-Valdes and A. J. Kastin; Successful induction of ovulation with synthetic luteinizing hormone-releasing hormone in anovulatory infertility, Fertil. & Steril., 22 188 (1971).
119) S. A. Phansey, M. A. Barnes, H. O. Williamson, J. Sagel and R. M. G. Nair; Combined use of clomiphene and intranasal luteinizing hormone-releasing hormone for induction of ovulation in chronically anovulatory women, Fertility and Sterility, 34(5) 448 (1980).
120) B. H. Vickery; Physiology and antifertility effects of LHRH and agonistic analogs in male animals in LHRH Peptides as Female and Male Contraceptives, (G. I. Zatuchni, J. D. Shelton and J. J. Sciarra, Eds.), Harper & Row, Publishers, Philadelphia (1976), pp. 275-290.
121) J. J. Nestor, T. L. Ho, R. A. Simpson, B. L. Horner, G. H. Jones, G. I. McRae and B. H. Vickery; Synthesis and biological activity of some very hydrophobic superagonist analogues of luteinizing hormone-releasing hormone, J. Med. Chem., 25 795 (1982).
122) S. T. Anik, G. McRae, C. Nerenberg, A. Worden, J. Foreman, J. Y. Hwang, S. Kushinsky, R. E. Jones and B. Vickery; Nasal absorption of nafarelin acetate, the decapeptide [D-NaI(2)^6] LHRH, in rhesus monkeys I., J. Pharm. Sci., 73 684 (1984).
123) A. Osol, Remington's Pharmaceutical Sciences, Mack Publishing Company, Easton, Pennsylvania, (1980) pp. 896.
124) J. Hofbauer and J. K. Hoerner; the nasal application of pituitary extract for the induction of labor, Am. J. Obstet. & Gynec., 14 137 (1927).
125) D. G. Morton; Induction of labor by means of artificial rupture of membranes, castor oil and quinine, and nasal pituitrin, ibid., 26 323 (1933).
126) R. A. Bartholomerv; Diagnostic and therapeutic uses of pituitary extracts in obstetrics, J. Med. Ass. Georgia, 34 110 (1945).
127) C. Hendricks and R. A. Gabel; Use of intranasal oxytocin in obstetrics I. laboratory evaluation, Am. J. Obstet. & Gynec., 79 780 (1960).

128) C. Hendricks; Use of intranasal oxytocin in obstetrics. II. A clinical appraisal, ibid., 79 789 (1960).
129) K. Baumgarten and W. Hofhansl; Induction of labor by means of oxytocin spray, Zbl. Gynäk, 83 154 (1961).
130) K. Baumgarten and W. Hofhansl; A modified oxytocin sensitivity test, Geburtsh U. Franenheilk, 21 10 (1961).
131) C. H. Hendricks and S. V. Pose; Intranasal oxytocin in obstetrics, J. Am. Med. Assoc., 175 384 (1961).
132) J. E. Clement, V. C. Harwell and J. R. McCain; Use of intranasal oxytocin for induction and/or stimulation of labor, Am. J. Obstet. & Gynec., 83 778 (1962).
133) N. E. Borglin; Intranasal administration of oxytocin for induction and stimulation of labour, Acta. Obstet. Gynec. Scand., 41 238 (1962).
134) J. Cohen, J. Danezis and M. S. Burnhill; Response of the gravid uterus at term to intranasal oxytocin as determined by intra-amniotic fluid pressure recordings, Am. J. Obstet. Gynec., 83 774 (1962).
135) F. C. Hinde; The value of intranasal oxytocin spray in obstetrics, Med. J. Aust., 1 268 (1963).
136) R. W. Stander, J. F. Thompson and C. P. Gibbs; Evaluation of intranasal oxytocin by amniotic fluid pressure recordings, Am. J. Obstet. Gynec., 85 193 (1963).
137) E. Talledo, S. F. Adams and F. P. Zuspan; Response of pregnant human uterus to oxytocin given intranasally, J. Am. Med. Assoc., 189 348 (1964).
138) A. Bradfield; Reservations on the safety of oxytocin nasal spray in obstetrics, Aust. N. Z. J. Obstet. Gynaec., 5 138 (1965).
139) C. Jones; Clinical experience with intranasal oxytocin spray, Med. J. Austri., 2 1099 (1966).
140) I. V. Gent, T. Eskes and J. C. Seelen; Changes in intrauterine pressure due to intranasal administration of oxytocin (partocon), Acta. Obstet. Gynec. Scand., 46 340 (1967).
141) K. Müller and M. Osler; Induction of labor: A comparison of intravenous, intranasal and transbuccal oxytocin, Acta. Obstet. Gyneco. Scand., 46 59 (1967).
142) K. Devoe, Jr., W. C. Rigsby and B. A. Mcdaniels; The effect of intranasal oxytocin on the pregnant uterus, Am. J. Obstet. Gynec., 97 208 (1967).
143) P. Bergsjö and H. Jenssen; Nasal and buccal oxytocin for the induction of labor: a clinical trial, J. Obstet. Gynec. Brit. Cwlth., 76 131 (1969).
144) S. Sjöstedt; Induction of labour: A comparison of intranasal and transbuccal administration of oxytocin, Acta. Obstet. Gynecol. Scand., 48 (Suppl 7) 1 (1969).
145) J. Laine; Experience of the use of intranasal, buccal and intravenous oxytocin as methods of inducing labor, Acta. Obstet. Gynec. Scand., 49 149 (1970).
146) R. T. Hoover; Intranasal oxytocin in eighteen hundred patients: A study on its safety as used in a community hospital, Am. J. Obstet. Gynec., 110 788 (1971).
147) L. E. Sandholm; The effect of intravenous and intranasal oxytocin on intrammary pressure during early lactation, Acta. Obstet. Gynec. Scand., 47 145 (1968).
148) M. Newton and G. E. Egli; The effect of intranasal administration of oxytocin on the let-down of milk in lactating women, ibid., 76 103 (1958).
149) R. Wenner; Galaktokinetische wirkung von synthetischem oxytocin bei nasaler anwendung, Schweiz. Med. Wchnschr., 89 441 (1959).
150) R. H. Stewart and R. N. Nelson; Synthetic oxytocin. II. Evaluation of its results in milk letdown, Obstet. & Gynec., 13 204 (1959).
151) C. Hollenbach; Lactagogue action of oxytocin (Oxytozin als LaKagoges Hormon.), Zbl. Gynäk., 81 1980 (1959).

152) B. Berde and A. Cerletti; Uber die wirkung pharmakologischer oxytocindosen auf die milchdruse, Acta. Endocrinologica (Kbh), 34 543 (1960).
153) E. A. Friedman and M. R. Sachtleben; Oxytocin in lactation: Clinical applications, Am. J. Obstet. Gynec., 82 846 (1961).
154) P. J. Huntingford; Intranasal use of synthetic oxytocin in the treatment of breast feeding, Brit. Med. J., 1 709 (1961).
155) U. Heckmann; Clinical experiences with intranasal oxytocin spray, Zbl. Gynäk., 83 2042 (1961).
156) N. Altszuler and J. Hampshire; Intranasal instillation of oxytocin increases insulin and glucagon secretion (41245), Proc. Soc. Exp. Biol. Med., 168 123 (1981).
157) A. Osol; Remington's Pharmaceutical Sciences, Mack Publishing Company, Easton, Pennsylvania (1980) p. 896.
158) R. Fraser and D. J. Scott; Nasal spray of synthetic vasopressin for the treatment of diabetes insipidus, Lancet, I 1159 (1963).
159) J. Pepys, P. A. Jenkins, P. J. Lachman and W. E. Mahon; An iatrogenic auto-antibody: immunological responses to "pituitary snuff" in patients with diabetes insipidus, J. Endocrinology, 33 viii (1965).
160) W. E. Mahon, D. J. Scott, G. Ansell, G. L. Manson and R. Fraser; Hypersensitivity to pituitary snuff with miliary shadowing in the lungs, Thorax, 22 13 (1967).
161) H. L. Blumgart; The antidiuretic effect of pituitary extract applied intranasally in a case of diabetes insipidus, Arch. Intern. Med., 29 508 (1982).
162) V. · U. Guhl; Die antidiuretische und pressorische von arginin^8-vasopressin, lysin^8-vasopressin, und phenylalanin^2-lysin^8-vasopressin, Schweiz. Med. Wchnschr., 91 798 (1961).
163) A. R. Spiegelman; Treatment of diabetes insipidus with synthetic vasopressin, J. Am. Med. Assoc., 184 657 (1963).
164) D. Barltrop; Diabetes insipidus treated with synthetic lysine vasopressin, Lancet I 276 (1963).
165) H. Sjöberg and R. Luft; Nasal spray of synthetic vasopressin for the treatment of diabetes insipidus, Lancet I 1159 (1963).
166) N. D. Fabricant; Nasal spray treatment of diabetes insipidus, the Eye, Ear, Nose and Throat Monthly, 42 64 (1967).
167) A. M. Moses; Synthetic lysine vasopressin nasal spray in the treatment of diabetes insipidus, Clin. Pharmacol. & Therap., 5 422 (1964).
168) A. M. Dashe, C. R. Kleeman, J. W. Czaczkes, H. Rubinoff and I. Spears; Synthetic vasopressin nasal spray in the treatment of diabetes insipidus, J. Am. Med. Assoc., 190 1069 (1964).
169) J. F. Dingman and J. H. Hauger-Klevene; Treatment of diabetes insipidus: Synthetic lysine vasopressin nasal solution, J. Clin. Endocri., 24 550 (1964).
170) S. B. Chirman and L. W. Kinsell; Diabetes insipidus: Treatment with 8-lysine vasopressin in a nasal spray, Calif. Med., 101 1 (1964).
171) F. I. R. Martin and T. H. Mathew; The treatment of diabetes insipidus with synthetic lysine-vasopressin by inhalation, Med. J. Aust., 2 984 (1964).
172) R. L. Fogel; Treatment of diabetes insipidus with lysine vasopressin spray, J. Med. Soc. New Jersey, 63 203 (1966).
173) W. Hung; Treatment of diabetes insipidus in children with synthetic lysine-8-vasopressin nasal spray, Med. Ann. Dis. Col., 36 400 (1967).
174) N. Mimica, L. C. Wegienka and P. H. Forsham; Lypressin nasal spray: Usefulness in patients who manifest allergies to other antidiuretic hormone preparation, J. Am. Med. Assoc., 203 802 (1968).
175) H. D. Green and J. B. Blumberg; The use of a synthetic analogue of posthypophysial vasopressin (PVL-2) for local hemostasis, Surgery, 58 524 (1965).

176) I. Vávra, A. Machová, V. Holeček, J. H. Cort, M. Zaoral and F. Sorm; Effect of a synthetic analogue of vasopressin in animals and in patients with diabetes insipidus, Lancet, I 948 (1968).
177) K. E. Andersson and B. Arner; Effects of DDAVP, a synthetic analogue of vasopressin, in patients with cranial diabetes insipidus, Acta. Med. Scand., 192 21 (1972).
178) C. R. W. Edwards, M. J. Kitau, T. Chard and G. M. Besser; Vasopressin analogue DDAVP in diabetes insipidus: Clinical and laboratory studies, Br. Med. J., 3 375 (1973).
179) J. P. Radó and J. Marosi; Prolongation of duration of action of 1-Deamino-8-D-Arginine Vasopressin (DDAVP) by ineffective doses of clofibrate in diabetes insipidus, Horm. Metab., 7 527 (1975).
180) A. Grossman, A. Fabbri, P. L. Goldberg and G. M. Besser; Two new modes of desmopressin (DDAVP) administration, Br. Med. J., 280 1215 (1980).
181) J. W. Wall and N. Shure; Intranasal Cortisone, Arch. Otolaryng., 56 172 (1952).
182) D. Myers; Experiences in the treatment of the allergic nasal polyp by the intrapolyp injection of prednisolone T.B.A., Laryngoscope, 58 1 (1958).
183) M. W. Simmons; Intranasal injection of corticosteroids, Calif. Med., 92 155 (1960).
184) D. C. Baker and R. B. Strauss; Intranasal injections of long-acting corticosteroids, Ann. Otol. Rhinol. Laryngol., 71 525 (1962).
185) R. J. Rowe, T. W. Dasler and A. M. Kinkella; Visual changes and triamcinolone, J. Am. Med. Assoc., 201 117 (1967).
186) D. McCleve, J. Goldstein and S. Silver, Corticosteroid injections of the nasal turbinates: Past experience and precautions, Otolaryngology, 86 851 (1978).
187) R. Mabry; Intranasal corticosteroid injection: Indications, technique, and complications, Otolaryngol. Head Neck Surg., 87 207 (1979).
188) D. C. Baker; Intranasal steroid injections: Indications, technique, results and complications, Laryngoscope, 89 998 (1979).
189) R. L. Mabry; Intranasal steroid injection during pregnancy, South. Med. J., 73 1176 (1980).
190) R. L. Mabry; Visual loss after intranasal corticosteroid injection: incidence, causes, and prevention, Arch. Otolaryngol., 107 484 (1981).
191) R. L. Mabry; Practical applications of intranasal corticosteroid injection, Ear, Nose & Throat J., 60(11) 506 (1981).
192) J. L. Dill and D. S. Bolstad; Observations on the local use of cortisone in the nose in allergic rhinitis, Laryngoscope, 61 415 (1951).
193) E. E. P. Seidmon and N. Schaffer; Cortogen nasal suspension with chlor-trimeton in the treatment of allergic rhinitis, Ann. Allergy, 12 85 (1954).
194) H. S. Tuft; Topical use of hydrocortisone alcohol in the treatment of ragweed hay fever, Ann. Allergy, 12 687 (1954).
195) T. T. Smith; Local use of hydrocortisone acetate in the nose, Arch. Otol., 60 24 (1954).
196) M. B. Rohen; The use of hydrocortisone suspension in nasal allergic and infectious conditions, Ann. Allergy, 113 109 (1955).
197) J. H. Burger and J. H. Shaffer; Controlled studies in the topical application of hydrocortisone in vasomoter rhinitis, Ann. N. Y. Acad. Sci., 61 566 (1955).
198) H. Herxheimer and M. McAllen; Treatment of hay-fever with hydrocortisone snuff, Lancet, I 537 (1956).
199) R. M. Morris-Owen and S. C. Truelove; Treatment of hay-fever with local hydrocortisone hemisuccinate sodium, Br. Med. J., 1 969 (1958).
200) C. F. Lake, G. B. Logan and G. A. Peters; Treatment of ragweed hay fever with powdered hydrocortisone applied intranasally, Staff Meetings of the Mayo Clinic, 32 641 (1957).
201) S. J. Taub and R. A. Hecht; Treatment of hay fever with intranasal hydrocortisone acetate powder, Amer. Pract. Digest Treat., 10 469 (1959).

202) L. Bagratuni; A comparative study of topical steroids, antihistamines and pollen vaccine in the treatment of hay fever and hay asthma, Ann. Allergy, 18 859 (1960).
203) J. R. Anderson and H. D. Ogden; Topical use of prednisolone in nasal allergy, Ann. Allergy, 14 44 (1956).
204) M. P. Godfrey and K. Maunsell; Prednisolone snuff in hay-fever: A controlled trial, Lancet, I 767 (1957).
205) H. T. Friedman and B. Hills; A double-blind study of triamcinolone acetonide nasal spray in allergic rhinitis, J. Allergy, 33 1 (1962).
206) T. H. Aaron and E. L. C. Muttitt; Intranasal dexamethasone phosphate in perennial allergic rhinitis, Ann. Allergy, 22 155 (1964).
207) P. S. Norman and W. L. Winkenwerder; Suppression of hay fever symptoms with intranasal dexamethasone aerosol, J. Allergy, 36 284 (1965).
208) T. H. Aaron and E. L. C. Muttitt; Effect of intranasal dexamethasone phosphate on the adrenal function of patients with perennial allergic rhinitis, Ann. Allergy, 23 100 (1965).
209) R. E. Smith; Dexamethasone nasal aerosol in nasal polyps and hypertrophic allergic rhinitis: A clinical and controlled evaluation, Ann. Allergy, 23 273 (1968).
210) P. S. Norman, W. L. Winkenwerder, G. W. Murgatroyd and J. W. Parsons; Evidence for the local action of intranasal dexamethasone aerosols in the suppression of hay fever symptoms, J. Allergy, 38 93 (1966).
211) M. I. Michels, R. E. Smith and E. M. Heimlich; Adrenal suppression and intranasally applied steroids, Ann. Allergy, 25 569 (1967).
212) S. J. Taub; Dexamethasone nasal aerosol vs. placebo in the treatment of nasal polyposis, The Eye, Ear, Nose and Throat Monthly, 47 80 (1968).
213) P. K. Champion; Cushing syndrome secondary to abuse of dexamethasone nasal spray, Arch. Intern. Med., 134 750 (1974).
214) A. W. Frankland and S. R. Walker; A comparison of intranasal betamethasone valerate and sodium cromoglycate in seasonal allergic rhinitis, Clin. Allergy, 5 295 (1975).
215) S. M. Harding and S. Heath; Intranasal steroid aerosol in perennial rhinitis: Comparison with an antihistamine compound, Clin. Allergy, 6 369 (1976).
216) N. Mygind; Local effect of intranasal beclomethasone dipropionate aerosol in hay fever, Br. Med. J., 4 464 (1973).
217) I. Hansen and N. Mygind; Local effect of intranasal beclomethasone dipropionate aerosol in perennial rhinitis, Acta. Allergologica, 29 281 (1974).
218) I. Gibson, D. J. Maberly, S. Lal, M. M. Ali and A. G. Butler; Double-blind cross-over trial comparing intranasal beclomethasone dipropionate and placebo in perennial rhinitis, Br. Med J., 4 503 (1974).
219) N. Mygind, C. B. Pedersen, S. Prytz and H. Sorenson; Treatment of nasal polyps with intranasal beclomethasone dipropionate aerosol, Clinical Allergy, 5 159 (1975).
220) J. M. Smith, R. T. Clegg, N. Cook and A. G. Butler; Intranasal beclomethasone dipropionate in allergic rhinitis, Br. Med. J., 2 255 (1975).
221) R. N. Brogden, R. M. Pinder, P. R. Sawyer, T. M. Speight and G. S. Avery; Beclomethasone dipropionate: II: Allergic rhinitis and other conditions, Drugs, 10 211 (1975).
222) H. Sørensen, N. Mygind, C. B. Pedersen and S. Prytz; Long-term treatment of nasal polyps with beclomethasone dipropionate aerosol: II. Clinical results, Acta. Otolaryngol., 82 256 (1976).
223) H. Sørensen, N. Mygind, C. B. Pedersen and S. Prytz; Long-term treatment of nasal polyps with beclomethasone dipropionate aerosol: III. Morphological studies and conclusions, Acta. Otolaryngol., 82 260 (1976).
224) D. W. Cockcroft, D. W. MacCormack, M. T. Newhouse and R. E. Hargreave; Beclomethasone dipropionate aerosol in allergic rhinitis, Can. Med. Assoc. J., 115 523 (1976).

225) L. Malm and J. A. Wihl; Intranasal beclomethasone dipropionate in vasomotor rhinitis, Acta Allergologica, 31 245 (1976).
226) D. Wheatley; A corticosteroid nasal spray in hay fever, Curr. Ther. Res. Clin. Exp., 19 612 (1976).
227) N. Mygind; Effects of beclomethasone dipropionate aerosol on nasal mucosa, Br. J. Clin. Pharmacol., 4 287S (1977).
228) D. Poynter; Beclomethasone dipropionate aerosol and nasal mucosa, Br. J. Clin. Pharmacol., 4 295S (1977).
229) N. Mygind, N. J. Johnsen and J. Thomsen; Intranasal allergen challenge during corticosteroid treatment, Clin. Allergy, 7 69 (1977).
230) N. Mygind, H. Sørensen and C. B. Pedersen; The nasal mucosa during long-term treatment with beclomethasone dipropionate aerosol, Acta. Otolaryngol., 85 437 (1978).
231) N. Mygind; Topical corticosteroids - beclomethasone dipropionate in Nasal Allergy, Blackwell Scientific Publications, Oxford, London, Edinburgh, Melbourne (1978), pp. 312-332.
232) J. Hillas, R. J. Booth, S. Somerfield, R. Morton J. Avery and J. D. Wilson; A comparative trial of intranasal beclomethasone dipropionate and sodium cromoglycate in patients with chronic perennial rhinitis, Clin. Allergy, 10 253 (1980).
233) E. Munch, G. Gomez, C. Harris R. P. Lack, V. A. Edwards, P. O'Connor, D. V. Snowden and N. Mygind; An open comparison of dosage frequencies of beclomethasone dipropionate in seasonal allergic rhinitis, Clin. Allergy, 11 303 (1981).
234) A. Toft, J. Å Wihl, J. Toxman and N. Mygind; Double-blind comparison between beclomethasone dipropionate as aerosol and as powder in patients with nasal polyposis, Clin. Allergy, 12 391 (1982).
235) N. Mygind; Intranasal corticosteroid treatment of rhinitis, Eur. J. Respir. Dis. [Suppl], 122 192 (1982).
236) M. Okuda, K. Sakaguchi and H. Ohtsuka; Intranasal beclomethasone mode of action in nasal allergy, Ann. Allergy, 50 116 (1983).
237) P. C. Turkeltaub, P. S. Norman and S. Crepea; Treatment of ragweed hay fever with an intranasal spray containing flunisolide, a new synthetic corticosteroid, J. Allergy Clin. Immun., 58 597 (1976).
238) P. Larochelle, P. Du Souich, E. Bolte, J. LeLorier and R. Goyer; Toxicortol pivalate, a corticosteroid with no systemic glucocorticoid effect after oral, intrarectal, and intranasal application, Clin. Pharmacol. Ther., 33 343 (1983).
239) T. C. Anand Kumar, G. F. X. David, K. Kumar, B. Umberkoman and M. S. Krishnamoorthy; A new approach to fertility regulation by interfering with neuroendocrine pathways. In Proceedings of international symmposium on neuroendocrine regulation of fertility (T. C. Anand Kumar, Ed.), Karger, Basel (1976), pp. 314-322.
240) T. C. Anand Kumar, G. F. X. David, B. Umberkoman and K. D. Saini; Uptake of radioactivity by body fluids and tissues in rhesus monkeys after intravenous injection or intranasal spray of tritium-labeled oestradiol and progesterone, Current Science, 43 435 (1974).
241) T. C. Anand Kumar, G. F. X. David and V. Puri; Nasal sprays for controlling ovulation in rhesus monkeys. In Recent Advances in Primatology (D. J. Chivers and E. H. R. Ford, Eds.), Academic Press (1978), Vol. 4.
242) L. Öhman, R. Hahnenberger and E. D. B. Johansson; Topical administration of progestational steroids in the eye and nose - a rapid absorption to the blood, Contraception, 18 171 (1978).
243) T. C. Anand Kumar, G. F. X. David and V. Puri; Nasal spray contraceptives. In Recent Advances in Reproduction and Regulation of Fertility (G. P. Talwar, Ed.), Elsevier/North-Holland Biomedical Press, Amsterdam, New York, Oxford (1979).
244) G. F. X. David, C. P. Puri and T. C. Anand Kumar; Bioavailability of progesterone enhanced by intranasal spraying, Experientia, 37 533 (1981).

245) A. A. Hussain, S. Hirai, and R. Bawarshi; Nasal absorption of natural contraceptive steroids in rats-progesterone absorption, J. Pharm. Sci., 70 466 (1981).
246) E. B. Brittebo; Metabolism of progesterone by the nasal mucosa in mice and rats, Acta Pharmacol. et. toxicol., 51 441 (1982).
247) T. C. Anand Kumar, G. F. X. David, A. Sankaranarayanan, V. Puri and K. R. Sundrani; Pharmacokinetics of progesterone after its administration to ovariectomized rhesus monkeys by injection, infusion, or nasal spraying, Proc. Natl. Acad. Sci., USA, 79 4185 (1982).
248) L. A. Rigg, B. Milanes, B. Villanueva and S. S. C. Yen; Efficacy of intravaginal and intranasal administration of micronized estradiol-17β, J. Clin. Endocr. Metab., 45 1261 (1977).
249) L. Öhman, R. Hahnenberger and E. D. B. Johansson; 17β-Estradiol levels in blood and cerebrospinal fluid after ocular and nasal administration in women and female rhesus monkeys (macaca mulatta), Contraception, 22 349 (1980).
250) T. C. Anand Kumar, A. Sehgal, G. F. X. David, J. S. Bajoj and M. R. N. Prasad; Effects of intranasal administration of hormonal steroids on serum testosterone and spermatogenesis in rhesus monkey (macaca mulatta), Biology of reproduction, 22 935 (1980).
251) A. A. Hussain, R. Kimura and C. H. Huang; Nasal absorption of testosterone in rats, J. Pharm. Sci., 73 1300 (1984).
252) H. Klostermeyer and R. E. Humbel; The chemistry and biochemistry of insulin, Angew. Chem. Intern. Ed., 5 807 (1966).
253) E. L. Smith, R. L. Hill and A. Borman; Activity of insulin degraded by leucine aminopeptidase, Biochim. Biophys. Acta, 29 207 (1958).
254) R. H. Engel, S. J. Riggi and M. J. Fahrenbach; Intestinal absorption as water-in-oil-in-water emulsion, Nature, 219 856 (1968).
255) C. W. Crane, M. C. Path and G. R. W. Luntz; Absorption of insulin from the human small intestine, Diabetes, 17 625 (1968).
256) G. A. Harrison; Insulin in alcoholic solution by mouth, Br. Med. J., 2 1204 (1923).
257) R. P. Walton and C. F. Lacey; Absorption of drugs through the oral mucosa, J. Pharm. Exp. Ther., 54 61 (1938).
258) E. P. McCullagh and L. A. Lewis; Comparison of effectiveness of various methods of administration of insulin, J. Clin. Endocri., 2 435 (1942).
259) M. P. Earle; Experimental use of oral insulin, Isr. J. Med. Sci., 8 899 (1971).
260) Y. Yamaski, M. Shichiri and R. Kawamori; The effectiveness of rectal administration of insulin suppository in normal and diabetic subjects, Diabetes Care, 4 454 (1981).
261) N. F. Fisher; The absorption of insulin from the intestine, vagina and scrotal sac, Am. J. Physiol., 67 65 (1923).
262) F. M. Wigley, J. H. Londono and S. H. Wood; Insulin across respiratory mucosa by aerosol delivery, Diabetes, 20 552 (1971).
263) B. K. Davis; Control of diabetes with polyacrylamide implants containing insulin, Experientia, 28 348 (1972).
264) R. T. Woodyatt; The clinical use of insulin, J. Metab. Res., 2 793 (1922).
265) W. Heubner, S. E. de Jough and E. Laquer; Ueber inhalation von insulin, Klin. Wchnschr., 3 2342 (1924).
266) M. Gänsslen; Ueber inhalation van insulin, ibid., 4 71 (1925).
267) W. S. Collens and M. A. Goldzieher; Absorption of insulin by nasal mucous membrane, Proc. Soc. Exp. Biol. Med., 29 756 (1932).
268) R. H. Major; The intranasal application of insulin, experimental and clinical experiences, Am. J. M. Sci., 192 257 (1936).
269) J. Hankiss and C. S. Hadhazy; Resorption on insulin und asthmolysin von der nasenschleimhaut, Acta. Med. Acad. Sci. Hung., 12 107 (1958).
270) M. Gibaldi; Role of surface-active agents in drug absorption, Fed. Proc., 29 1343 (1970).

271) M. Gibaldi and S. Feldman; Mechanisms of surfactant effects on drug absorption, J. Pharm. Sci., 59 579 (1970).
272) C. J. Kreutler and W. W. Davis; Normal and promoted GI absorption of water-soluble substances. III. Absorption of antibiotics from stomach and intestine of the rat, J. Pharm. Sci., 60 1835 (1971).
273) W. W. Davis and C. J. Kreutler; Normal and promoted GI absorption of water-soluble substances. II. Absorption of vitamin B_{12} from ligated stomach and intact intestine of the rat, ibid., 60 1651 (1971).
274) I. Utsurm, K. Kohno and Y. Takeuchi; Surfactant effects on drug absorption III: Effects of sodium glycocholate and its mixtures with synthetic surfactants on absorption of thiamine disulfide compounds in rat, ibid., 63 676 (1974).
275) N. Khalafallah, M. W. Gouda and S. Khalil; Effect of surfactants on absorption through membranes IV: Effect of dioctyl sodium sulfosuccinate on absorption of a poorly absorbable drugs, phenolsulfonphthalein, in humans, ibid., 64 991 (1975).
276) M. W. Gouda, N. Khalatallah and S. A. Khalil; Effect of surfactant on absorption through membrane V: Concentration-dependent effect of a bile salt (sodium deoxycholate) on absorption of a poorly absorbable drug, phenolsulfonphthalein, in humans, ibid., 66 727 (1977).
277) D. Birkett and W. Silen; Alteration of the physical pathways through the gastric mucosa by sodium taurocholate, Gastroenterology, 67 1131 (1974).
278) J. T. Harries and G. E. Sladen; The effects of different bile salts on the absorption of fluid, electrolytes, and monosaccharides in the small intestine of the rat in vivo, Gut, 13 596 (1972).
279) K. Ichikawa, I. Ohata, M. Mitomi, S. Kawamura, H. Maeno and H. Kawata; Rectal absorption of insulin suppositories in rabbits, J. Pharm. Pharmacol., 32 314 (1980).
280) Y. Nishioka and T. Kawamura; Effect of surface active agent on insulin absorption upon rectal administration of insulin suppository to rabbits, Yakuzaigaku, 37 119 (1977).
281) T. Yokosuka, Y. Omori, Y. Hirata and S. Hirai; Nasal and sublingual administration of insulin in man, J. Japan Diab. Soc., 20 146 (1977).
282) S. Hirai, T. Ikenaga and T. Matswzawa; Nasal absorption of insulin in dogs, Diabetes, 27 296 (1978).
283) S. Hirai, T. Yashiki and H. Mima; Effect of surfactants on the nasal absorption of insulin in rats, Int. J. Pharm., 9 165 (1981).
284) S. Hirai, T. Yashiki and H. Mima; Mechanisms for the enhancement of the nasal absorption of insulin by surfactants, ibid., 9 173 (1981).
285) A. E. Pontiroli, M. Alberetto, A. Secchi, G. Dossi, I. Bosi and G. Pozza; Insulin given intranasally induces hypoglycaemia in normal and diabetic subjects, Br. Med. J., 284 303 (1982).
286) A. C. Moses, G. S. Gordon, M. C. Carey and J. S. Flier; Insulin administered intranasally as an insulin-bile salt aerosol: Effectiveness and reproducibility in normal and diabetic subjects, Diabetes, 32 1040 (1983).
287) J. H. Childrey and H. E. Essex; Absorption from the mucosa of the frontal sinus, Arch. Otolaryngol., 14 564 (1931).
288) O. E. V. Alyea and A. Donnelly; Intranasal medication with vasoconstrictors, Arch. Otolaryngol., 49 234 (1941).
289) D. W. Empey and K. T. Medder; Nasal decongestants, Drugs, 21 438 (1981).
290) M. G. Myers and J. J. Iazzetta; Intranasally administered phenylephrine and blood pressure, Can. Med. Assoc. J., 127 365 (1982).
291) W. W. Lindsay; Tobispray in nasal surgery, Med. J. Aust., 1 751 (1977).
292) L. Hamilton, Effect of topical decongestants on nasal airway resistance, Curr. Ther. Res., 24 261 (1978).
293) L. H. Hamilton; Effect of xylometazoline nasal spray on nasal conductance in subjects with coryza, J. Otolaryngol., 10(2) 109 (1981).

294) B. Petruson and H. A. Hansson; Function and structure of the nasal mucosa after 6 weeks use of nose-drops, Arch. Otolargngol., 94 563 (1982).
295) R. T. Jackson and J. E. Birnbaum; A comparison of a synthetic prostaglandin and xylometazoline hydrochloride as nasal decongestants, Otolaryngol. Head Neck Surg., 90 594 (1982).
296) J. Tonndorf, H. I. Chinn and J. E. Lett; Absorption from nasal mucous membrane: Systemic effect of hyoscine following intranasal administration, Ann. Otol. Rhinol. Laryngol., 62 630 (1953).
297) R. W. Hyde, J. Tonndorf and H. E. Chinn; Absorption from the nasal mucous membrane, Ann. Otol. Rhinol. Laryngol., 62 957 (1953).
298) R. T. Jackson; Low-dose topical atropine for rhinorrhea, Arch. Otolaryngol., 107 288 (1981).
299) P. Borum and N. Mygind; Nasal methacholine challenge and ipratropium therapy: Laboratory studies and a clinical trial in perennial rhinitis, Acta Otol-Rhinol-Laryngologica Belgica., 33(4) 528 (1979).
300) P. Borum, L. Olsen, B. Winther and N. Mygind; Ipratropium nasal spray: A new treatment for rhinorrhea in the common cold, Ann. Rev. Respir. Dis., 123 418 (1981).
301) J. M. Ritchie and P. J. Cohen, in The Pharmacological Basis of Therapeutics (L. S. Goodman and A. Gilman, Eds.), New York (1975), p. 379.
302) D. J. Stewart, T. Inaba, M. Lucassen, and W. Kalow; Cocaine metabolism: cocaine and norcocaine hydrolysis by liver and serum esterases, Clin. Pharmacol. Ther., 25 464 (1979).
303) D. J. Stewart, T. Inaba, B. K. Tang and W. Kalow; Hydrolysis of cocaine in human plasma by cholinestrase, Life Sci., 20 1557 (1977).
304) R. Byck, P. Jatlow, P. Barash, and C. V. Dyke; Cocaine: blood concentration and physiological effect after intranasal application in man. In Cocaine and other stimulants (E. H. Ellinwood and M. M. Kilbey, Eds.), Plenum Press, New York (1976), pp. 629-646.
305) C. V. Dyke, P. G. Barash, P. Jatlow and R. Byck; Cocaine: Plasma concentrations after intranasal application in man, Sciences, 195 859 (1977).
306) R. B. Resnick, R. S. Kestenbaum and L. K. Schwartz; Acute systemic effects of cocaine in man: a controlled study of intranasal and intravenous route of administration. In Cocaine and other stimulants (E. H. Ellinwood and M. M. Kilbey, Eds.), Plenum Press, New York (1976), pp. 615-628.
307) R. B. Resnick, R. S. Kestenbaum and L. K. Schwartz; Acute systemic effects of cocaine in man: a controlled study by intranasal and intravenous routes, Sciences, 195 696 (1977).
308) C. V. Dyke, P. Jatlow, J. Ungerer, P. G. Barash and R. Byck; Oral cocaine: Plasma concentrations and central effects, ibid., 200 211 (1978).
309) C. V. Dyke, P. Jatlow, J. Ungerer, P. Barash and R. Byck; Cocaine and lidocaine have similar psychological effects after intranasal application, Life Sciences, 24 271 (1979).
310) P. Wilkinson, C. V. Dyke, P. Jatlow, P. Barash and R. Byck; Intranasal and oral cocaine kinetics, Clin. Pharmacol. Ther., 27(3) 386 (1980).
311) C. V. Dyke, J. Ungerer, P. Jatlow, P. Barash and R. Byck; Intranasal cocaine: Dose relationships of psychological effects and plasma levels, Int. J. Psychiatry Med., 12(1) 1 (1982).
312) H. L. Lippton, B. M. Chapnick and P. J. Kadowitz; Influence of prostaglandins on vasoconstrictor responses in the hindquarters vascular bed of the cat, Prostaglandins Med., 6 183 (1981).
313) P. Hedquist; Basic methods of prostaglandin action on autonomic transmission, Ann. Rev. Pharmacol. Toxicol., 17 259 (1977).
314) A. Änggard; The effect of prostaglandins on nasal airway resistance in man, Ann. Otol. Rhinol. & Laryngol., 78 657 (1969).

315) R. T. Jackson; Prostaglandin E_1 as a nasal constrictor in normal human volunteers, Curr. Ther. Res., 12 711 (1970).
316) S. M. M. Karim, P. G. Adaikan and N. Kunaratnam; Effect of topical prostaglandins on nasal patency in man, Prostaglandins, 15 457 (1978).
317) S. M. M. Karim, P. G. Adaikan and N. Kunaratnam; Effect of 17-phenyl-PGF$_{2\alpha}$ on nasal patency in man, Prostaglandins and Medicine, 3 33 (1979).
318) R. T. Jackson and J. E. Birnbaum; A comparison of a synthetic prostaglandin and xylometazoline hydrochloride as nasal decongestants, Otolaryngol. Head Neck Surg., 90 594 (1982).
319) G. Greenwood, R. E. Pittenger, G. A. Constant and A. C. Ivy; Effect of zephiran chloride, tyrothricin, penicillin and streptomycin on ciliary action, Arch. Otolaryngol., 43 623 (1946).
320) T. Bergan; Penicillins, Antibiotics chemother., 25 1 (1978).
321) J. M. Brogard, F. Comte and M. Pinget; Pharmacokinetics of cephalosporin antibiotics, Antibiotics Chemother., 25 123 (1978).
322) S. Hirai, T. Yashiki, T. Matswzawa and H. Mima; Absorption of drugs from the nasal mucosa of rat, Int. J. Pharm., 7 317 (1981).
323) A. Rubinstein, E. Rubinstein, E. Toitum and M. Donbrow; Increase of intestinal absorption of gentamicin and amitracin by nonionic surfactant, Antimicrob. Agents Chemother., 19 696 (1981).
324) A. Rubinstein; Intranasal administration of gentamicin in human subjects, Antimicrob. Agents Chemother., 23 778 (1983).
325) R. A. Bucknall; Why aren't antivirals effective when administered intranasally? In: Chemotherapy and control of influenza (J. S. Oxford and J. D. Wiliams, Eds.), Academic Press Inc., New York (1976), pp. 77-80.
326) D. C. Delong and S. E. Reed; Inhibition of rhinovirus replication in organ cultures by a potential antiviral drug, J. Infect. Dis., 141 87 (1980).
327) R. A. Levandowski, C. T. Pachucki, M. Rubenis and G. G. Jackson; Topical enviroxime against rhinovirus infection, Antimicrob. Agents Chemother., 22 1004 (1982).
328) J. T. Connell; A novel method to assess antihistamine and decongestant efficacy, Ann. Allergy, 42 278 (1979).
329) L. Wong, L. Hendeles and M. Weinberger; Pharmacologic prophylaxis of allergic rhinitis: relative efficacy of hydroxyzine and chlorpheniramine, J. Allergy Clin. Immunol., 67 273 (1981).
330) S. West, B. Brandon, P. Stolley and R. Rumrill; A review of antihistamines and the common cold, Pediatrics, 56 100 (1975).
331) J. H. Childrey and H. E. Essex; Absorption from the mucosa of the frontal sinus, Arch. Otolaryngology, 14 564 (1931).
332) L. K. Gundrum; Experimental investigations on action of antihistaminic nasal solutions, Calif. Med., 75 207 (1951).
333) N. Schaffer and E. E. Seidmon; The intranasal use of prophenpyridamine maleate and chlorprophenpyridamine maleate in allergic rhinitis, Ann. Allergy, 10 194 (1952).
334) C. Secher, J. Kirkegaard, P. Borum, A. Maansson, P. Osterhammel and N. Mygind; Significance of H_1 and H_2 receptors in the human nose: rationale for topical use of combined antihistamine preparations, J. Allergy Clin. Immunol., 70 211 (1982).
335) O. Resta, M. P. F. Barbars and N. Carnimeo; A comparison of sodium cromoglycate nasal solution and powder in the treatment of allergic rhinitis, Br. J. Clin. Pract., 36 94 (1982).
336) R. G. Cuddihy and J. A. Ozog; Nasal absorption of CsCl, $SrCl_2$, $BaCl_2$ and $CeCl_3$ in syrian hamsters, Health Physics Pergamon Press, 25 219 (1973).
337) A. Czerniawska; Experimental investigations on the penetration of ^{198}Au from nasal mucous membrane into cerebrospinal fluid, Acta Otolaryng., 70 58 (1970).

338) P. G. Gopinath, G. Gopinath and T. C. A. Kumar; Target site of intranasally sprayed substances and their transport across the nasal mucosa: a new insight into the intranasal route of drug delivery, Curr. Ther. Res., 23 596 (1978).

Transnasal Systemic Medications, edited by Y.W. Chien
Elsevier Science Publishers B.V., Amsterdam, 1985 – Printed in The Netherlands

NASAL PHYSIOLOGY IN INTRANASAL DRUG ADMINISTRATIONS

DONALD F. PROCTOR
Schools of Hygiene and Public Health and of Medicine
The Johns Hopkins University
Baltimore, Maryland 21205

Certain considerations are necessary if we are to approach the practicality of intranasal administration of therapeutic drugs through the nasal mucosa. Among these are:

1) What is the normal physiology of the nose, which makes it an especially useful site for drug administration?
2) In what circumstances might such intranasal drug administration be detrimental to nasal function?
3) What are the nasal conditions which may interfere with the intranasal drug administration?
4) What may be the most effective means for the intranasal administration of drugs?

Although, phylogenetically, the olfactory function of the nose is of major importance, physiologically, the nasal structure and function in man are primarily related to the modification of inspired air (ref. 1-4). It happens that the mechanisms, which enable the nasal passage to play that role, can also be of use in the transmission of pharmacologically-active agents into the circulation. In a way, this may seem paradoxical. The nasal modification of inspired air includes the entrapment of many air pollutants and their dispatch to the stomach before they can make contact with nasal epithelial cells. Therefore, one could expect the same fate for the drugs introduced into the inspired air. One of the problems we must address is: what factors determine the nasal surface clearance or nasal absorption.

NORMAL NASAL PHYSIOLOGY

Even from a brief look at some aspects of the nasal morphology and physiology, it becomes immediately obvious that the nasal passage is quite different, in the shape, from the remainder of the airways (Figure 1).

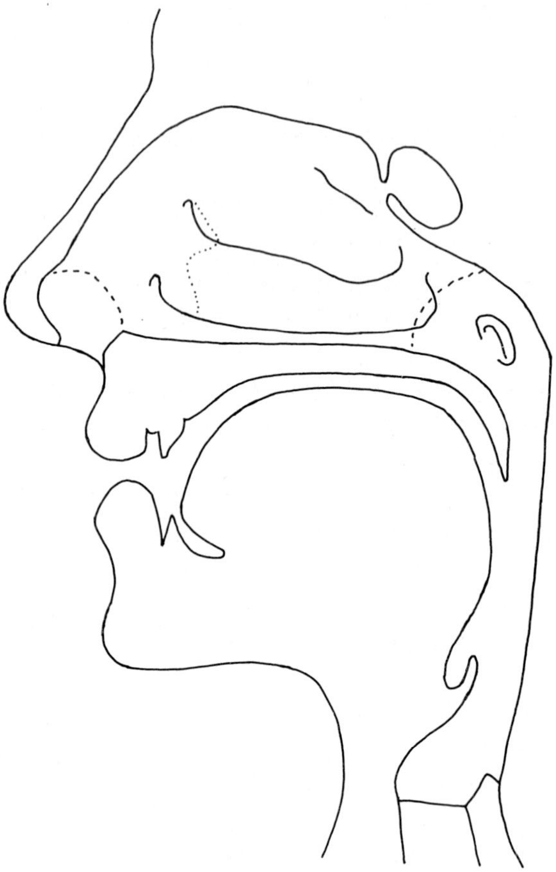

Figure 1: The upper airways seen from the midline. The dashed line just beyond nostril marks the beginning of nasal valve, while the dotted line shows approximately the beginning of ciliated epithelium region. Large aerosol particles largely deposit in the zone between the dashed and dotted lines. The dashed line near the nasopharynx indicates the posterior termination of nasal septum. Materials applied topically to conjunctiva will enter the nose through the nasolacrimal duct just beneath the anterior end of inferior turbinate. (Reproduced with permission from copyright owner - Elsevier Biomedical Press, Ref. 3).

Whereas the other conducting airways provide conduits to permit the passage of respired air with a minimum resistance to the airflow, the nasal airway accounts for as much of that resistance as all the rest of the respiratory tract to the alveoli. This results from the division of the nose into two halves by the nasal septum, each in turn convoluted by the folds of the turbinates, an arrangement which, at the cost of added resistance to the air flow, permits an intimate contact between the air stream and the mucosal surfaces (Figure 2).

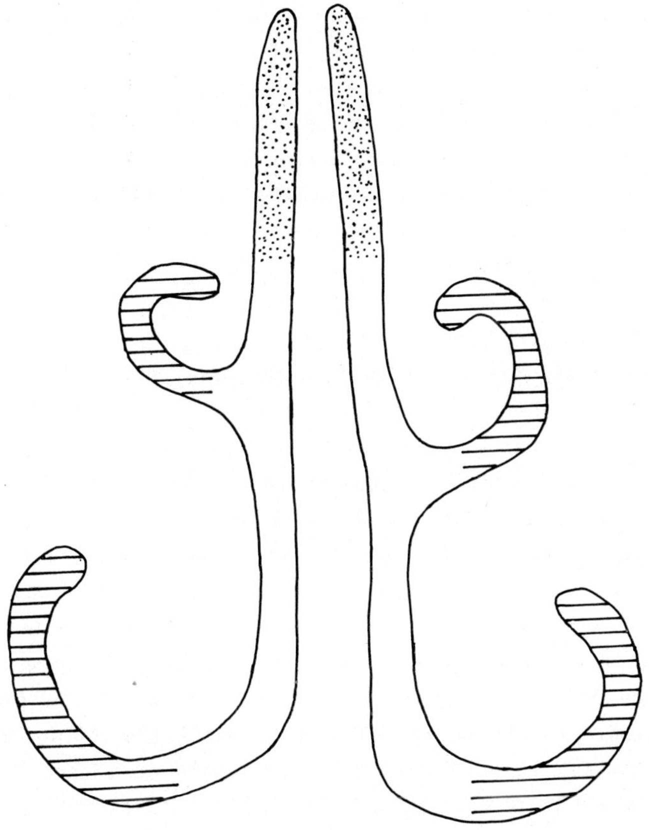

Figure 2: Section through the main nasal passage showing nasal septum, folds of the turbinates, and airway. The stippled area indicates the olfactory region, which is generally free of inspiratory airflow. Horizontal lines mark the meatal spaces, through which there is very little airflow, but in which there exist the communications with the paranasal sinuses and nasolacrimal duct. The clear areas mark the zone of inspiratory airflow and the region lined with richly vascular erectile tissue. This is the site primarily reached by the medications applied intranasally as nose drops or fine aerosol sprays. (Reproduced with permission from the copyright owner - Elsevier Biomedical Press, Ref. 3).

The modification of inspired air, which is of vital importance even in breathing a perfectly clean air, includes the adjustment of the temperature and the water vapor content of the ambient air entering the nose. This adjustment becomes possible because of the close contact between the narrow air streams and mucosal surfaces, and also because of the nature of the circulatory and mucociliary systems, which are quite different in the nose from those systems in the tracheobronchial airways. The nasal vascular system is extremely rich and highly adjustable (ref. 5-15).

The mucociliary system consists of a great number of submucosal glands and goblet cells, which provide the surface fluids, and the cilia, which transport these fluids to the nasopharynx whence they are swallowed (ref. 10, 16-22). Of special importance is the fact that both the circulatory and secretory mechanisms are susceptible to profound effects from a variety of influences. If the influences have yielded a sufficient vasoconstriction, the capability of the nose to transmit surface materials to the blood stream could be significantly reduced.

Since a drug may be introduced into the nose, not only in a liquid form as nose drops, but also as a nasal spray form, such as a liquid aerosol or a dry powder, it is therefore necessary to understand the factors influencing the fate of inhaled aerosols or dusts (ref. 23). In the anterior area of the nose there is a constriction known as the nasal valve (Figure 1). The air stream must flow at a high linear velocity to pass through this constriction, and just beyond that point the stream undergoes a sharp bend in direction. These two characteristics of the nasal airflow result in deposition of most aerosols or dusts in the anterior nose. The larger particles lodge far enough anteriorly to be in front of the exchange region of the nose and, therefore, not subject to nasal absorption into the body. Insoluble particles, even if they pass this point and deposit in the main passage, are likely to be carried backward in the ciliary stream and dispatched to the stomach. If the drug is introduced as a vapor or a soluble particle, it may readily pass into the lining secretions and thence through them for absorption into the blood.

EFFECTS OF INTRANASAL DRUG ADMINISTRATION ON NASAL PHYSIOLOGY

Before introducing a drug nasally we should determine whether or not it has the potential of damaging either the mucociliary system or the underlying epithelium, or of increasing the nasal airflow resistance to a degree that affects oronasal breathing. Such potential injurious effects can be readily tested and the rate of nasal mucociliary transport can be measured with considerable accuracy, whereas the nasal airflow resistance can also be determined through nasal rhinometry.

EFFECT OF NASAL CONDITIONS ON NASAL ABSORPTION

Nasal obstruction as a result of extensive nasal polyposis would reduce the capacity of nasal absorption. In addition, atrophic rhinitis or severe vasomotor rhinitis could also reduce the usefulness of the nose to absorb a drug. In some persons, an excessive response of the secretory system to some irritants could drain away whatever is introduced prior to its absorption. Such a tendency may exist in persons with severe nasal allergies.

EFFECTIVE MEANS OF INTRANSAL DRUG ADMINISTRATION

First, one should ask if the drug is available in a water-soluble form. If not, its likelihood of effective nasal absorption is very small. If a drug is available in water-soluble form, should it be used in solution and, if so, as drops, aerosols or vapors, or perhaps as a dust? This problem was recently studied (ref. 24). It was found that if a dust is to be used, it should be introduced through a device which holds the nostril open, thus at least part of the applied dose will be able to pass most of the anterior portion of the nose. If an aqueous solution is the vehicle of choice, nose drops may be most appropriate. An aerosol nebulizer, which is also introduced by a device holding the nostril open, can be effective too; but, it was observed that when one uses the nebulizer, it is best to administer each nostril at least twice.

It has become apparent that more research is needed if we are to discover which drugs may be administered safely by nasal route, and in what manner they should be given. The following questions require further investigation:

1) To what degree and in what circumstances may a nasal vasoconstrictor facilitate or impair the intranasal administration of drugs?
2) Which drugs may have some detrimental local effects that may outweigh the benefits of intranasal administration?
3) For each drug, what is the best mode of intranasal administration?

It is becoming obvious that the intranasal administration of certain systemically effective drugs is both feasible and desirable.

REFERENCES

1) N. Mygind, F. V. Rasmussen and F. Mølgaard; Cellular and Neurogenic Mechanisms in Nose and Bronchi, Eur. J. Respir. Dis., 64 (Suppl 128) 483-554 (1983).
2) D. F. Proctor; The upper airways I. Nasal physiology and defense of the lungs, Am. Rev. Respir. Dis., 115 97-130 (1977).
3) D. F. Proctor and I. Anderson; The Nose, Upper Airway Physiology and the Atmospheric Environment, Elsevier, Amsterdam (1982).
4) D. F. Proctor and J. C. F. Chang; Comparative anatomy and physiology of the nasal cavity. In Nasal Tumors in Animals and Man (G. Reznik and S. F. Stinson, Eds.), C R C Press, Boca Raton (1983) Volume I, Chapter 1.

5) O. V. Batson; The venous networks of the nasal mucosa, Ann. Otol. Rhinol. Laryngol., 63 571-580 (1954).
6) N. Cauna; Blood and nerve supply of the nasal lining. In The Nose, Upper Airway Physiology and the Atmospheric Environment (D. F. Proctor and I. Anderson, Eds.), Elsevier, Amsterdam (1982), Chapter 3, pp. 45-70.
7) J. D. K. Dawes and M. N. L. Prichard; Studies of the vascular arrangements of the nose, J. Anat., 87 311-322 (1953).
8) R. Eccles; Neurological and pharmacological considerations. In The Nose, Upper Airway Physiology and the Atmospheric Environment (D. F. Proctor and I. Anderson, Eds.), Elsevier, Amsterdam (1982), Chapter 8, pp. 191-214.
9) L. J. Hall and R. T. Jackson; Effects of alpha and beta adrenergic agonists on nasal blood flow, Ann. Otol. Rhinol. Larnygol. 77 1120-1130 (1968).
10) T. Ishii and M. Toriyama; Acetylcholinesterase activity in the vasomotor and secretory fibers of the nose, Arch. Klin. Ohr. Nas. Kehlk. Heilk., 201 1-10 (1972).
11) R. T. Jackson and J. H. Burson; Effect of inflammatory mediators on nasal mucosa, Arch. Otolaryngol., 103 441-444 (1977).
12) L. Malm; Vascular and secretory effects of adrenoceptor agonists and peptides in man, Eur. J. Respir. Dir., 64 (Suppl. 128, Part 1) 139-142 (1983).
13) R. Stovall and R. T. Jackson; Prostaglandins and nasal blood flow, Ann. Otol. Rhinol. Laryngol., 76 1051-1060 (1967).
14) P. F. Swindle; The architecture of the blood vascular networks in the erectile and secreting lining of the nasal passages. Ann. Otol. Rhinol. Laryngol., 44 913-932 (1935).
15) K. Watanabe; Y. Saito, I. Watanabe and V. Mizuhriva, Characteristics of capillary permeability in nasal mucosa, Ann. Otol. Rhinol. Laryngol., 89 377-382 (1980).
16) P. M. Andrews; A scanning electron microscopic study of the extrapulmonary respiratory tract, Am. J. Anat., 139 399-424 (1974).
17) A. Anggard; Parasympathetic influence on the nasal mucosa, Acta Otolaryngol., 83 22-24 (1977).
18) A. Anggard; Nasal autonomic innervation with special reference to peptiderdic nerves, Eur. J. Respir. Dis., 64 (Suppl 128, Part 1) 143-149 (1983).
19) N. Mygind, H. Sørensen and C. B. Pedersen; The nasal mucosa during long-term treatment with beclamethasone dipropionate aerosol, Acta. Otolaryngol., 85 437-443 (1978).
20) N. Mygind, M. Pedersen and M. H. Nielsen; Morphology of the upper airway epithelium. In The Nose, Upper Airway Physiology and the Atmospheric Environment (D. F. Proctor and I. Anderson, Eds.), Elsevier, Amsterdam (1982), Chapter 4, pp. 71-98.
21) D. Pavia, P. P. Sutton, M. T. Lopez-Vidriero, J. E. Agnew and S. W. Clarke; Drug effects on mucociliary function, Eur. J. Respir. Dis., 64 (Suppl. 128, Part I) 304-317 (1983).
22) D. F. Proctor and G. K. Adams; Physiology and pharmacology of nasal function and mucus secretion, Pharmac. Ther. B., 2 492-509 (1976).
23) J. D. Brain and P. A. Valberg; Deposition of aerosol in the respiratory tract, Am. Rev. Respir. Dis., 120 1325-1373 (1979).
24) N. Mygind and S. Vesterhauge; Aerosol distribution in the nose, Rhinology, 16 1-10 (1978).

Transnasal Systemic Medications, edited by Y.W. Chien
Elsevier Science Publishers B.V., Amsterdam, 1985 – Printed in The Netherlands

PHARMACOKINETICS OF INTRANASAL DRUG ADMINISTRATION

JOHN L. COLAIZZI
College of Pharmacy
Rutgers-The State University of New Jersey
Piscataway, New Jersey 08854

ABSTRACT

The pharmacokinetic profiles of drugs administered for systemic effect by intranasal instillation can be expected to be influenced by the peculiar physiology of the nasal cavity and membranes. In addition, the elimination of possible metabolism in the gastrointestinal tract or tissues as well as pre-systemic metobolism in the liver represents important characteristics of the pharmacokinetics of intranasal drug administration.

Detailed information on the pharmacokinetic profiles of intranasally administered drugs has been published for only a relatively few drugs. This chapter intends to review some pertinent literature, with particular emphasis on the important pharmacokinetic implications. Comparisons with other mucosal and non-mucosal routes of administration are employed to illustrate differences in absorption characteristics.

INTRODUCTION

The principal pharmacokinetic rationale for employing the nasal route is to accommodate drugs that are extensively metabolized in the gut wall or that are subject to an extensive first-pass elimination in the liver when administered orally. Another important reason is to provide a suitable route of administration for drugs such as peptides or proteins, which are destroyed by the gastrointestional fluids, and not capable of being adequately absorbed into the systemic circulation following oral administration. Since drugs of a peptide, polypeptide or protein nature are expected to increase in number and importance in the years to come, it will be an important potential application for the nasal route.

COMPARISON AMONG VARIOUS ROUTES OF ADMINISTRATION

Of course, the parenteral routes also offer these same pharmacokinetic advantages, but for simplicity, convenience and other non-pharmacokinetic reasons, non-oral, non-parenteral routes such as transdermal have been pursued in recent years as a means of overcoming problems with pre-systemic metabolism (ref. 1). Many drugs with short half-life, like many peptides, for example, would necessitate the inconvenience and impractiality of frequent injections.

Of all of the parenteral routes, intravenous administration can serve as the reference standard for establishing the basis for nasal bioavailability. In fact, it is the standard of comparison for all the other routes of drug administration, since it is the only route which completely bypasses the absorption process. Therefore, it defines the base line for absolute bioavailability. Not only does it bypass the absorption process, but it results in no pre-systemic metabolism. Because of the elimination of these variables, the intravenous route produces the most predictable values for plasma concentration, peak plasma level, and area under the curve (AUC) as a function of dose, of any route. For drugs with potent pharmacologic effects or possible toxicity, the somewhat exaggerated concentration spikes that one finds with bolus IV injection can be problematic. However, these problems can often be eliminated by use of constant-rate intravenous infusion. Any other disadvantages of intravenous administration are related to matters of convenience, not pharmacokinetics.

Intramuscular (IM) injection, unlike intravenous, does not always ensure rapid or complete absorption. With IM injection, the rate of absorption is generally more variable than the extent of absorption. For most drugs, the fraction of dose absorbed (F) usually approaches 1 (100% absorbed) with the IM route. However, there are a greater number of variables than with intravenous injection. As in the case of intranasal administration, the degree of vascularity of the administration site becomes a factor, although there are a greater number of possible sites to choose from with IM than with intranasal.

Like IM and intranasal, subcutaneous (SC) administration also depends upon the vascularity and blood supply at the administration site, and these factors can influence the rate and/or extent of absorption. For most drugs, the rate and extent of absorption with the SC route is either less than or equal to what can be achieved by IM administration.

The inhalation route takes advantage of the permeability and rich blood perfusion that is associated with the lung tissue. This leads to a rapid absorption, and, as with the parenteral routes, there is also no first pass effect. Most studies with the inhalation route have involved the use of gases, vapors, mists, smokes or aerosols, and there is not much information on the absorption of drugs presented in traditional solution form. Also, there are many technical problems associated with the dosage forms for the inhalation route, such a particle size control and loss of drug in the mouth and throat. Therefore, in contrast to intranasal administration, inhalation is not often intended for systemic administration of drugs in general, but, in practice, it is limited to those drugs used in the treatment of respiratory disorders. The technical problems associated with the inhalation of drugs lead to potential problems of patient compliance.

Buccal and sublingual forms of drug administration are of interest, because some studies have compared them to intranasal. They provide for rapid absorption and, generally, avoid any pre-systemic metabolism. As with intranasal, this route of administration, like inhalation, has been used for the absorption of hormones, such as oxytocin (ref. 2, 3). As with the intranasal route, pH-partition principles apply to absorption, with the usual salivary pH of 6, expected to have a potential effect on the absorption of some weak acids and bases, depending on their pKa values. Some drugs have been found to be stored in the buccal tissues and may not be rapidly absorbed. In general, however, absorption is rapid and more extensive than with the oral route for drugs like methyltestosterone.

The relatively recent and intense interest in the transdermal route results from the fact that systemic absorption through the skin is more general than was previously thought. Transdermal systems of drug administration have to be regarded as a potential alternative non-oral route to intranasal administration. Like intranasal, the transdermal route also avoids first-pass elimination through the liver. However, the transdermal route is only applicable to those drugs with dosages and molecular weights low enough to permit the passage of a therapeutic level through the skin. The intranasal route does not pose such severe restrictions in that regard. Since the skin is a much larger anatomical entity than the intranasal cavity, the skin provides for much more variability in absorptive capacity. While the condition of the skin may alter the absorptive capacity, irritation or tissue damage in the nasal cavity can also influence the rate and extent of absorption by the nasal mucosa. Hydration and occlusion effects are specific to transdermal administration, but the chemical form of the drug and the nature of the vehicle can influence absorption by either the transdermal or intranasal route.

In some parts of the world, the rectal route has been frequently used as a means of systemic drug delivery. However, a serious limitation is that absorption is generally slow and more variable than with oral administration. The extent of absorption is also usually less complete with rectal administration. Variations are caused by formulation effects and by fecal materials in the rectum. Also, the rectal route only partially avoids the first-pass effect, and the extent to which it occurs depends on how far along in the rectal chamber or large intestine the drug is actually absorbed. Peptides and proteins are poorly absorbed through the rectal epithelium, because there is neither a carrier-mediated transport system nor a large absorptive surface area. Although surfactants and other absorption promoters may stimulate the absorption of such macromolecular drugs, the intranasal route offers a much more favorable opportunity for the absorption of such large bioactive molecules.

Absorption of drugs through the vaginal vault, as with rectal absorption, has many limitations and variables associated with it. Its absorptive capacity changes with age and as a function of the estrus cycle.

ADVANTAGES OF INTRANASAL DELIVERY

In comparison with the more traditional non-oral routes of administration of drugs intended for systemic effect, the intranasal route is experiencing increasing interest, especially for hormones, peptides, vaccines, and other drugs. There is a clear advantage for drugs that undergo either extensive hepatic first-pass elimination, gut wall metabolism or destruction in GI fluids. Also, for some drugs, like propranolol, it has been shown that the rate and extent of absorption, and the plasma level-time profile with intranasal administration can be made to be quite comparable to the I.V. profile if the proper dosage regimen and formulation are employed. The rich vasculature and numerous microvilli structures in the nasal tissue make it an absorption site with great potential for a variety of drugs. Therefore, the intranasal route shows great promise for increasing therapeutic applicability. In some cases, such as with influenza vaccine, a large population of individuals will be more willing to accept intranasal rather than parenteral administration, and this could have significant public health implications.

There are two widely-used nasal dosage forms for trans-nasal systemic medication today - Desmopressin Acetate and Oxytocin. Desmopressin is a synthetic polypeptide used intranasally to control polydipsia and polyuria. It is destroyed in the gastrointestinal tract, but 10-20% of the dose is absorbed by intranasal administration whereby drug effects are evident in 1 hour, with a peak at 1 to 5 hours. Oxytocin is an octapeptide hormone, which is given exogenously to induce labor usually by the IV route. It is destroyed by GI enzymes. Applied intranasally, it has limited use in the regulation of milk ejection.

INTRANASAL PHARMACOKINETICS

The bioavailability of drugs administered by the intranasal route may be expressed in terms of the absolute efficiency of absorption, F, where, for plasma levels (C) determined following intravenous and intranasal administration.

$$F = \frac{(\text{Dose})_{IV} \, [\int_0^\infty C \, dt]_{nasal}}{(\text{Dose})_{nasal} \, [\int_0^\infty C \, dt]_{IV}} \qquad \text{(Eq. 1)}$$

where $\int_0^\infty C\,dt$, represents the area under the curve (AUC), extrapolated to infinite time, for the administration of a single intravenous or intranasal dose. If the same dose is given by each route of administration, then the (dose) terms cancel out of Equation 1, and it reduces to a ratio of AUC values.

F can also be calculated from the urinary excretion data following a single-dose administration of known doses of drug by intranasal and intravenous routes. From a knowledge of the total amount of drug ultimately excreted in the urine in the unmetabolized form (Au^∞), F may be determined from

$$F = \frac{(\text{Dose})_{IV} \, (Au^\infty)_{nasal}}{(\text{Dose})_{nasal} \, (Au^\infty)_{IV}} \qquad \text{(Eq.2)}$$

Equation 2 is valid only when the fraction of drugs reaching the circulation after administration, which is excreted in the urine, is the same for both the IV and the intranasal route.

If the body is considered to act as a single compartment from a pharmacokinetic viewpoint, the pharmacokinetic behavior of a drug administered by the intranasal (IN) route may be considered according to the model:

$$X_{IN} \xrightarrow{\text{absorption}} \boxed{X_B, V} \xrightarrow{\text{elimination}} X_E$$

where X_{IN} represents the amount of drug administered to the intranasal site, X_B represents the amount of drug in the body compartment, V is the apparent volume of distribution, and X_E is the amount of drug eliminated. From this single compartment model, the biexponential differential equation can be shown as follows,

$$\frac{dX_B}{dt} = \frac{dX_{IN}}{dt} - \frac{dX_E}{dt} \qquad \text{(Eq. 3)}$$

Equation 3 reveals that changes in the amount of drug in the central compartment (X_B) are a function of input (absorption) rate and output (elimination rate).

A) Intranasal Absorption - Zero Order

In cases in which the absorption from the intranasal site is zero order (e.g., a controlled release formulation), the pharmacokinetic model may be described as

$$\frac{dX_B}{dt} = k_o - kX_B \qquad \text{(Eq. 4)}$$

in which k_o is the zero-order absorption rate constant, which also is the actual rate of absorption or input, and k is the overall elimination rate constant, which can also be expressed as $0.693/t_{1/2}$. Converting to plasma concentration (C_p), Equation 4 may be expressed as

$$C_p = \frac{k_o}{Cl}(1 - e^{-kt}) \qquad \text{(Eq. 5)}$$

where Cl is the total body clearance and t represents any specified time following drug administration. In the type of pharmacokinetic profile described by Equations 4 and 5, plasma levels would increase to a steady-state plateau level, and then begin to decline exponentially at time T, which is the time when no further absorption from the intranasal cavity is occurring. If X^o_{IN} is the amount of drug at the intranasal absorption site at time zero (beginning of absorption), then

$$T = \frac{X^o_{IN}}{k_o} \qquad \text{(Eq. 6)}$$

B) Intranasal Absorption - First Order

The pharmacokinetic pattern for the more common case of first-order drug absorption from the intranasal site can be described by

$$\frac{dX_B}{dt} = F\, k_a\, X_{IN} - kX_B \qquad \text{(Eq. 7)}$$

In Equation 7, k_a is the first-order absorption rate constant, and the single compartment model is assumed to apply. The amount of drug at the absorption site (X_{IN}), at any time t, can be described by

$$X_{IN} = X^o_{IN}\, e^{-k_a t} \qquad \text{(Eq. 8)}$$

where X^o_{IN} is the initial dose applied to the site at time zero. Equation 8 indicates that the more rapidly drug is absorbed, the less will remain at the intranasal site. By substituting Equation 8 into Equation 7, we obtain

$$\frac{dX_B}{dt} = Fk_a X^o_{IN} e^{-k_a t} - kX_B \qquad \text{(Eq. 9)}$$

By integration of Equation 9, the plasma level, C_p, at any time following intranasal administration of the dose (X^o_{IN}) of a drug that undergoes first-order absorption, may be calculated:

$$C_p = \frac{F\, k_a\, X^o_{IN}}{V(k_a - k)} (e^{-kt} - e^{-k_a t}) \qquad \text{(Eq. 10)}$$

After absorption has ended, the term $e^{-k_a t}$ may be eliminated from Equation 10, and the post-absorptive state may be described as

$$C_p = \frac{F\, k_a\, X^o_{IN}}{V(k_a - k)}\, e^{-kt} \qquad \text{(Eq. 11)}$$

For methods to determine k_a or to consider situations in which multi-compartment behavior applies, standard textbooks in pharmacokinetics may be consulted (refs. 5 and 6).

AVOIDANCE OF FIRST-PASS EFFECT

One of the major advantages of intranasal drug administration is the avoidance of pre-systemic metabolism, particularly the first-pass effect. The rate of drug extraction across the liver that can occur during first-pass metabolism may be described as follows:

$$\text{Rate of Extraction} = Q\,(C_A - C_V) \qquad \text{(Eq. 12)}$$

where Q is the rate of blood flow to the liver, C_A is the concentration in the arterial plasma being presented to the liver, and C_V is the concentration of drug in the venous plasma exiting from the liver. The extraction ratio, E, may then be defined as:

$$E = \frac{\text{Rate of Extraction across liver}}{\text{Rate of Presentation to liver}} \qquad \text{(Eq. 13)}$$

$$E = \frac{Q\ (C_A - C_V)}{Q\ C_A} \quad \frac{C_A - C_V}{C_A} \qquad \text{(Eq. 14)}$$

When E is equal to 1, this would indicate that all of the drug was metabolized during the first pass through the liver. When there is no first-pass effect, E is equal to 0 during the first pass through the liver.

Since clearance can be regarded as a rate of elimination term divided by a concentration term,

$$Cl = \frac{Q\ (C_A - C_V)}{C_A} = Q\ E \qquad \text{(Eq. 15)}$$

If one considers the fraction of an oral dose of drug that reaches the circulation as F, assuming 100% absorption from the gastrointestinal tract, then

$$F = 1 - E \qquad \text{(Eq. 16)}$$

If we consider propranolol, with an E value of 0.64, then

$$F = 1 - 0.64 = 0.36 \qquad \text{(Eq. 17)}$$

which indicates that only 36% of the absorbed dose would survive the pre-systemic metabolic effects of the first pass through the liver. If the same dose were administered intranasally, the 64% reduction in dose reaching the systemic circulation would not occur, assuming similar extents of absorption by the oral and intranasal routes.

Similar considerations would apply in the case of drugs which undergo gut wall metabolism.

LITERATURE REVIEW OF INTRANASAL PHARMACOKINETIC STUDIES

In 1967, Muller and Osler (ref. 3) did a comparative study of intransasl, constant-rate IV infusion and buccal administrations of oxytocin. Their work noted that the use of the intranasal route for oxytocin can be dated back as far as 1927. When the three routes were compared, the relative rates of success for the induction of labor were close. Intranasal was 60% relative to 73% of the success rate with the intravenous route, but toxicity problems did not differ between intravenous and intranasal.

In 1969, Agosti and Bertaccini published a study on the decapeptide caerulein with cholecystokinetic effects (ref. 7). Intranasal and intravenous responses were the same if doses above a certain threshold level were given. This study also showed that nasal congestion or chronic rhinitis interfered with absorption via the intranasal route.

In 1973, the nasal absorption of inorganic chloride salts of cesium, strontium and barium was investigated in hamsters (ref. 8). The extent of absorption was found to be more than 50% greater for the intranasal route than for the gastrointestinal route. It was noted that the diameter of the aerosolized fluids of the salt solutions is an influencing factor and so is the flow rate of aerosol through the nose during respiration. It was also found that nasal absorption is also complicated by "mechanical clearance", defined as loss of drug solution into the esophagus.

A study by Fink et al. (ref. 9), published in 1974, determined the concentrations of Luteinizing Hormone Releasing Hormone (LHRH) by radioimmunoassay in the blood of males after the administration of different doses of synthetic LHRH by the intravenous and intranasal route. The results revealed that peak concentrations occurred within 15 to 30 minutes following a nasal dose of the hormone. Peak concentrations were dose-dependent for both intravenous and intranasal routes. The linearity of C_{max} versus dose relationships for LHRH suggested that nasal absorption is a first-order process.

Reports on intranasal administration stimulated publication of an editorial in the British Journal of Clinical Pharmacology in 1976 (ref. 10). The editorial provided an interesting summary of the factors affecting pharmacokinetic profiles with the intranasal route of administration. These factors were summarized as follows:

1) Physiological conditions of nasal vascularity.
   a. speed of mucus flow
   b. presence of infection
   c. atmospheric condition
2) Dosage form factors.
   a. Concentration
   b. physico-chemical properties of active drug
   c. density/viscosity properties

   d. pH-tonicity
   e. excipients
3) Techniques and devices of administration.
   a. droplet size
   b. site of deposition
   c. mechanical loss into the esophagus
   d. mechanical loss to other sites
   e. mechanical loss anteriorly from nose

A publication describing the comparative pharmacokinetic profile of nasal and sublingual administration of insulin in man was published by Yokosuka et al. in 1977 (ref. 11). Blood glucose and immunoreactive insulin levels were determined in 18 healthy adults. Sodium glycocholate, 1%, as an absorption promoter, significantly enhanced the ability to obtain a reduction in glucose levels within 15 minutes of intranasal administration. The nasal route produced a peak almost as quickly as the intravenous route, and certainly much more rapidly than the subcutaneous route. Intranasal administration also produced a higher peak than the subcutaneous. However, the peak level obtained with the nasal route was not as high as that achieved by the intravenous bolus injection of the same dose. Intranasal administration produced peak insulin concentrations within 15 minutes or less in most cases. When the sodium glycocholate was not included, essentially no intranasal absorption of insulin was observed. Also, there was no appreciable effect from sublingual administration. This article showed that intranasal administration of insulin could produce plasma-time insulin profiles that are somewhat intermediate, in terms of C_{max} and T_{max}, between intravenous and subcutaneous administrations, and with AUC values sufficient to make it appear that the nasal route may be a clinically suitable alternative to parenteral insulin administration. A surfactant-type absorption promoter was essential, and provided F values of approximately 0.3 (Equation 16).

Another Japanese study (ref. 12) also investigated the nasal absorption of insulin in dogs, but, in general, the results were supportive of the findings of Yokosuka et al. in humans (ref. 11). The effect of pH on intranasal insulin administration showed that absorption is minimal at the pH_{iso} of insulin (6.1), with maximal absorption on the acidic side of the pH_{iso}.

A series of studies by Hussain et al. have provided additional pharmacokinetic insights concerning nasal absorption. In a 1979 publication (ref. 13), it was showed that propranolol, a drug which undergoes a substantial first-pass elimination and some gastrointestinal metabolism, produces a pharmacokinetic profile from nasal absorption in rats that is quite similar to intravenous. The AUC from intranasal administration was directly proportional to dose, with a attainment of peak blood levels within about 5 minutes. The profile from oral administration was much lower in levels and more delayed than either intranasal or intravenous. These results with propranolol were later confirmed in dogs as well as in rats (ref. 14). In these experiments, F values for the intranasal route (using intravenous data as the standard) were nearly 1.00, whereas by the oral route the values of F were 0.068 in dogs and 0.190 in rats. These investigators subsequently investigated the nasal absorption of propranolol in adult males (ref. 15). At the same dose, the intranasal route provided a serum level-time profile that was very similar to IV administration. Nasal bioavailability (absolute efficiency of absorption), as based on serum level AUC's, was 1.09 for intranasal and 0.25 for oral administration. In these investigations the solution of propranolol was administered in a 2% methylcellulose gel, as in the other propranolol studies, but no absorption promoter was used. Recently, Hussain et al. also studied the nasal absorption of progesterone in rats (ref. 16). A 1% polysorbate 80 solution was used as the absorption promoter. F was essentially equal to 1 at 3 different doses, while F for intraduodenal administsrations was 0.012, due to GI metabolism and the first-pass effect.

Javaid et al. (ref. 17) investigated the kinetics of cocaine in humans after intravenous and intranasal administration. In their 1983 publication, intranasal cocaine was administered in a powdered form diluted with lactose, and the dose was sniffed through a straw. The pharmacokinetics of intranasally administered cocaine was found to follow the classical one-compartment open model with first-order absorption and first-order elimination kinetics. First-order absorption rate constants were calculated and values of 3.54 and 3.68 hr^{-1} were reported, based on averages of four subjects, at 64 mg and 96 mg doses of cocaine, respectively. The absorption rates showed a considerable degree of intersubject variability, and individual peak times ranging from 15 minutes to 1 hour were obtained following a single dose. One-compartment behavior was observed at all three doses used in this study: 32 mg (intravenous); and 64 and 96 mg (intranasal). However, it was reported that cocaine may also follow two-compartment pharmacokinetics at higher doses. Calculated values for average elimination half-life of cocaine in this study were as follows:

Dose	Route	$t_{1/2}$
32 mg	intravenous	0.58 h.
64 mg	intranasal	0.75 h.
96 mg	intranasal	1.54 h.

The authors (ref. 17) noted that other studies have also shown this increase in half-life with increasing dose. However, it appeared that in the current study, the differences in half-life are not statistically significant, and in light of the small number of subjects used (n=4), this is not surprising. The average values for F were 0.28 for the 64 mg dose and 0.57 for the 96 mg dose. Although no clear explanation for the difference in F values was offered by Javaid et al., it may be concentration related. In this instance, it is reasonable to assume that with the higher nasal dose, a more concentrated solution of cocaine forms within the nasal fluids with a resultant greater concentration flux effect during the absorption process, leading to a greater bioavailability at the higher dose.

SUMMARY

Survey of the literature of the intranasal route of drug administration indicates that intranasal administration is a suitable non-parenteral alternative form of administration for drugs which are subject to degradation in the luminal fluids of the GI tract, or which are subject to pre-systemic metabolism in the liver or gut wall.

Plasma levels following intranasal administration show a concentration-time profile more similar to intravenous bolus injection than can be achieved with other non-parenteral forms. The rate of absorption is generally quite rapid, with peak concentrations often occurring within 15 minutes of a dose.

The value of F varies from 1 for drugs like propranolol to much lower values for other drugs. For some drugs, there is a linear relationship between area under the curve (AUC) or peak plasma concentration (C_{max}) and the dose. For other drugs, however, linearity is not observed, and this non-linearity may be associated with the absorption phase in the nasal cavity, where the limited volume of nasal fluids leads to a situation in which differences in drug concentration in the solutions applied at the absorption site result in differences in flux sufficient to alter absorption. Such non-linearity could also be related to metabolism in the nasal tissues that differ as a function of concentration.

REFERENCES

1) M. Gibaldi, Biopharmaceutics and Clinical Pharmacokinetics, 3rd edition, Lea and Febiger, Philadelphia, (1984), pp. 85-112
2) N. E. Borglin, Intranasal Administration of Oxytocin for Induction and Stimulation of Labor, Acta Obstet. Gynecol. Scand., 41 238-252 (1962).
3) K. Muller and M. Osler, Induction of Labor: A comparison of Intravenous, Intranasal and Transbuccal Oxytocin, Acta Obstet. Gynecol. Scand., 46 59-67 (1967).

4) P. Bergsjo and H. Jenssen, Nasal and Buccal Oxytocin for the Induction of Labor: A Clinical Trial, J. Obstet. Gynal. Brit. Comm., 76 131-145 (1969).
5) J. G. Wagner, Fundamentals of Clinical Pharmacokinetics, Drug Intelligence Publications, Inc., Hamilton, Il, (1975), pp. 82-119 and 173-200.
6) M. Gibaldi and D. Perrier, Pharmacokinetics, Second Edition, Marcel Dekker, Inc., New York, (1982), pp. 45-111 and 145-167.
7) A. Agosti and G. Bertaccini, Nasal Absorption of Caerulein, Lancet, 1 580 (1969).
8) R. G. Cuddihy and J. A. Ozog, Nasal Absorption of Cs, Cl, $SrCl_2$, $BaCl_2$, and Ce Cl_3 in Serian Hamsters, Health Physics, 25 219-224 (1973).
9) G. Fink, G. Gennser, P. Liedholm, J. Thorell, and J. Mulder, Comparison of Plasma Levels of Luteinizing Hormone Releasing Hormone in Men After Intravenous or Intranasal Administration, J. Endocr., 63 351-360 (1974).
10) D. S. Freestone and A. L. Weingerg, The Administration of Drugs and Vaccines by the Intranasal Route, Brit. J. Clin. Pharmacol., 3 827-830 (1976).
11) T. Yokosuka, Y. Omori, Y. Hirata and S. Hirai, Nasal and Sublingual Administration of Insulin in Man, J. Japan. Diab. Soc., 20 (2) 146-152 (1977).
12) S. Hirai, T. Ilenaga and T. Matsuzawa, Nasal Absorption of Insulin in Dogs, Diabetes, 27 296-299 (1978).
13) A. Hussain, S. Hirai, and R. Bawarshi, Nasal Absorption of Propranolol in Rats, J. Pharm. Sci., 68 1196 (1979).
14) A. Hussain, S. Hirai, and R. Bawarshi, Nasal Absorption of Propranolol from Different Dosage Forms by Rats and Dogs, J. Pharm. Sci., 69 1411-1413 (1980).
15) A. Hussain, T. Foster, S. Hirai, T. Kashihara, R. Batenhorst and M. Jones, Nasal Absorption of Propranolol in Humans, J. Pharm. Sci., 69 1240 (1980).
16) A. Hussain, S. Hirai, and R. Bawarshi, Nasal Absorption of Natural Contraceptive Steroids in Rats - Progesterone Absorption, J. Pharm. Sci. 70 466-467 (1981).
17) J. I. Javaid, M. N. Musa, M. Fischman, C. R. Schuster, and J. M. Davis, Kinetics of Cocaine in Humans After Intravenous and Intranasal Administsration, Biopharmaceutics and Drug Disposition, 4 9-18 (1983).

Transnasal Systemic Medications, edited by Y.W. Chien
Elsevier Science Publishers B.V., Amsterdam, 1985 – Printed in The Netherlands

PHYSICOCHEMICAL CONSIDERATIONS IN INTRANASAL DRUG ADMINISTRATIONS

A. A. HUSSAIN, R. BAWARSHI-NASSAR and C. H. HUANG
College of Pharmacy
University of Kentucky
Lexington, Kentucky 40536-0053

ABSTRACT

For the past few years, research efforts have been directed toward finding a non-parenteral route, other than the oral, for the administration of drugs. In recent years, the nasal absorption has received a great deal of attention as a convenient and reliable method for the administration of certain drugs. Although this route is currently being used for the systemic administration of drugs, such as Oxytocin and DDAVP, it has only recently been quantitatively studied. .

This chapter will deal with the importance of the physical and chemical properties of drugs on the rate and extent of their nasal absorption.

INTRODUCTION

In recent years the nasal route has received a great deal of attention as a convenient and reliable method for the administration of drugs. Although this route is currently being utilized for the systemic administration of drugs, such as oxytocin or 1-desamino-8-arginine-vasopressin (DDAVP), (ref. 1, 2), it has only recently been quantitatively studied.

In the case of lipophilic drugs, such as propranolol, the intranasal administration in rats (ref. 3), dogs (ref. 4) and humans (ref. 5) has resulted in blood levels similar to those observed following the intravenous administration (Figure 1). It is apparent from this figure that nasal absorption of this drug was very rapid and complete. Such rapid and complete absorption was also observed in rats after the intranasal administration of progesterone (ref. 6) and 17β-estradiol (ref. 7). These drugs are metabolized in the gastrointestinal tract or by hepatic first-pass elimination, consequently their oral bioavailabilities are low, ranging from 25% in the case of propranolol to less than 1% in the case of progesterone. Furthermore, studies on the narcotic antagonist, naloxone, and the male hormone, testosterone, showed that these drugs are also rapidly and completely absorbed from the nasal cavity, whereas their oral bioavailability is less than 3% (ref. 8).

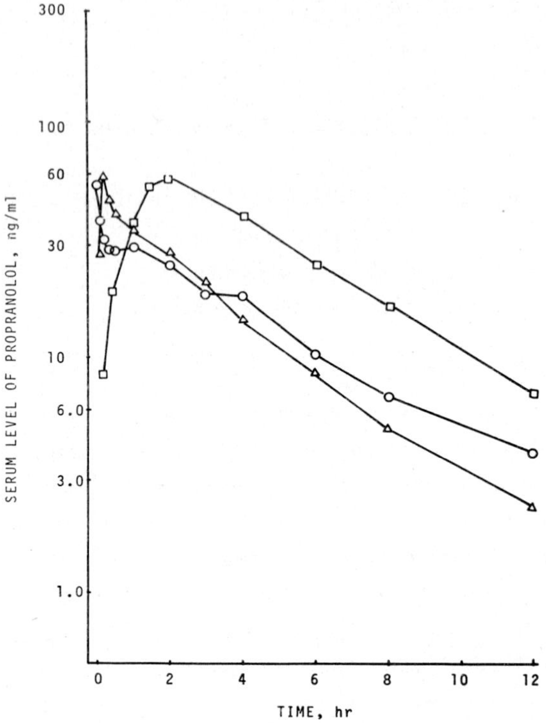

Figure 1: Time course for the average serum propranolol levels in six male subjects following intranasal administration of 10 mg/subject (△), intravenous administration of 10 mg/subject (○), and oral administration of 80 mg/subject (□).

Peptides, on the other hand, are poorly absorbed nasally. For example, in the case of insulin and nafarelin acetate (an LHRH analog), a nasal dose, which is considerably greater than the parenteral dose, is needed to produce a similar effect (ref. 9-12). The nasal bioavailability of nafarelin acetate in monkeys was found to be only 1% of that from the intravenous administration (ref. 12). Similarly, the tripeptide, L-pyro - 2 - aminodipyl-L-histidyl-L-thiazolidine-4-carboxamide, although it consists of fewer amino acids than insulin and nafarelin acetate, has a poor nasal bioavailability, which is about 7% of that from the intravenous injection (ref. 8). Intuitively, one may attribute the poor bioavailability of peptides to the polarity of their molecules. However, recent studies in rats using a polar quaternary ammonium compound, clofilium tosylate (I), showed that the blood levels after intranasal administration are similar to those observed after the intravenous administration, while the oral bioavailability was found to be only 1.3% of that from the intravenous injection (See the Chapter by Su and Campanale).

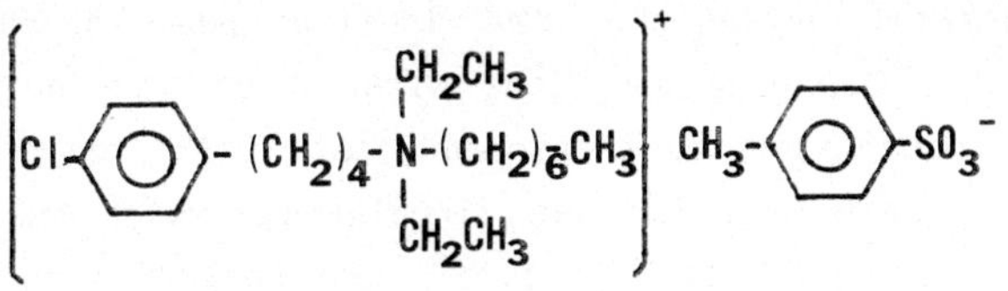

(I)

It appears from the discussions above that the mechanism of nasal absorption of drugs, such as peptides, is not fully understood. In order to gain an insight into this mechanism, a convenient and reliable method for studying nasal absorption is needed. The in situ rat nasal technique has been shown to be a satisfactory method for studying the rate and extent of absorption of drugs (ref. 7, 13). This technique involves the perfusion of drug solution through the nasal cavity of the rat at a constant rate for a certain period of time. The extent of nasal absorption is obtained by analyzing the concentration of the drug remaining in the perfusing solution.

This chapter deals with the effects of physico-chemical parameters on the rate and extent of nasal absorption of drugs. In particular, the following topics will be discussed:

a) Effect of the rate of perfusion and the volume of perfusate on the rate and extent of nasal absorption of drugs.
b) Effect of pH and partition coefficient on the rate and extent of nasal absorption of drugs.
c) Stepwise approach to study the factors that contribute to the low bioavailability of peptides.

STUDIES ON NASAL ABSORPTION

A) In-Situ Nasal Perfusion Experiments

The surgical procedure for the in situ nasal absorption experiments was carried out according to the method by Hirai et al (ref. 13). Sprague-Dawley male rats, weighing approximately 300 gm each, were used. The animals were anesthetized by sodium pentobarbital injection (50 mg/kg). An incision was made in the neck of the rat, and the trachea was cannulated with a polyethylene tube. Another tube, which served to introduce the perfusion solution into the nasal cavity, was inserted through the esophagus to the posterior part of the nasal cavity. The nasopalatine was sealed with an adhesive agent to prevent the drainage of the drug solution from the nasal cavity into the mouth.

The experimental set-up for the in-situ nasal perfusion experiments is shown in Figure 2. Drug solutions with volume ranging from 3 to 20 ml were placed in a water-jacketed beaker and kept at 37°C by means of a circulating water bath. Each solution was circulated through the nasal cavity of the rat by means of a polystaltic pump. The perfusing solution passed out from the nostrils through the funnel and into the beaker again. The extent of drug absorption was determined over a period of one hour by analyzing periodically the amount of drug remaining in the perfusing solution.

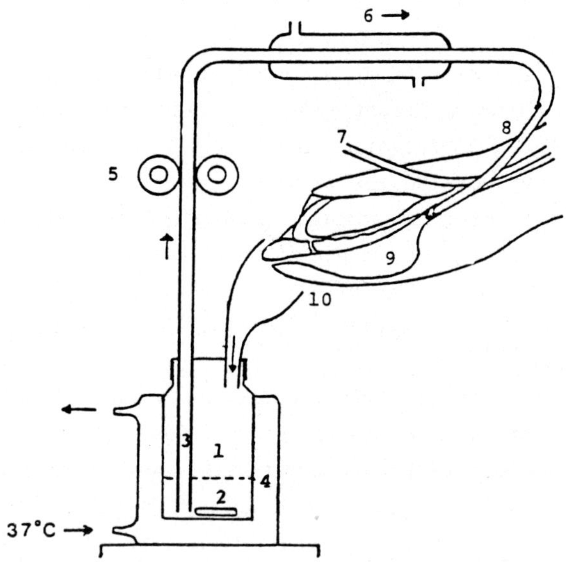

Figure 2: Experimental set-up for the in-situ nasal perfusion experiment.

Key:
1. Drug reservoir
2. Magnetic stirring bar
3. Tygon tube
4. Water-jacketed beaker
5. Polystaltic pump
6. Water bath
7. Trachea cannulation
8. Esophagus cannulation
9. Nasal cavity
10. Funnel

B) Physico-Chemical Parameters

1. Effect of Rate of Perfusion and Volume of Perfusate on Nasal Absorption

The dependency of the apparent first-order rate constant of absorption (k_{obs}) of phenobarbital on the rate of perfusion of the nasal solution is shown in Figure 3.

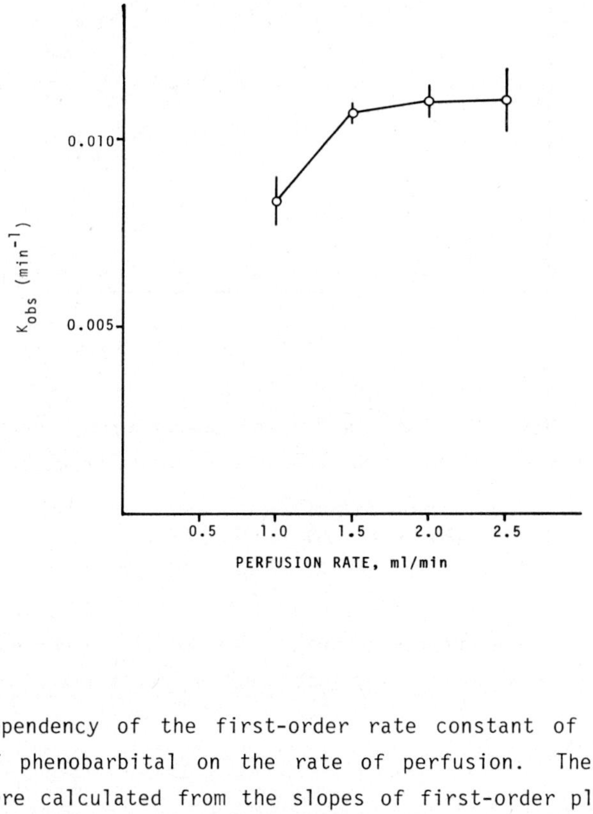

Figure 3: Dependency of the first-order rate constant of absorption (k_{obs}) of phenobarbital on the rate of perfusion. These rate constants were calculated from the slopes of first-order plots of the amount of drug remaining in the perfusion solution as a function of time.

The results indicate that for phenobarbital, the rate of nasal absorption becomes independent of the rate of perfusion at rates higher than 2 ml/min.

The effect of varying the volume of perfusion solution on the apparent rate of absorption was also studied using phenobarbital, L-tyrosine, propranolol and phenol red. Figure 4 shows a representative plot of the amount remaining versus time using four different volumes of a solution containing 0.46 mg/ml of phenobarbital at pH 6.0.

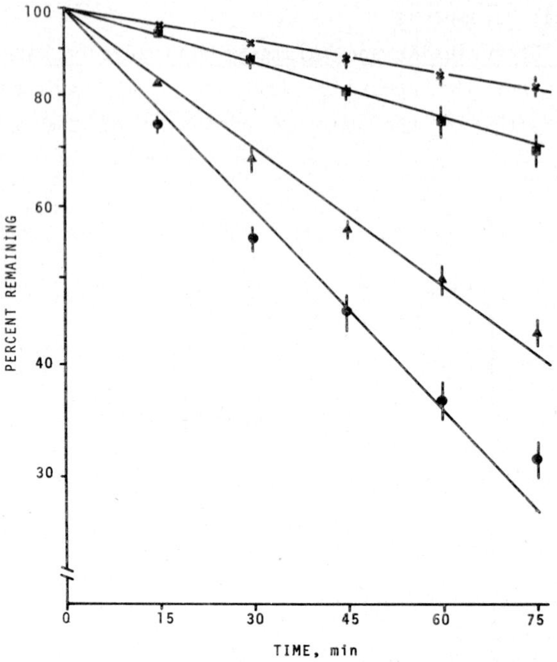

Figure 4: Percent (Mean ± S.E.M., n=3-5) of phenobarbital remaining in the in-situ perfusing solution versus time as a function of different perfusion volumes at pH 6.0, 37°C.
Key: (x) 20 ml; (■) 10 ml; (▲) 5 ml; (●) 3 ml.

The apparent first-order rate constants, calculated from the slope of the lines in Figure 4, are dependent upon the volume of the perfusion solution. Such dependency can be mathematically described by Fick's law of diffusion:

$$\frac{dm}{dt} = V\frac{dC}{dt} = -DA\frac{dC}{dx} \qquad \text{(Eq. 1)}$$

where m is the amount of the drug in the perfusion solution with a volume V, dC/dx is the concentration gradient across the nasal membrane with a thickness of h, D is the diffusion coefficient, and A is the surface area of the nasal mucosa. Equation 1 can be rearranged to give Equation 2.

$$\frac{dC}{dt} = \frac{-DA}{Vdx}(dC) \simeq \frac{-DA}{h} \cdot \frac{1}{V} \cdot (C_d - C_r) \qquad \text{(Eq. 2)}$$

$(C_d - C_r)$ could be approximated by the concentration in the donor side (C_d) when sink conditions are maintained in the receptor side $(C_r \simeq o)$.

From Equation 2, a relationship between k_{obs} and volume could be obtained as shown in Equation 3.

$$k_{obs} = \frac{DA}{h} \cdot \frac{1}{V} = \frac{k_a}{V} \qquad \text{(Eq. 3)}$$

where k_a represents the intrinsic rate constant for nasal absorption. By integrating Equation 2 and incorporating Equation 3, a first-order kinetic rate equation could be obtained as in Equation 4.

$$\ln C_d = \ln C_d^{o} - k_{obs} \cdot t \qquad \text{(Eq. 4)}$$

where C_d^{o} represents the initial concentration of the drug in the donor side, i.e., perfusing solution. A plot of k_{obs} versus 1/V (Equation 3) resulted in straight lines with slopes of k_a. The intrinsic nasal absorption rate constants, k_a, calculated for phenobarbital, phenol red, L-tyrosine and propranolol are shown in Table 1.

TABLE 1: Intrinsic nasal absorption rate constants (k_a)

Compound	k_a, min^{-1} ml
Propranolol	0.054
Phenobarbital	0.048
L-Tyrosine	0.012
Phenol red	0.007

In order to establish whether these rate constants can be correlated to the *in vivo* rate constants of absorption, the results for propranolol and L-tyrosine were used and compared. The *in vivo* first-order nasal absorption rate constants calculated for these compounds, following the administration of 0.1 ml of the drug solution to the rats, were found to be 0.4 min^{-1} and 0.12 min^{-1}, respectively. The predicted rate constants calculated from the data in Table 1 were found to be 0.54 min^{-1} and 0.11 min^{-1} for propranolol and L-tyrosine, respectively. It is apparent from the comparison that the *in situ* nasal absorption studies can be used to predict approximately the *in vivo* nasal absorption rate constant of drugs.

2) Effect of pH and Partition Coefficient on Nasal Absorption

The effect of pH on the nasal absorption of benzoic acid was examined in the pH range of 2 to 7.1. The results apparently indicated that the extent of absorption depends on the pH of the perfusion solution (Figure 5). For example, at pH 2.5 the amount absorbed in sixty minutes was found to be 44%, whereas within the same period of time the amount absorbed at pH 7.19 was 13%. If one assumes that benzoic acid is absorbed only in its unionized form, then at pH 7.19, where the drug exists to the extent of 99.9% in its ionized form, the rate of absorption would be negligible. However, as seen from Figure 5, 13% of benzoic acid is also absorbed from the nasal mucosa.

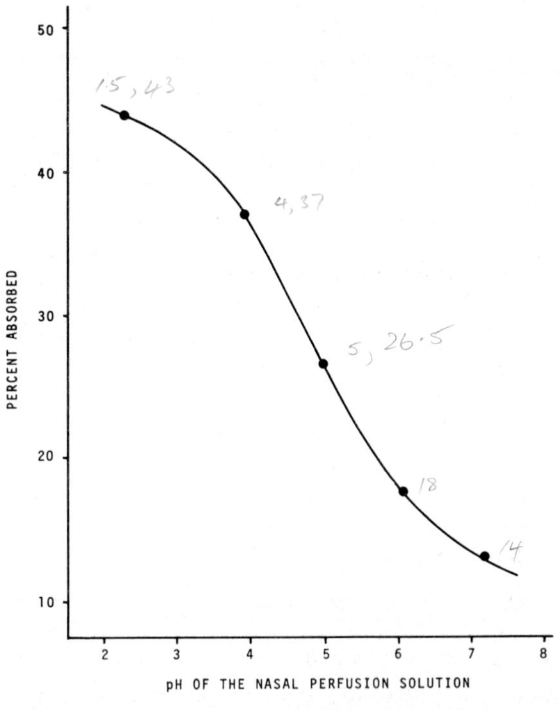

Figure 5: The percent of benzoic acid absorbed in sixty minutes as a function of pH.

The overall rate of absorption of benzoic acid at any given pH can be described according to Equation 5.

$$\frac{-d[\text{Benzoic acid}]_{\text{Total}}}{dt} = k_{HA}[HA] + k_{A^-}[A^-] \qquad \text{(Eq. 5)}$$

where k_{HA} and k_{A^-} are first-order absorption rate constants for the nonionized and ionized species of benzoic acid, HA and A^-, respectively.

Substituting for the species involved in terms of the ionization constant of benzoic acid ($K_a = 6.3 \times 10^{-5}$) and pH, and assigning k_{obs} to be the observed overall first-order absorption rate constant, then

at low pH:

$$k_{obs} = (k_{HA}) \frac{H^+}{H^+ + K_a} \qquad \text{(Eq. 6)}$$

at high pH:

$$k_{obs} = (k_{A^-}) \frac{K_a}{H^+ + K_a} \qquad \text{(Eq. 7)}$$

Using the values of k_{obs} at pH 2.4 and 7.19, where benzoic acid exists either entirely in its nonionized or ionized form, respectively, k_{HA} and k_{A^-} were calculated to be 9.75×10^{-3} and 2.4×10^{-3} min^{-1}, respectively. Thus, it appears that both the nonionized and ionized species of benzoic acid can be.absorbed through the nasal mucosa. However, the nonionized species is absorbed at a rate which is four times faster than the ionized species. Such pH dependency is similar to that observed in the gastrointestinal absorption of salicylic acid (ref. 14).

Since the rate and extent of absorption of drugs through a biological membrane is influenced by the lipophilicity of the compound, the effect of lipid solubility on the extent of nasal absorption was also studied using a series of barbituates at pH 6.0. At this pH the barbituates exist almost entirely in their nonionized form (pK_a 7.6). As seen in Table 2 the extent of absorption was related to the (chloroform/water) partition coefficient. However, a forty-fold difference in the partition coefficient between secobarbital and barbital resulted in only four-fold difference in the rates of nasal absorption. Furthermore, the insensitivity of the rate of nasal absorption to partition coefficient could also be seen by comparing the *in vivo* absorption rate constants of propranolol and L-tyrosine. Large difference between the (octanol/pH 7.4) partition coefficients of propranolol and L-tyrosine (propranolol 15.1, L-tyrosine 0.02) resulted in only a very little difference in the absorption rate constants for these compounds. Based on the above results and the additional data obtained in this laboratory coupled with the fact that polar quaternary ammonium compounds are also efficiently absorbed from the nasal cavity, it appears that the mechanism of absorption of drugs through the nasal membrane may be different from that observed through other biological membranes.

TABLE 2: Comparison of the extent of nasal absorption of barbiturates[a] and partition coefficient (chloroform/water) of the undissociated drug

Barbiturate	PC_{CHCl_3/H_2O}[b]	Percent Absorbed	
		Nasal	Gastro-intestinal[b]
Barbital	0.7	5.0 ± 3.00[c]	12
Phenobarbital	4.8	10.6 ± 3.88[c]	20
Pentobarbital	28.0	20.3 ± 4.65[d]	30
Secobarbital	50.7	23.9 ± 3.38[c]	40

[a]in rats at pH 6 for 60 min.
[b]Shanker, L. S., J. Med. Pharm. Chem., 2 343 (1960).
[c]Mean ± Standard Deviation (n = 3)
[d]Mean ± Standard Deviation (n = 4)

STUDIES ON THE MECHANISM OF NASAL ABSORPTION OF PEPTIDES

As mentioned earlier in the introduction, the nasal absorption of peptides is considerably lower than that observed for other drugs administered nasally. Furthermore, such poor absorption was shown to be unrelated to the size of the peptide. These authors believe that the low nasal bioavailability of peptides can be attributed to one of the following factors:

1) High polarity
2) Possible absorption by a carrier-mediated mechanism.
3) Possible hydrolysis in the nasal cavity.
4) Combination of the above factors.

In order to investigate the importance of the first and second factors, it was decided to examine the nasal absorption of a model amino acid, L-tyrosine. This amino acid was chosen because it has three polar functional groups, each of which can have a significant effect on its nasal absorption.

A) The Effect of Structural Modification on the Nasal Absorption of L-Tyrosine

In situ perfusion studies showed that the nasal absorption of L-tyrosine was pH independent in the range of 4 to 7.4, in which the extent of absorption after 60 minutes was found to be 12.7-14.2%. On the other hand, the nasal absorption of L-tyrosine was found to be concentration-dependent in the range of 0.28×10^{-3}M to 2.22×10^{-3}M. If one assumes that the mechanism of nasal absorption follows the Michaelis-Menten process, then the following relationship

$$\frac{1}{\text{Initial Rate}} = \frac{k_m}{V_{max} \cdot S} + \frac{1}{V_{max}} \quad \text{(Eq. 8)}$$

is valid, and a plot of the reciprocal of the initial rate for the disappearance of L-tyrosine versus the reciprocal of the initial concentration of the amino acid should result in a straight line. This is shown in Figure 6.

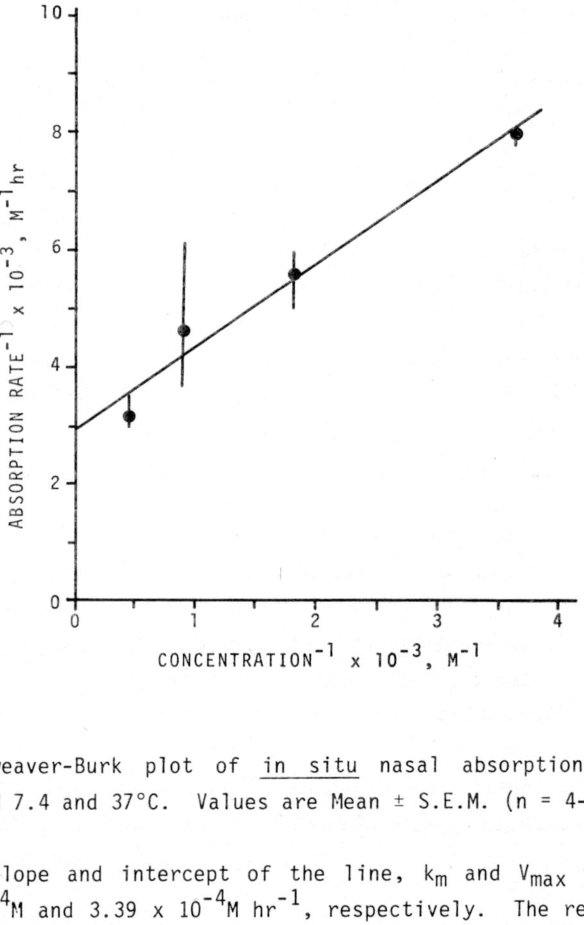

Figure 6: Lineweaver-Burk plot of <u>in situ</u> nasal absorption of L-tyrosine at pH 7.4 and 37°C. Values are Mean ± S.E.M. (n = 4-5).

From the slope and intercept of the line, k_m and V_{max} were calculated to be 4.8×10^{-4}M and 3.39×10^{-4}M hr^{-1}, respectively. The results indicated that L-tyrosine is absorbed from the nasal cavity in its zwitterionic form, and that its absorption is a carrier-mediated process. It may be possible that peptides are also absorbed by such a mechanism.

In view of the fact that any one of the various polar functional groups of L-tyrosine can have a significant effect on its nasal absorption, a stepwise approach of isolating the effect of each group was followed. This was accomplished by selective esterification of each functionality in the L-tyrosine molecule. Table 3 shows the various derivatives of L-tyrosine that were studied.

TABLE 3: Derivatives of L-tyrosine used in the in situ nasal perfusion studies

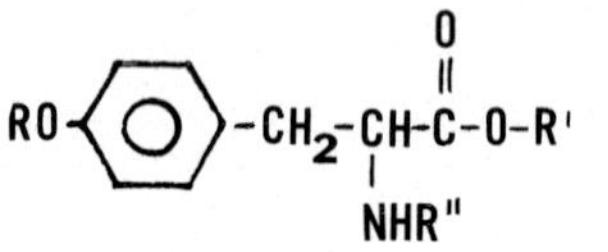

Compound	R	R'	R"
O-Acetyl-L-tyrosine	CH_3CO	H	H
O-Valeryl-L-tyrosine	C_4H_9CO	H	H
O-Hexanoyl-L-tyrosine	$C_5H_{11}CO$	H	H
L-Tyrosine methyl ester	H	CH_3	H
L-Tyrosine ethyl ester	H	C_2H_5	H
L-Tyrosine n-propyl ester	H	C_3H_7	H
L-Tyrosine t-butyl ester	H	C_4H_9	H
N-Acetyl-L-tyrosine	H	H	CH_3CO

In order to determine the contribution of the hydroxyl group, O-acyl derivatives of L-tyrosine were prepared and their nasal absorption was studied. Furthermore, their partition coefficients, non-enzymatic as well as enzymatic hydrolysis were also determined. The O-acyl-L-tyrosine esters were found to be relatively stable in the perfusate, since only 1-3% of tyrosine was detected after 60 minutes. However, these esters were found to generate L-tyrosine in the presence of pseudocholinesterase and 4% human plasma.

The rate of nasal absorption of these esters was not significantly different from that of L-tyrosine despite the fact that their (octanol/pH 7.4) partition coefficients were considerably greater than that of the parent amino acid (Table 4).

TABLE 4: Apparent partition coefficients and observed nasal absorption rate constants of L-tyrosine and its O-acyl derivatives

Compound	Apparent Partition Coefficient	k_{obs}, min^{-1} (Mean ± S.E.M.)
L-Tyrosine	0.0256	0.0023
O-Acetyl-L-tyrosine	0.0468	0.0026
O-Valeryl-L-tyrosine	1.17	0.0029

The insignificant difference in the rates of nasal absorption between L-tyrosine and its more lipophilic O-acyl derivatives may be attributed to the similarity in the ionic character of these compounds. It should be pointed out that L-tyrosine and its O-acyl esters exist in zwitterionic form in the pH range studied. One approach to verify the validity of this assumption was to reduce the ionic characteristic of L-tyrosine via the masking of the carboxylic and/or amino groups in the molecule.

The nasal absorption of the carboxylic acid esters of L-tyrosine and N-acetyl-L-tyrosine was studied (Table 3). Acylation of the amino functional group of L-tyrosine did not enhance its nasal absorption. After 60 minutes, ~6% of N-acetyl-L-tyrosine was absorbed, whereas ~15% of L-tyrosine was absorbed in the same period of time. It should be pointed out that the N-acetyl derivative has a similar (octanol/pH 7.4) partition coefficient to that of L-tyrosine.

Esterification of the carboxylic acid functional group of L-tyrosine, however, resulted in derivatives that possessed higher partition coefficients than the parent amino acid (Table 5).

TABLE 5: Calculated nasal absorption rate constants[a)] of L-tyrosine carboxylic acid esters and N-acetyl-L-tyrosine[b)]

Compound	Apparent Partition Coefficient[c)]	k_a, Min^{-1}
L-Tyrosine Methyl Ester	1.97	0.0116
L-Tyrosine Ethyl Ester	5.20	0.0254
L-Tyrosine n-Propyl Ester	20.79	0.0230
L-Tyrosine t-Butyl Ester	62.50	0.0105
N-Acetyl-L-Tyrosine	0.0256	0.0024

a) Perfusate volume, 5 ml.
b) At pH 7.4 and 37°C
c) Octanol/pH 7.4

Using L-tyrosine ethyl ester as a model compound, the esters were found to generate L-tyrosine enzymatically in the presence of pseudocholinesterase and human plasma. Furthermore, these compounds were also found to undergo hydrolysis in the nasal perfusate.

Using Equations 9 and 10, the nasal absorption rate constants for the esters were determined from the overall rate of loss of the ester as well as from the rate of appearance of L-tyrosine and are also shown in Table 5. It is apparent that the rate of nasal absorption of these esters is about 4 to 10 times faster than that of L-tyrosine.

$$-\frac{dA}{dt} = k_a[A] + k_{hyd}[A] \qquad \text{(Eq. 9)}$$

and

$$k_{obs} = k_a + k_{hyd} \qquad \text{(Eq. 10)}$$

where A is the concentration of the compound, k_{obs} is the overall apparent first-order rate constant for the loss of the drug, k_a is the apparent first-order rate constant for nasal absorption and k_{hyd} is the apparent pseudo-first-order rate constant of hydrolysis.

The enhancement in the rate of nasal absorption observed for the carboxylic acid esters cannot be rationalized only based on the difference in the partition coefficients between these derivatives and L-tyrosine. For example, the O-valaryl-L-tyrosine exhibited an approximately similar magnitude of partition coefficient as that of the methyl ester of L-tyrosine (1.17 vs. 1.97), yet there was four-time difference in their rates of absorption (0.0029 vs. 0.0116 min^{-1}).

Based on the results above, one can conclude that the greater enhancement in the nasal absorption of the carboxylic acid esters of L-tyrosine was the result of masking the negative charge on the carboxylate ion. It is the result of this negative charge that L-tyrosine, O-acyl-L-tyrosine and N-acetyl-L-tyrosine have a similar rate of nasal absorption, despite the significant difference in their partition coefficients (Tables 4 & 5).

B) Nasal Absorption of Peptides - L-tyrosyl-L-tyrosine

It was shown in the previous section that L-tyrosine is absorbed by a carrier-mediated process and that its nasal absorption is enhanced via the acylation of the carboxyl group. In an attempt to determine whether a similar modification can enhance the absorption of peptides, the nasal absorption of L-tyrosyl-L-tyrosine (II) and its methyl ester derivative (III) was studied. Using a specific HPLC method, the intact compounds as well as their hydrolysis products were determined as a function of time.

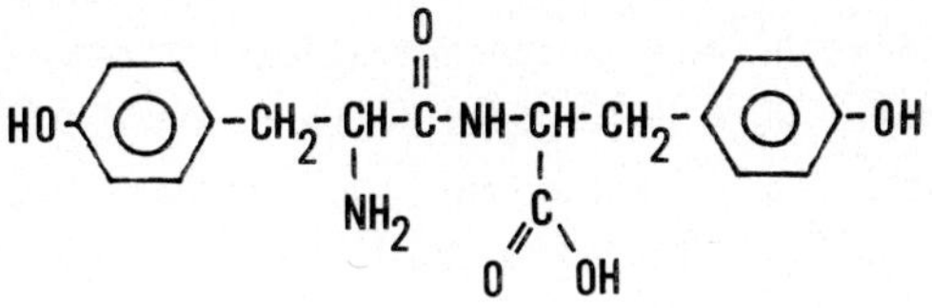

(II)

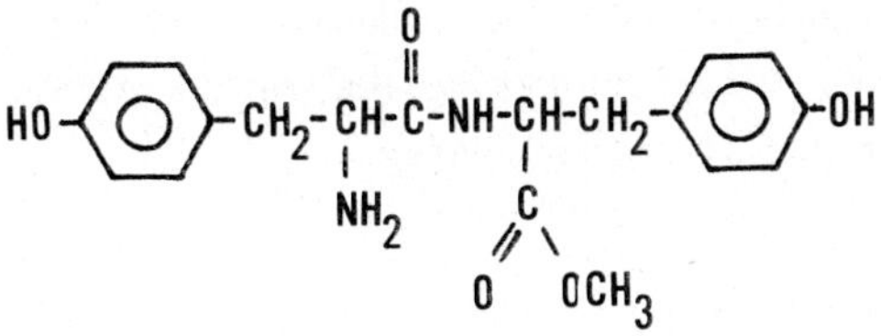

(III)

L-Tyrosyl-L-tyrosine was found to undergo considerable hydrolysis in the perfusate. This must be due to the presence of the enzyme, peptidase, in the nasal cavity, since the peptide was shown to be stable in the perfusion medium at pH 7.4. It was also found that the concentration of L-tyrosine formed in the perfusate is dependent upon the initial concentration of L-tyrosyl-L-tyrosine (Table 6).

TABLE 6: Concentrations of L-tyrosine formed during the in situ nasal absorption studies with different initial concentrations of L-tyrosyl-L-tyrosine[a].

Time (min)	Concentration of L-tyrosine formed ($\times 10^3$M) (Mean ± S.E.M.)		
	1.18×10^{-3}M	2.22×10^{-3}M	4.89×10^{-3}M
2	----	0.032 ± 0.003	0.036 ± 0.004
15	0.104 ± 0.042	0.110 ± 0.023	0.148 ± 0.029
30	0.197 ± 0.086	0.220 ± 0.055	0.287 ± 0.060
45	0.297 ± 0.122	0.322 ± 0.085	0.444 ± 0.087
60	0.388 ± 0.224	0.412 ± 0.113	0.597 ± 0.109
N[b]	3	3	4

[a] Isotonic phosphate buffer (0.1M, pH 7.4) at 37°C.

[b] Number of rats studied.

Using the material balance of all the species formed, it can be shown that the loss of the dipeptide from the perfusate is mainly due to its hydrolysis to L-tyrosine. For example, for the peptide at an initial concentration of 1.18×10^{-3}M, the concentrations of L-tyrosine and the intact peptide after 15 minutes were determined to be 0.104×10^{-3}M and 1.12×10^{-3}M, respectively. The calculated value for the residual amount of the peptide is equal to $1.18 \times 10^{-3} - [(0.104 \times 10^{-3})/2] = 1.13 \times 10^{-3}$M, which agrees fairly well with the experimentally determined concentration of 1.12×10^{-3}M.

Since the rate of nasal absorption of L-tyrosine was enhanced via formation of its methyl ester, the same rationale was examined in the case of the peptide, L-tyrosyl-L-tyrosine. However, it was found that the more lipophilic derivative, L-tyrosyl-L-tyrosine methyl ester, is also hydrolyzed rapidly to L-tyrosine and its methyl ester.

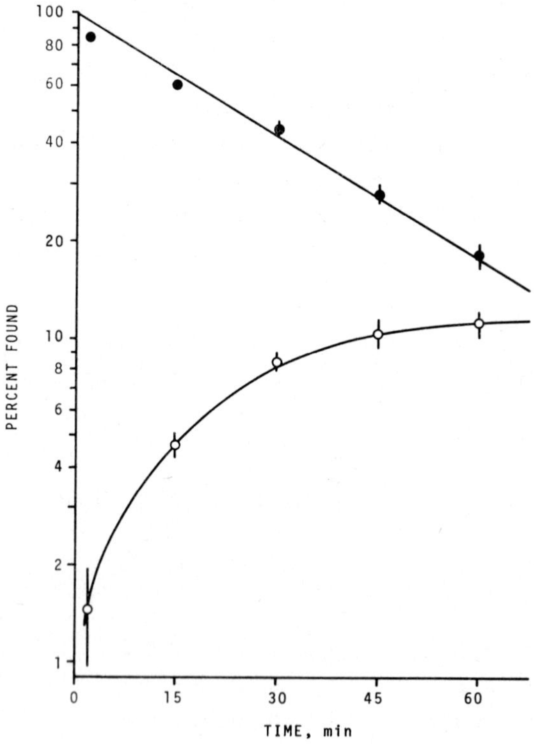

Figure 7: Disappearance of L-glycyl-L-tyrosinamide, and the appearance of L-tyrosinamide in the perfusate (Percent ± S.E.M., n = 3) at pH 7.4 and 37°C.
Key: (•) L-glycyl-L-tyrosinamide; (o) L-tyrosinamide.

In order to further establish that the enzymatic hydrolysis observed during the nasal absorption studies is not necessarily specific for L-tyrosyl-L-tyrosine, the nasal absorption of L-glycyl-L-tyrosine and L-glycyl-L-tyrosinamide was also studied. It was found that the two peptides also cleave enzymatically in the perfusate (Figure 7).

It appears from this study that one reason for the poor bioavailability of peptides is their hydrolysis in the nasal cavity during the absorption process.

REFERENCES

1) The United States Pharmacopeia; 20th rev., U. S. Pharmacopeial Convention, Inc., Rockville, Maryland, (1980), pp. 579-580.
2) Physician's Desk Reference; 37th ed., Medical Economics Company, Inc., Oradell, New Jersey, (1983) pp. 592-593.
3) A. Hussain, S. Hirai and R. Bawarshi; Nasal Absorption of Propranolol in Rats, J. Pharm. Sci., 68 1196 (1979).
4) A. Hussain, S. Hirai and R. Bawarshi; Nasal Absorption of Propranolol from Different Dosage Forms by Rats and Dogs, J. Pharm. Sci., 69 1411-1413 (1980).
5) A. Hussain, T. Foster, S. Hirai, T. Kashihara, R. Batenhorst and M. Jones; Nasal Absorption of Propranolol in Humans, J. Pharm. Sci., 69 1240 (1980).
6) A. Hussain, S. Hirai and R. Bawarshi; Nasal Absorption of Natural Contraceptive Steroids in Rats - Progesterone Absorption, J. Pharm. Sci., 70 466-467 (1981).
7) R. Bawarshi; Ph.D. Thesis, University of Kentucky, Lexington, Kentucky (1981).
8) A. Hussain; College of Pharmacy, University of Kentucky, Lexington, Kentucky, Private Communication.
9) S. Hirai, T. Ikenaga and T. Matsuzawa; Nasal Absorption of Insulin in Dogs, Diabetes, 27 296-299 (1978).
10) S. Hirai, T. Yashiki and H. Mima; Mechanisms for the Enhancement of the Nasal Absorption of Insulin by Surfactants, Int. J. Pharm., 9 173-184 (1981).
11) S. Hirai, T. Yashiki and H. Mima; Effect of Surfactants on the Nasal Absorption of Insulin in Rats, Int. J. Pharm. 9 165-172 (1981).
12) S. Anik, G. McRae, C. Nerenberg, A. Worden, J. Foreman, H. J. Yu, S. Kushinsky, R. Jones and B. Vickery; Nasal Absorption of Nafarelin Acetate, the Decapeptide [D-N_a1(2)^6]LHRH, in Rhesus Monkeys I, J. Pharm. Sci., 73 684-685 (1984).
13) S. Hirai, T. Yashiki, T. Matsuzawa and H. Mima; Absorption of Drugs from the Nasal Mucosa of Rat, Int. J. Pharm., 7 317-325 (1981).
14) H. Nogami and T. Matsuzawa; Absorption and Excretion of Drugs. I. Kinetics of Penetration of an Acidic Drug, Salicylic Acid, through the Intestinal Barrier In Vitro, Chem. Pharm. Bull. (Tokyo), 9 532 (1961) through Chem. Abstract, 4042h (1962).

Transnasal Systemic Medications, edited by Y.W. Chien
Elsevier Science Publishers B.V., Amsterdam, 1985 – Printed in The Netherlands

NASAL DRUG DELIVERY SYSTEMS
REQUIREMENTS, DEVELOPMENT AND EVALUATIONS

K. S. E. SU and K. M. CAMPANALE
Pharmaceutical Research Department
Lilly Research Laboratories
Eli Lilly and Company
Indianapolis, Indiana 46285

ABSTRACT

The physicochemical properties of drugs and additives and other parameters needed for consideration in the development of nasal drug delivery systems are discussed. In this chapter, the use of *in situ* and *in vivo* nasal absorption kinetics, drug deposition in the nasal cavity and tissue distribution after nasal administration will be demonstrated and compared. The application of aerosol technology in the development of nasal drug delivery devices, such as the pressurized aerosol system and mechanical pump system, will be illustrated. All aspects of aerosol formulation, including basic techniques, propellant practice, quality control, and regulations will be outlined. The toxicological and pharmacological effects related to the use of a particular aerosol system as well as the histological study of nasal mucosa and the evaluation procedures will also be reviewed.

INTRODUCTION

The intranasal route of administration is probably one of the most overlooked methods of drug administration for systemic medication. However, in recent years, the possibility of using intranasal administration for the delivery of compounds, which are not bioavailable orally, has received a great deal of attention. For instance, for the orally poorly absorbed drugs, such as sulbenicillin, cefazolin, and other antibiotics, the nasal absorption has yielded a bioavailability which is about 50% of the intramuscular dose (ref. 1). The excellent bioavailability of propranolol when administered by nasal route has been reported in rats, dogs, and humans (ref. 2, 3). Other compounds, such as hydralazine (ref. 4), progesterone (ref. 5, 6), 17β- estradiol (ref. 7), and clofilium tosylate (ref. 8) have also demonstrated a good nasal bioavailability by several investigators.

The nasal absorption of polypeptides, such as oxytocin (ref. 9), synthetic lysine vasopressin (ref. 10), synthetic LH-RH and its analogues (ref. 11-14), insulin (ref. 15, 16), enkephalins analogues (ref. 17), interferon (ref. 18), and growth hormone releasing factor (ref. 19) was also reported.

Other types of compounds, such as hyoscine (ref. 20), nitroglycerin (ref. 21), α_1- and α_2-adrenoceptor agonists (ref. 22), and antiviral enviroxime (ref. 23), had their nasal absorption studied also.

This chapter aims to review and to outline the strategies and options in the design of nasal drug delivery systems. Based on the fundamental knowledge of pharmaceutical sciences and the research results reported in the literature so far, the approaches used in the development of nasal drug delivery systems can be outlined as follows:

I. PHYSICOCHEMICAL PROPERTIES OF DRUGS

Like any dosage form development, the first consideration in the development of a new nasal drug delivery system is to evaluate the physicochemical properties of the drug through preformulation studies. Various physicochemical properties need to be determined, such as the solubility in the commonly used solvents, possibility of polymorphism, sensitivity to possible degradative conditions of pH, heat, light, moisture, oxidants, catalysts, and others. The preformulation data forms the basis for the development of a final formulation with maximum stability and optimum bioavailability. Since a drug is often formulated in either a solution or a solid state, the stability studies can be pursued from the following two approaches.

A. Kinetic Studies on Chemical Stability of Drug at Solution State

The data generated from a short-term accelerated degradation study are very useful, since they provide the advance information on the stability and possible degradation products of the drug investigated. To illustrate this approach, the study on an antirhinovirus compound, enviroxime, is given as an example. Enviroxime is a benzimidazole derivative and has been shown to be a highly specific inhibitor to the multiplication of rhinoviruses in tissue culture (ref. 24). Two isomers have been known to exist, i.e. the anti-oxime isomer (LY122772, enviroxime) and the syn-oxime isomer (LY122771, znviroxime). The antirhinovirus activity of the former is more potent than that of the latter. The scheme for the accelerated degradation of enviroxime is shown in Figure 1.

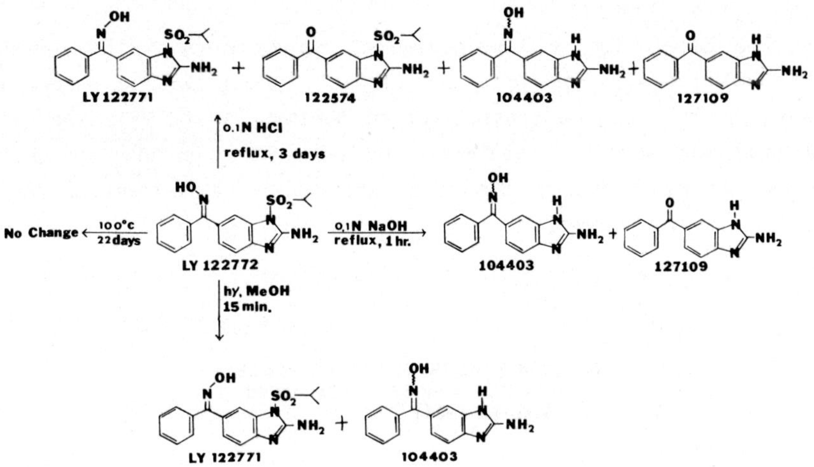

Figure 1: Reaction scheme for the accelerated degradation of enviroxime

Apparently, the compound is quite stable chemically at solid state; however, in solution state, it is sensitive to pH and the major degradation product appears to be the compound LY104403. The results also suggested that the formation of degradation product LY104403 is more favorable under the alkaline conditions. A series of experiments were then initiated to study the formation of LY104403 as a function of moisture, alcohol, temperature, and acid-base catalysis. Based on these data, a stable formulation can be designed for the nasal delivery system.

B. Kinetic Studies on Physical Stability of Drug at Solid State

Physical characteristics, such as polymorphism and particle size distribution, should be considered in the physical stability of a drug at solid state. It will be discussed in more detail later.

II. METHODS FOR ENHANCING NASAL ABSORPTION

To improve the nasal absorption of a drug, the following three methods could be considered:

A. Structure Modification

The chemical modification of a drug molecule, such as the synthesis of analogues, is commonly used to improve the physicochemical properties of the drug and to enhance its nasal absorption. However, it should be aware that the product may be considered as a new chemical entity.

B. Salt or Ester Formation

In some cases, the drug molecule may be modified by the formation of salts or esters. Although in a dry aerosol system, the base form is more preferable due to its low sensitivity to humidity (ref. 25), the salt form of the drug has several advantages, including the improved solubility of a drug, which could enhance the nasal absorption significantly. A typical example is shown in Figure 2.

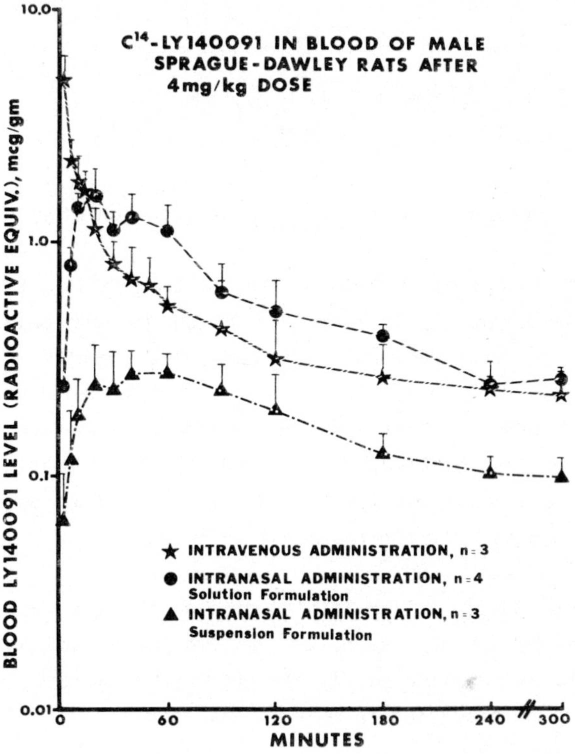

Figure 2: The plasma profiles of C^{14}-LY140091 in Male Sprague-Dawley Rats after intranasal administration of C^{14}-LY140091 as sodium salt (4 mg/Kg) in a solution formulation or as parent drug (4 mg/Kg) in a suspension formulation. The intravenous administration was run for comparison.

The results indicated that the nasal bioavailability of the antiasthma compound, LY140091, is essentially equivalent to that of the intravenous dose when administered as the sodium salt, whereas only about 35% of the intravenous level was achieved when administered as the parent compound (Table 1).

TABLE 1: COMPARISON IN NASAL BIOAVAILABILITY OF COMPOUND ^{14}C-LY140091

Formulation	Route of Administration	No. of Animals	AUC[3] ± S.E.	Bioavailability[4]
Solution[1]	I.V.	3	142.98 ± 45.13	-
Solution[1]	Nasal	4	142.08 ± 42.84	99.4%
Suspension[2]	Nasal	3	50.03 ± 14.71	35.0%

1. LY140091 sodium salt dissolved in saline.
2. LY140091 suspended in saline.
3. mcg min/gm, calculated from 0 to 5 hours
4. calculated from the ratio of $(AUC)_{nasal}$ over $(AUC)_{i.v.}$

C. Formulation Design

Proper manipulation of the excipients in the formulation can also be effective in enhancing the nasal absorption of a drug. It will be illustrated later.

III. SCREENING OF COMPOUNDS AND FORMULATIONS

A. Animal Models

Review of literature has shown that there are two types of animal models which could be utilized for nasal absorption studies.

1. In situ nasal perfusion

Figure 3 shows the experimental set-up for *in-situ* nasal perfusion studies (ref. 1). The surgical procedure is outlined as follows: The rats are anesthetized by i.p. injection of sodium pentobarbital. After an incision is made in the neck, the trachea is cannulated with a polyethylene tube. Another tube is inserted through the esophagus toward the posterior part of the nasal cavity. This second tube serves to introduce the perfusion solution into the nasal cavity. The nasopalatine tract, which connects the nasal cavity to the mouth, is sealed with an adhesive to prevent the drainage of the drug solution from the nasal cavity into the mouth. A funnel is carefully placed between the nose and the reservoir to minimize the loss of solution. Drug solution is placed in the reservoir, which is water jacketed and kept at 37°C. The solution is circulated through the nasal cavity of the rat using a polystaltic pump. The perfusion solution passes out from the nostrils, through the funnel, and into the reservoir again. The drug solution in the reservoir is stirred continously, using a stirring magnet. The extent of drug absorption was determined over a period of time by analyzing, periodically, the drug concentration remaining in the perfusing solution.

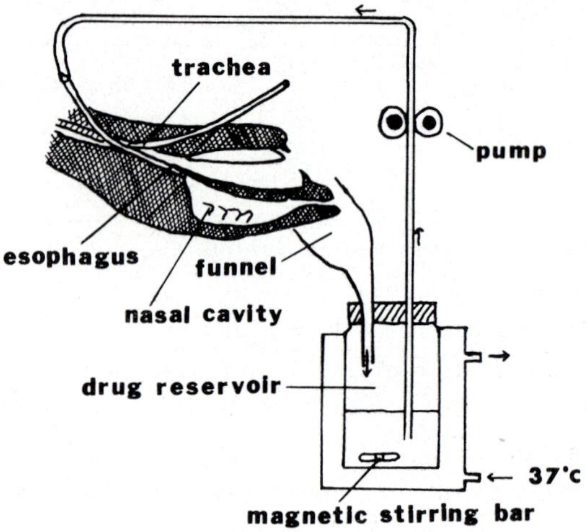

Figure 3: The experimental setup for in situ nasal perfusion studies.

Since the assay of the samples does not involve any biological fluids, such as blood, the analytical procedure for analyzing the drug concentration is relatively simple. However, because of the use of a rather large volume of the solution, the assay sensitivity may be limited, if the nasal absorption is extremely poor. Nevertheless, the in situ perfusion model has the following applications:

a. To screen the nasal absorption potential of a drug candidate.
b. To predict the in vivo rate of nasal absorption.

2. In vivo model

As shown in Figure 4, the surgical procedure for in vivo studies in the rats is similar to that described for the in situ nasal perfusion studies. The drug solution was delivered to the nasal cavity through the esophagus cannulation tubing or the nostril with a syringe. The blood samples were then collected periodically from the femoral vein (ref. 2).

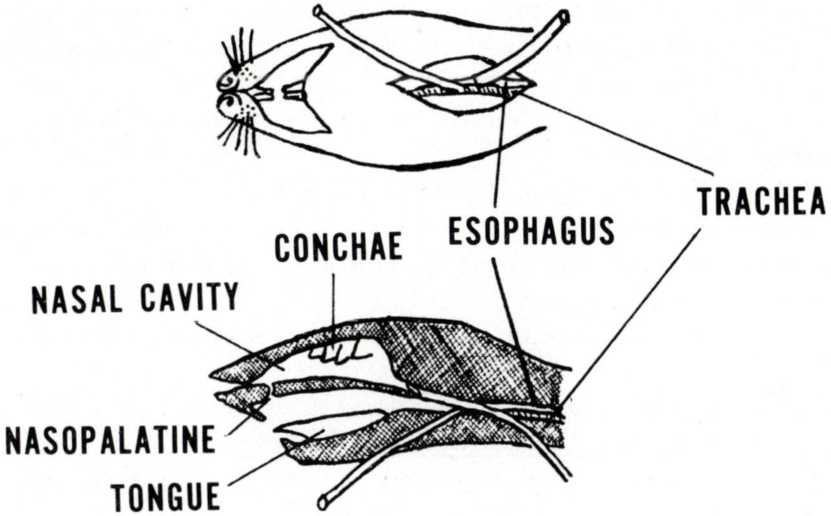

Figure 4: The top and side views of the cannulation arrangement in the rat model.

Since all the possible outlets in the in vivo rat model are blocked after surgical preparation, the only possible passage for the absorption of a drug into the systemic circulation is penetration through the nasal mucosa. It is a well-controlled animal model for screening the nasal absorption potential of drug candidates and can also be utilized for other applications, which will be discussed shortly.

B. Assay Methodology

During the process of screening drugs for possible nasal absorption, development of a sensitive analytical method for assaying the drug and its possible metabolites in the biological fluids is essential. Based on the nature of the drug selected, the methodology can be outlined as follows:

1. For radiolabeled drugs

a. Acid digestion technique

Samples are weighed and then acid digested in 0.2 ml of 70% $HClO_4$ and 0.4 ml of 30% H_2O_2 at 70°C in scintillation vials for one hour. The samples are then cooled down to room temperature and counted after the addition of scintillation fluid.

b. Combustion technique

Samples are weighed and combusted in a Hewlett Packard Tri-Carb model 306 sample oxidizer with a Carbosorb/Permafluor (8:13 v/v) mixture to trap $^{14}CO_2$ and then counted on a Searle Mark III scintillation spectrometer. Urine samples can be analyzed by liquid scintillation counting.

2. For unlabeled drugs

a. High performance liquid chromatography method

After sample extraction, samples are analyzed by HPLC equipped with an ultraviolet, electrochemical, or fluorescent detector.

b. Gas chromatography method

If a drug is volatile, a gas chromatography assay might be preferable.

C. Application of animal model

1. Studies of Nasal Absorption and Tissue Distribution

The utilization of the *in vivo* model for studying the nasal absorption and tissue distribution after the intranasal administration can be illustrated by the studies on clofilium tosylate (ref. 8). Clofilium tosylate is a newly synthesized quaternary ammonium compound (Figure 5) for antiarrhythmia (ref. 26).

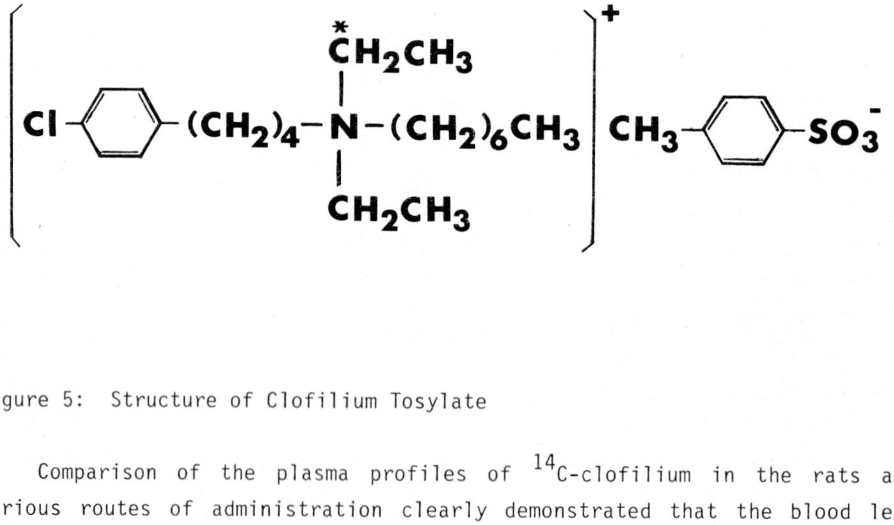

Figure 5: Structure of Clofilium Tosylate

Comparison of the plasma profiles of ^{14}C-clofilium in the rats after various routes of administration clearly demonstrated that the blood levels following oral administration of clofilium is erratic and low. While nasal administration of the drug resulted in a much higher level of radioactivity (Figure 6).

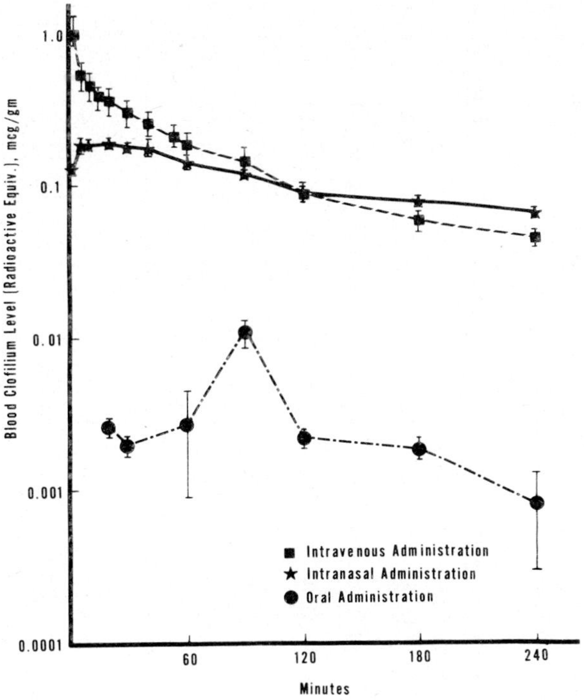

Figure 6: Plasma profiles of the radioactivity in the rats following various routes of administration of ^{14}C-clofilium tosylate [Reproduced with permission of the copyright owner - J. Pharm. Sci.]

At various time intervals after intranasal administration of clofilium tosylate, tissues were dissected, rinsed, blotted, weighted, and analyzed. The distribution kinetics of the radioactivity in the blood circulation showed a great contrast with that from some tissues (Table 2). One hour after intranasal administration, high levels of radioactivity, as compared to that in the blood, were observed in the heart, lung, liver, and kidney tissues. There was a gradual accumulation of the drug in the heart. By 6 hours after intranasal administration, the total radioactivity in the heart was about 18 folds greater than that in the blood. It was reported that the biological response of clofilium tosylate correlates with the levels of radioactivity in the heart (ref. 27). Based on the results of tissue distribution, the blood levels may not be an accurate index of cardiac levels or biological response of clofilium tosylate after nasal absorption.

TABLE 2 - TISSUE DISTRIBUTION OF [^{14}C]CLOFILIUM TOSYLATE IN RATS[1] AFTER INTRANASAL ADMINISTRATION

	Distribution profiles (ng equivalent of ^{14}C/Gm of Tissue)[2]				
Tissue	0.5 Hour[3]	1 Hour	2 Hours	4 Hours	6 Hours
Blood	12.06 ± 1.80	9.30 ± 0.34	14.88 ± 1.44	11.80 ± 1.20	14.40 ± 3.80
Heart	82.12 ± 12.54	88.09 ± 4.10	175.16 ± 23.10	227.80 ± 22.50	263.70 ± 27.00
Lung	58.95 ± 8.42	49.47 ± 4.69	83.88 ± 8.90	97.06 ± 15.20	112.10 ± 15.00
Liver	221.31 ± 29.19	218.24 ± 12.20	328.60 ± 36.30	482.90 ± 39.80	271.90 ± 36.00
Kidney	475.13 ± 87.60	609.42 ± 20.59	944.40 ± 85.50	1116.00 ± 106.80	813.00 ± 110.00

1. Species: Harlan Sprague-Dawley, males, N=3.
2. Each value represents the mean ± S.E.M. of three animals.
3. The time after intranasal administration of 0.3 mg/Kg dose.

2. Studies of drug deposition in the nasal cavity

The *in vivo* model is also useful for studying the drug deposition in the nasal cavity. Using the results from the antirhinovirus compound, enviroxime, as the example, different levels of nasal bioavailability, relative to the I.V. administration, were observed following the intranasal administration of enviroxime in various nasal formulations. Specifically, one of the suspension formulations evaluated in the rats showed the best combination of physical, chemical, and biological characteristics, in terms of wettability, stability, acceptability, and absorption profile. Subsequently, a satisfactory clinical result, in terms of virus shedding, was also reported. It is assumed that the better the nasal absorption, the greater the antirhinovirus activity develops in the nasal epithelia. The results suggested that the *in vivo* model should allow one to determine whether a drug molecule is capable of penetrating the mucosa barrier and reaching the respiratory cells. Therefore, the phenomenon of nasal absorption and the deposition of a drug in the nasal cavity can be indirectly manifested from the data. In summary, the *in vivo* rat model can be utilized for the following purposes:

a. To screen the potential candidate for nasal absorption from a series of drug entities.
b. To evaluate the effect of vehicle and/or formulation on the deposition in the nasal cavity.
c. To generate the information on the tissue distribution of a drug after the intranasal administration.

IV. NASAL DRUG DELIVERY DEVICES

In the exploration of nasal drug delivery devices, the following two systems will be discussed:

- mechanical pump system
- pressurized aerosol system.

Because both systems are capable of delivering drug accurately, they are widely used in the industry and clinics. The selection of either the mechanical pump system or the pressurized aerosol system as the delivery system for the intranasal drug administration entirely depends upon the nature of the product. In general, the mechanical pump system is simpler than the pressurized aerosol system. Once the final formulation has been assured to be stable, chemically and physically, and is compatible with all the components of the delivery device, the use of a pump system should be straightforward. However, the pressurized aerosol system could be more complicated than expected, because of the presence of the propellants in the formulation. Nevertheless, as we discuss the nasal delivery devices, we will review these two system together since they all contain a valve, actuator, and container. We have to constantly remember that, whether utilizing a mechanical pump or an aerosol system, the device operates as a unit. Therefore, the formulation ingredients and packaging components need to be studied all together.

In general, five areas should be included in the consideration of the requirements for a pharmaceutical aerosol and/or pump system.

A. Formulation Aspects

1. If an ingredient to be incorporated in the formulation is required to be dissolved or dispersed, the physicochemical compatibility of the ingredient with the propellant (if a pressurized aerosol system is used), co-solvents and/or dispersing agents will require evaluation.
2. During the course of formulation assessments, it is essential to know that each formula type presents its own specific requirements. If an active ingredient has the problems of solubility and stability in an aqueous system, a non-aqueous solvent system should be considered alternatively. Otherwise, an aqueous system would certainly be the first choice and then its used with a mechanical pump system as a nasal drug delivery device, should be straightforward. Once a specific formulation is decided, three basic systems can be considered, i.e., solution system, suspension system, and emulsion system (ref. 28).

   If a drug is not totally soluble in an acceptable nonaqueous solvent and a small amount of water is required to make it soluble; in such a system, the drug, water, cosolvents and propellants in the formulation must be maintained at balance to achieve the stability required. Otherwise, a phase separation or the precipitation of the active ingredient might occur. Ratio of propellants will also affect the physical stability of an aerosol system, mainly, the phase separation. The vapor pressure of the combination of propellants could also determine the patient's acceptance. The particle size distribution is always an important factor, since it affects the degree and rate of drug absorption by the nasal mucosa. As reported in the literature (ref. 29), with nasal breathing nearly all particles with an aerodynamic size of 5 to 10 microns are deposited in the nose. In general, the extent of nasal deposition increases with the increase in particle size. There are three methods commonly used in the determinations of particle size distribution for aerosol systems, i.e. cascade impactor method, laser light scattering technique, and holography method (ref. 30).

3. When a formulation is finalized, it is essential to evaluate how the product will maintain its stability under the variable conditions of time, temperature and pressure. Accelerated stability testings, in which the final formulation is subjected to the stability evaluations under more extreme conditions, will generate some advance information on the stability of the nasal drug delivery devices developed.

   The stability studies, in addition to assaying the active ingredient, should also include testings for weight loss, delivery rate, tail-off, pressure, pH, and physical examination of any unexpected changes. The studies must be conducted with the formulation in a glass container to permit the observation of any physical changes, if the final package is to be in metal.

   During storage, the adsorption of drug by the plastic components could occur, leading to a reduction in the drug concentration delivered to the patient. An appropriate analytical procedure needs to be developed to assess this possibility.

   Although the aerosol products, like oral dosage forms, need not be sterile, they should be free from any bacterial contamination. A variety of preservatives are available for incorporation into the formulation to minimize any potential growth of microorganisms.

   With regard to the evaluation of the physical stability of aerosol system, the pertinent parameters include polymorphism, crystal growth, phase separation, dispersibility, dose distribution, and the like. Products are subjected to stability testing at the temperatures of -8°C, 4°C, room temperature, and a cycling temperature range from -8°C to 40°C to mimic the shipping conditions. A wrong choice of polymorph can result in some physical instability. Furthermore, the presence of a less stable crystal form may cause the crystal growth at a later stage, which will subsequently affect the aerosol performance. One should keep in mind that since the propellant content in the formulation can vary once the product is in use, the dose distribution from the first dose could be significantly different from the last dose. Therefore, the dose distribution must be fully studied.

B. Valve Requirements

The valve perhaps plays the most important role in any aerosol product. It must mechanically function upon each use and must also repeatedly deliver the drug in the specified quantity. Therefore, the components in the valve have to be compatible with the formulation. Plastic parts used in the valve could be subject to swelling, softening, and cracking; and the metal parts of the valve could also be corroded depending upon the formula involved. Dip tube growth, for instance, is a common problem in the aerosols. Swelling, due to incompatibility with the formula, is also often observed. Therefore, separate testing for each valve part by the total immersion technique should be conducted to detect any incompatibility problems in advance.

The plasticizers and lubricants required in the molding of the plastics may be extracted by various solvents used in the formulation. These materials should not have any adverse effects on the physiological properties of the drug and its efficacy. For example, the pumps and/or the aerosol systems employ at least one rubber gasket which comes in contact with the content of the product. These gaskets almost always contain plasticizers, antioxidants, lubricants, and other substances. Compatibility of these gaskets with the formula must be evaluated. The gaskets fabricated from the rubbers, such as buna and neoprene, are commonly utilized in the aerosol industry because of their acceptable compatibility with most products.

It is well known that no matter how well a valve is designed, variation in the volume dispensed will exist from one valve to another and from one actuation to another even with the same valve. The limits of acceptable variation depends entirely on the formulation to be dispensed and the safety of the medication to be administered. Therefore, a good quality control program should be established.

C. Container Requirements

The type of container to be used is also important, because each type presents different problems. Among all the containers, the most popular one is probably the aluminum container, due to its low cost, light weight, and high strength. Issues, such as plasticizers, antioxidants, corrosion and coating material used in the linings, all require testing and evaluation.

D. Actuator Requirements

Mostly, there is a potential for the buildup of residual material in the actuator during the course of use. The accumulated material can eventually affect the spraying volume in the subsequent usage, which may, in turn, affect the amount of drug dispensed and the efficacy of a product. The residual buildup can be minimized by proper design of an actuator.

E. General Quality Control Requirements

Like other dosage forms, a good quality control procedure for issues, such as methodology of determining active material and other ingredients, statistical control procedure, microbiological test, etc., should be established.

V. DRUG DISTRIBUTION IN NASAL CAVITY

There is no doubt that the drug distribution in the nasal cavity is an important factor for nasal medication. Because the mode of administration will affect the drug distribution in the nose, it will, in turn, determine the efficacy of a medication. Mygind et al demonstrated that a significant difference in the drug distribution in a cast of the human nose was observed following the intranasal drug administration by different drug delivery devices, like drop bottle, plastic bottle nebulizer, automized pump, and metered-dose pressurized aerosol (ref. 31, 32). The results also suggested that for a pressurized aerosol system, dosage should be delivered twice in each nostril, i.e., one puff in the upper direction and one puff in the lower direction, in order to yield a reasonably good distribution of drug (Figures 7 and 8).

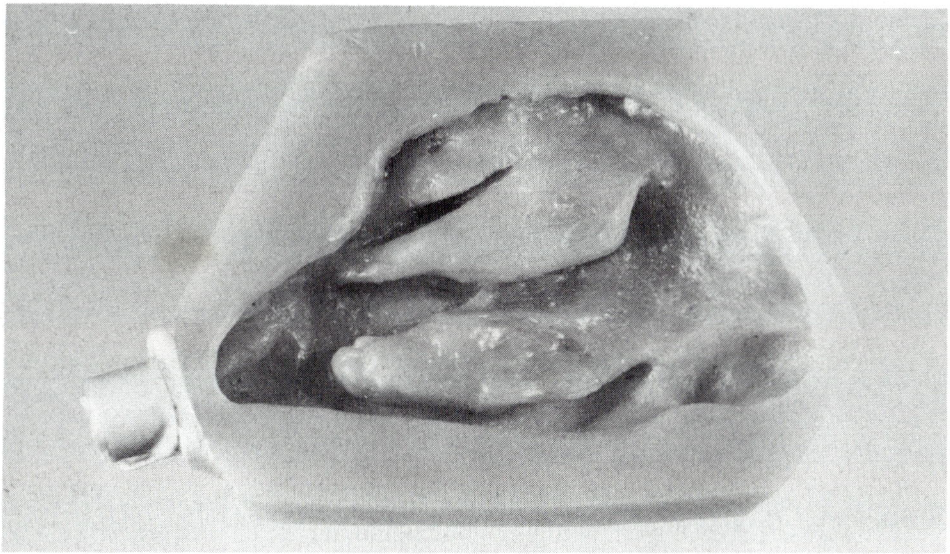

Figure 7: A cast of the artificial human nose.

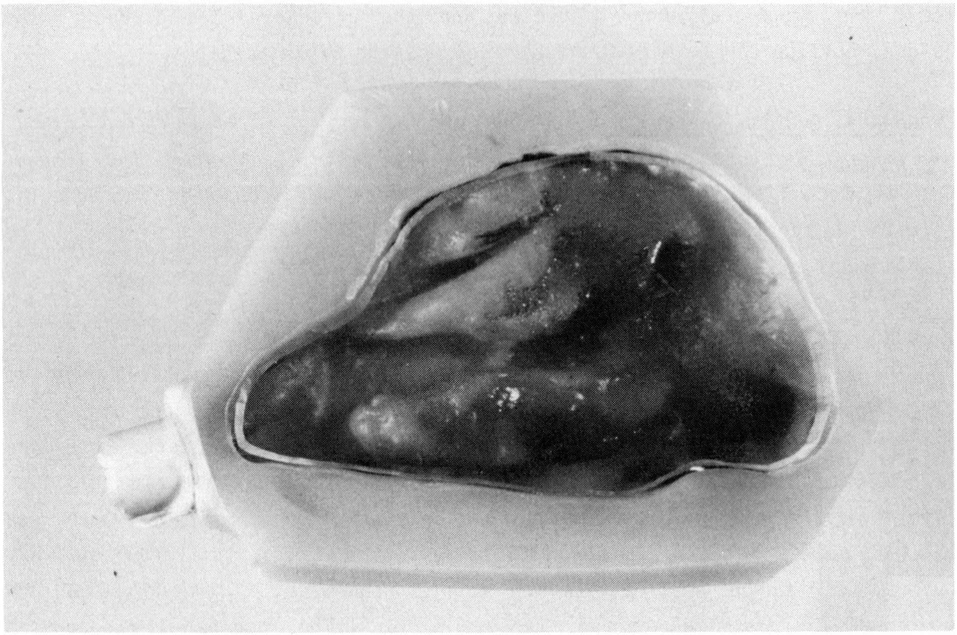

Figure 8: The drug distribution in the artificial human nose after spraying with a metered-dose aerosol

VI. TOXICOLOGICAL AND HISTOLOGICAL ASPECTS

The drug and the final dosage form must be submitted to both acute and chronic toxicity evaluations. Most of the ingredients used in the aerosol formulation are presumably of GRAS substances, i.e., generally regarded as safe, so that no major toxicity issues should be concerned. With regard to the active compound, the acute toxicity is fairly easy to evaluate, since the toxic manifestations show up within a very short period of time. Moreover, the data should be available in time for starting preformulation and designing dosage forms. The chronic toxicity presents a greater problem, because of the long waiting time required for determination of the toxicity under the normal conditions of exposure and use. Nevertheless, like other dosage form products, a 30-day toxicity program on the finished product should be sufficient for the single-dose clinical trials and a 90-day toxicity program for the multiple-dose clinical trials.

The nasal mucosa of the experimental animals needs to be examined histologically to ensure that absorption is not the result of a damage to the absorptive cells in the nasal mucosa. A gross examination of the nasal cavity should be conducted by an E.N.T. specialist during the clinical study.

For the histopathological examination of the rat model, a general procedure has been developed (ref. 33) and is outlined as follows:

1) Preparation of necropsy
2) Decalcification
3) Trimming
4) Processing
5) Embedding
6) Sectioning
7) Staining

Typical lesions observed in the exposed nasal mucosa specimens of rat after an intranasal administration study of clofilium tosylate are shown in Figures 9 - 11.

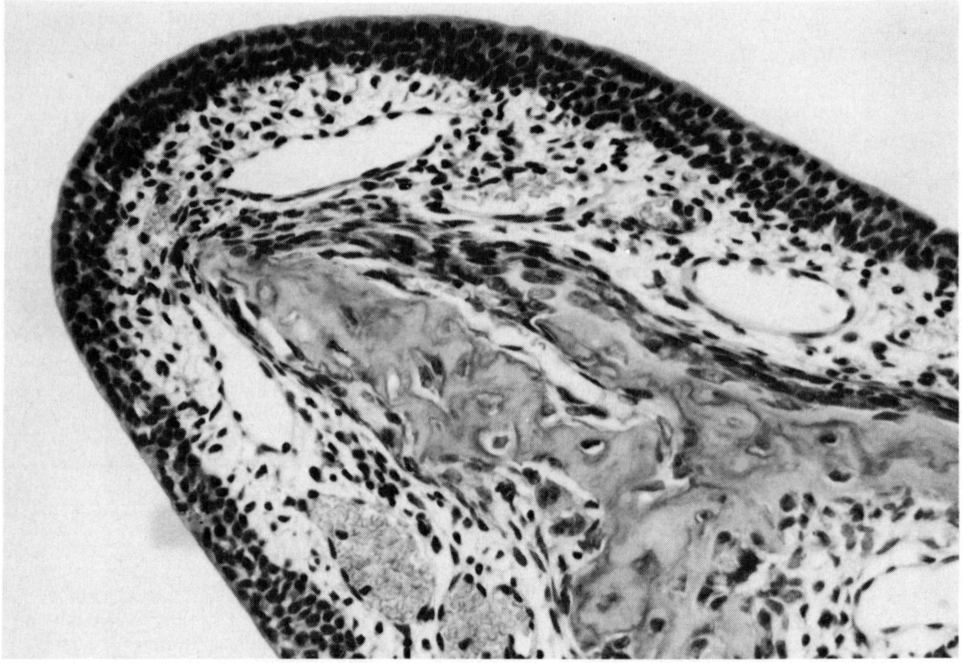

Figure 9: Nasal mucosa of necropsy from the control rat (Reproduced with permission of the copyright owner - J. Pharm. Sci.)

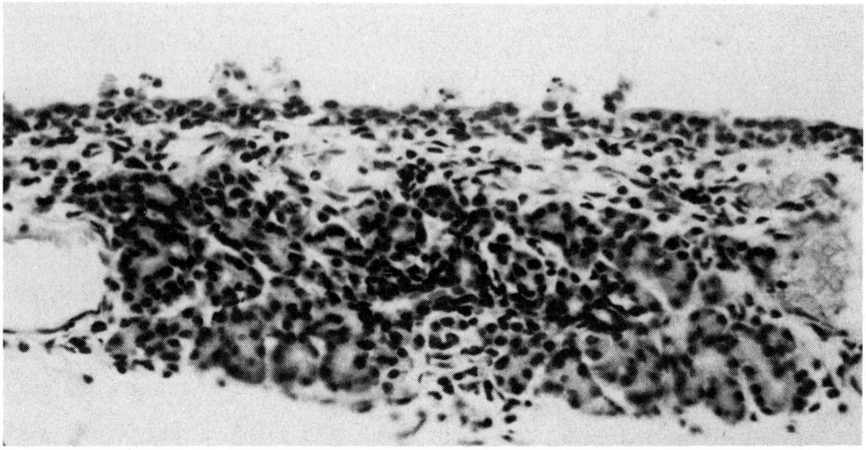

Figure 10: Nasal mucosa of necropsy after the rat was given a 0.6 mg/kg dose. (Reproduced with permission of the copyright owner - J. Pharm. Sci.)

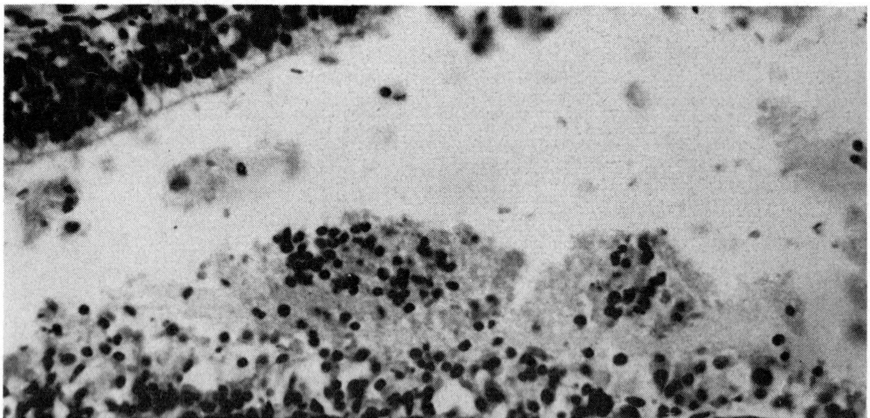

Figure 11: Nasal mucosa of necropsy after the rat was given a 1.2 mg/kg dose. (Reproduced with permission of the copyright owner - J. Pharm. Sci.)

In general, large portions of the mucosa, which was in contact with the higher dose of clofilium tosylate, became necrotic (Figure 11). At the lower dose, only a small fraction of the epithelial cells was necrotic (Figure 10), while large areas of the mucosa were still not affected. The control group, which was exposed to the vehicle, showed no damage of the nasal mucosa.

VII. CONCLUSIONS

In conclusion, we can state that:

1. Preformulation studies need to be conducted to ensure the conditions required for the maximum stability of a drug.
2. Biopharmaceutical studies may shed some light on whether a drug is deposited in the nasal cavity and its possible effect on the nasal mucosa as well as the establishment of nasal absorption profiles.
3. In the development of nasal delivery devices, regardless of whether it is a mechanical pump or a pressurized aerosol, all formulation ingredients and packaging components must be studied and evaluated with respect to one another.
4. The biological compatibility is obviously one of the essential parameters to be evaluated in the clinical trials.
5. The results generated so far on the nasal absorption of drugs suggest that it could be a useful route of systemic administration for many compounds, such as polypeptides, polar compounds, and products produced by genetic engineering.

ACKNOWLEDGMENTS

The authors wish to thank Drs. A. J. Cutie, C. L. Gries, N. Mygind, J. J. Sciarra, and J. J. Tai as well as Pechiney/Valois Corporation for their technical assistance and helpful discussions.

REFERENCES

1) S. Hirai, T. Yashiki, T. Matsuzawa and H. Mima; Absorption of drugs from the nasal mucosa of rat, Int. J. Pharm., 7 317-325 (1981).
2) A. Hussain, S. Hirai and R. Bawarshi; Nasal absorption of propranolol from different dosage forms by rats and dogs, J. Pharm. Sci., 69 1411-1413 (1980).
3) A. Hussain, T. Foster, S. Hirai, T. Kashahara, R. Batenhorst and M. Jones; Nasal absorption of propranolol in humans, J. Pharm. Sci., 69 1240 (1980).
4) Y. Kaneo; Absorption from the nasal mucous membrane, I. Nasal absorption of hydralazine in rats, Acta Pharm. Suec, 20 379-388 (1983).
5) G. F. X. David, C. P. Puri and T. C. Anand Kumar; Bioavailability of progesterone enhanced by intranasal spraying, Experientia, 37 533-534 (1981).
6) A. Hussain, S. Hirai and R. Bawarshi; Nasal absorption of natural contraceptive steroids in rats - progesterone absorption, J. Pharm. Sci., 70 466-467 (1981).

7) L. A. Rigg, B. Milanes, B. Villanueva and S. S. C. Yen; Efficacy of intravaginal and intranasal administration of micronized estradiol-17 , J. Clin. Endocr. Metab., 45 1261-1264 (1977).

8) K. S. E. Su, K. M. Campanale and C. L. Gries; Nasal drug delivery system of a quaternary ammonium compound: clofilium tosylate, J. Pharm. Sci., 73 1251-1254 (1984).

9) E. Talledo, S. F. Adams and F. P. Zuspan; Response of pregnant human uterus to oxytocin given intranasally, J. Am. Med. Assoc., 189 348-350 (1964).

10) A. M. Moses; Synthetic lysine vasopressin nasal spray in the treatment of diabetes insipidus, Clin. Pharmacol. Ther., 5 422-427 (1964).

11) G. Fink, G. Ginnser, P. Liedholm, J. Thorell and J. Mulder; Comparison of plasma levels of luteinizing hormone releasing hormone in men after intravenous or intranasal administration, J. Endocr., 63 351-360 (1974).

12) C. Berquist, S. J. Nillius and L. Wide; Intranasal gonadotropin-releasing hormone agonist as a contraceptive agent, Lancet, II 215-216 (1979).

13) G. Gennser and P. Liedholm; Intranasal administration of luteinizing-hormone releasing factor, Lancet, I 865 (1974).

14) S. T. Anik, G. McRae, C. Nerenberg, A. Worden, J. Foreman, J. Y. Hwang, S. Kushinsky, R. E. Jones, and B. Vickery; Nasal absorption of nafarelin acetate, the decapeptide, [D-Nal $(2)^6$]LHRH, in rhesus monkeys I, J. Pharm. Sci., 73 684-685 (1984).

15) A. C. Moses, G. S. Gordon, M. C. Carey and J. S. Flier; Insulin administered intranasally as an insulin-bile salt aerosol: effectiveness and reproducibility in normal and diabetic subjects, Diabetes, 32 1040-1047 (1983).

16) S. Hirai, T. Yashiki, and H. Mima; Effect of surfactants on the nasal absorption of insulin in rats, Int. J. Pharm., 9 164-172 (1981).

17) K. S. E. Su, K. M. Campanale, L. G. Mendelsohn, G. A. Kerchner and C. L. Gries; Nasal delivery of polypeptides, I: nasal absorption of enkephalins in rats, J. Pharm. Sci., Submitted.

18) S. B. Greenberg, M. W. Harmon, P. E. Johnson, and R. B. Couch; Antiviral activity of intranasally applied human leukocyte inteferon, Antimicrob. Agents and Chemoth., 14 596-600 (1978).

19) W. S. Evans, J. L. C. Borges, D. L. Kaiser, M. L. Vance, R. P. Sellers, R. M. MacLeod, W. Vale, J. Rivier and M. O. Thorner; Intranasal administration of human pancreatic tumor GH-releasing factor-40 stimulates GH release in normal men, J. Clin. Endocr. Metab., 57 1081-1083 (1983).

20) R. W. Hyde, J. Tonndorf and H. I. Chinn; Absorption from nasal mucous membrane, Ann. Otol. Rhinol. Laryngol., 62 957-968 (1953).

21) A. B. Hill; Intranasasl administration of nitroglycerin, Anesth., 51 67 (1979).

22) K. E. Anderson and M. Bende; Adrenoceptors in the control of human nasal mucosal blood flow, Ann. Otol Rhinol. Laryngol., 93 179-182 (1984).

23) K. S. E. Su and K. M. Campanale; Simple animal model for assessing nasal delivery of an antirhinovirus compound, Antiviral Res., in preparation.

24) D. C. DeLong and S. E. Reed; Inhibition of rhinovirus replication in organ culture by a potential antiviral drug, J. Infect. Dis., 141 87-91 (1980).

25) E. Galambos; Formulation Des Formes Pulsees, Therapie Woche., 29 5881 (1979). Cited from the proceeding of Les Formes Pharmaceutiques Pulsees; le 6 mai 1982, pg. 89.

26) M. I. Steinberg and B. B. Molloy; A new antifibrillatory agent that selectively increases cellular refractoriness, Life Sci., 25 1397-1406 (1979).

27) T. D. Lindstrom, P. J. Murphy, J. K. Smallwood, S. A. Wiest, and M. I. Steinberg; Correlation between the disposition of [^{14}C] clofilium and its cardiac electrophysiological effect, J. Pharmacol. Exp. Ther., 221 584-589 (1982).

28) J. J. Sciarra and L. Stoller; The Science and Technology of Aerosol Packaging, Wiley and Sons, Inc., New York, N. Y. (1974), Chapter 13.
29) D. F. Proctor; The upper airways, I. Nasal physiology and defense of the lungs, Amer. Rev. Respir. Dis., 115 97-129 (1977).
30) J. J. Sciarra and L. Stoller; The Science and Technology of Aerosol Packaging, Wiley-Interscience Publication, John Wiley and Sons, Inc., New York, N. Y., (1974), Chapter 19.
31) N. Mygind and S. Vesterhauge; Aerosol distribution in the nose, Rhinol., XI 79-88 (1978).
32) N. Mygind; Nasal Allergy, Blackwell Scientific Publications, Oxford, Great Britain (1979), pp. 257-270.
33) J. T. Young; Histopathologic examination of the rat nasal cavity, Fund. Appl. Toxicol., 1 309-312 (1981).

Transnasal Systemic Medications, edited by Y.W. Chien
Elsevier Science Publishers B.V., Amsterdam, 1985 – Printed in The Netherlands

DEVELOPMENT OF A METERED-DOSE NEBULIZER FOR INTRANASAL PEPTIDE ADMINISTRATION

W. PETRI, R. SCHMIEDEL and J. SANDOW
Hoechst AG, D-6230 Frankfurt 80, Germany F.R.

SUMMARY

Dosage pumps are nowadays supplied by many pharmaceutical manufacturers as part of a finished product pack. The dosage pump, which unlike a metered-dose aerosol, operates by mechanical means and is both a device for dispensing the individual doses by spraying and also as an application aid.

Among the finished products, the largest group of preparations, in terms of numbers, are the nasal preparations. This chapter will discuss the development of a metered-dose nebulizer and its applications for the intranasal administration of three Hoechst/peptide products: LHRH, TRH and buserelin.

During the development of this metered-dose nebulizer, the contribution of (1) spraying process and droplet size, (2) metering accuracy, (3) sterility, and (4) storage stability to the overall performance of the nasal dispensing system was evaluated. It was found that, at the present stage of technical development, the metered-dose nebulizers developed are equivalent to the metered-dose aerosols with regard to metering accuracy. It should be pointed out that a metered-dose nebulizer is not simply part of a primary pack for the pharmaceuticals in question, but, essentially a precision device for equally dispensing the drug formulation in individual spray doses, which must ensure an exact metering over the entire shelf life of the preparation.

INTRODUCTION

Since a few years ago, more and more pharmaceutical products marketed in Europe and in the U. S. have supplied a metered-dose nebulizer as an application aid. The metered-dose nebulizer, also referred to as the dosage pump, is both a general application aid and also a precise metering device.

Unlike a metered-dose aerosol, the nebulizer operates by mechanical actuation. When a patient presses the actuator, a predetermined amount of the formulation is delivered to the oral or nasal cavity. The dose of each respective active ingredient administered depends upon the concentration of the active ingredient in the formulation, and upon the volume of solvent delivered at each actuation. The metering accuracy of the nebulizer thus represents a very important parameter of the finished product, especially when one considers the dosage accuracy over the shelf life of the product.

Some examples of the nebulizers, which have been used in the finished products for dermatologicals, cardiovascular agents, antimycotics, and mouth and throat preparations, are shown in Figure 1.

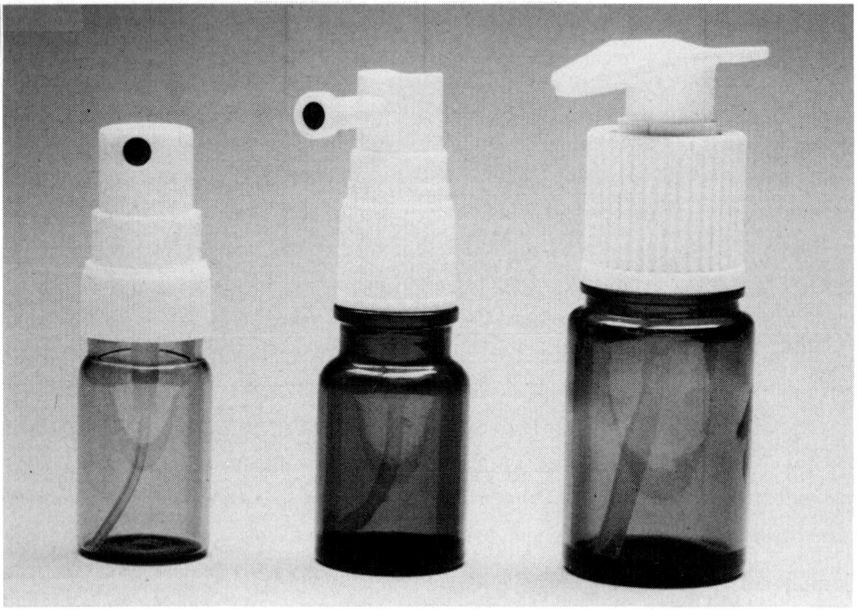

Figure 1: A collection of dispensers for horizontal application of different drug preparations (antimycotics, mouth and throat preparation, dermatologic ointment).

It is practical to classify the nebulizers into two groups:

1. The typical nebulizer that releases a cohesive quantity of pharmaceutical agent (e.g. cream, lotion).
2. The metered-dose nebulizer that delivers a specified dose of pharmaceutical solution. During delivery, the solution is dispersed into fine mist.

Among those pharmaceutical products that use a mechanical metering device, the nasal preparations are the largest group. Figure 2 shows a selection of metered-dose nebulizers used for nasal application.

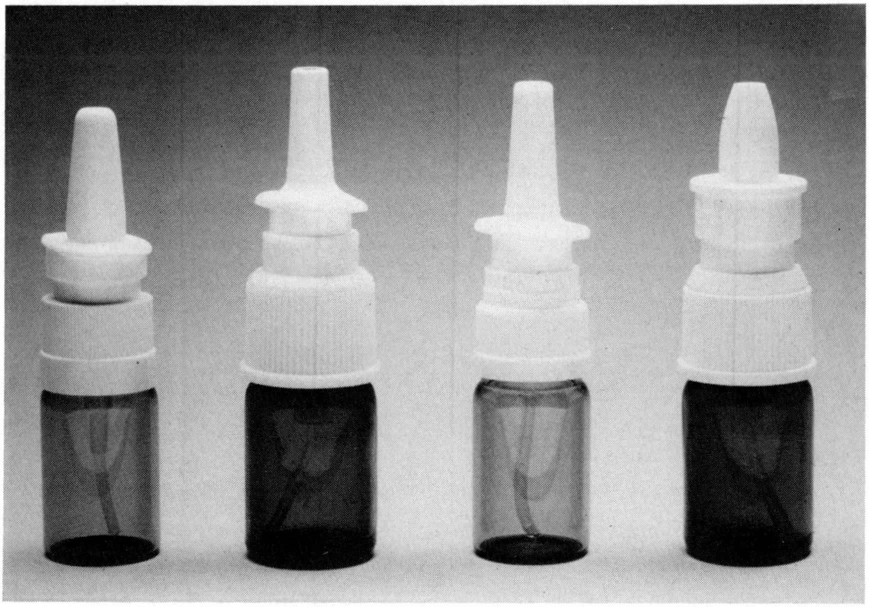

Figure 2: A collection of metered-dose nebulizers for the vertical application of drug solutions into the nose.

EXPERIMENTAL

In this investigation, the metered-dose nebulizers, designed and fabricated for nasal application by six European firms were evaluated. They were obtained directly from the manufacturers or by purchasing the finished product on the market.

A) Initial Evaluations of metered-dose nebulizers

1) Experimental products - The bottles of the metered-dose nebulizers to be tested were filled with a 1% aqueous benzyl alcohol solution. For the purpose of filling the dosage compartment prior to the commencement of actual testing, each metered-dose nebulizer was primed 5-10 times until the emergence of a uniform spray mist that is clearly visible to the eye. Testing then commenced. The quantity of solvent dispensed during each spray application was determined by reweighing the nebulizer by SARTORIUS model 2022 balance (which is connected to a data storage unit with computer and plotter). On the first day of the testing, 20 spray applications were removed from each metered-dose nebulizer, which was individually weighed to determine the quantity dispensed and to

evaluate the reproducibility. Ten consecutive spray doses were weighed on the 2nd day, in order to assess the change in the spraying rate and the reproducibility. Such variations could be caused, for example, by the swelling or shrinkage of different polymer parts used in the pump during a repeated use. A further test was conducted on the 5th day - again weighing was done following 10-spray applications, which were evaluated to assess whether the pumps were leak-tight or not. For each metered-dose nebulizer, 40 values were obtained and used in the analysis of the intra- and inter-individual frequency distributions.

2) Commercial products - The following commercial pharmaceutical products on the German market, which also utilize the metered-dose nebulizers for drug administration, were also evaluated: Extracort^{TM}, a corticoid preparation; Rhinospray^{TM}, a nasal decongestant; and Syntaris^{TM}, another corticoid spray. Tests were done in triplicate, using the finished products in three original packs from the same production batch.

B) Metered-dose nebulizers for intranasal peptide administration

1) Sterilization by Gamma-irradiation

During the development of metered-dose nebulizers, the feasibility of using gamma-irradiation, as a method of sterilization for the empty nebulizer before the filling of peptide solution, was evaluated.

Samples of the empty metered-dose nebulizers were irradiated at 20°C with a total dose of 0.5, 1.0, 1.5 or 2.0 Mrad, using a Cobalt-60 source with a rate of irradiation at 2×10^4 rad/h.

2) Development and evaluation

The metered-dose nebulizers, which were either an experimental or a commercial product, were filled with a nasal solution containing either the luteinizing hormone-releasing hormone (LHRH), thyrotropin-releasing hormone (TRH), or an LHRH agonist analog (named as buserelin). The development work on these three nasal solutions was facilitated by the excellent aqueous solubility of these three peptides and their adequate stability in the buffered solution. The question, which was proved to be problematic and required a great deal of work, was found to be the accuracy of dispensing of the nasal solutions. Dosage application by pipetting technique, such as the one which is normally used with the nose drops, was ruled out, because of the inexactness of the dosage dispensed.

As the first attempt for a technical solution of the problem, a metered-dose aerosol, using nitrogen as the propellant, was developed for the clinical testing of nasal LHRH solution. It soon became evident that a system of this type is not only subject to a relatively wide variation in individual dosage, ranging from up to 50% in most cases to 100% in some extreme cases, but that it also shows a frequent tendency to leak. An accurate dispensing of the solution was thus not possible.

In order to eliminate the leakage problem, the prototype of a spray system, which does not use compressed nitrogen, was developed. Using the commercial perfume spray as the model, a vertical spray head, by precision engineering, was fitted in place of a horizontal nebulizer. This prototype of metered-dose nebulizer is shown in Figure 3.

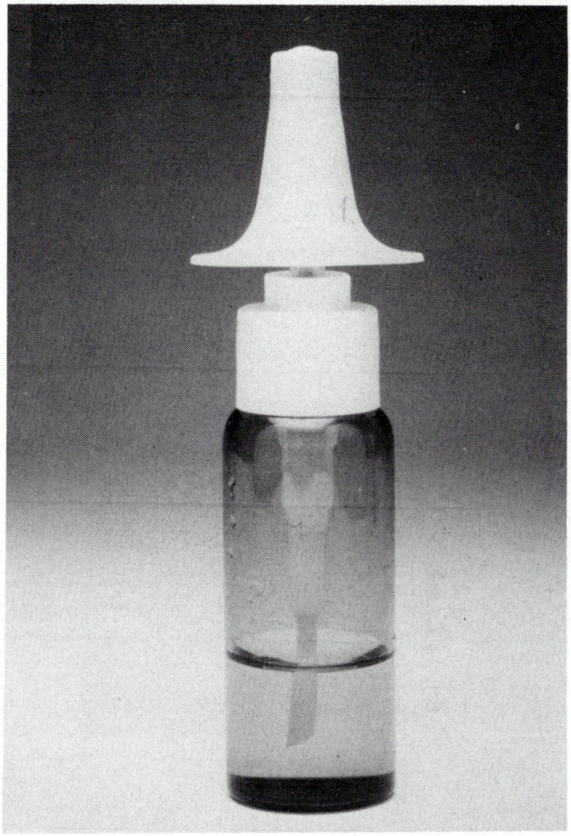

Figure 3: The first prototype of a metered-dose nebulizer developed at Hoechst AG for the nasal application of peptides.

This metered-dose nebulizer was used on a fairly wide scope during the initial clinical trials. However, this nebulizer had an inherent weakness in its design; a severe friction of the internal moving parts occurred, when tilted against one another during the spraying. As reported by the clinic investigators, this weakness led to an inexactness in the dosage delivered. This prototype was, therefore, quickly abandoned and we designed another improved version of the metered-dose nebulizer (Figure 4), which has a great improvement in the reliability over the first prototype.

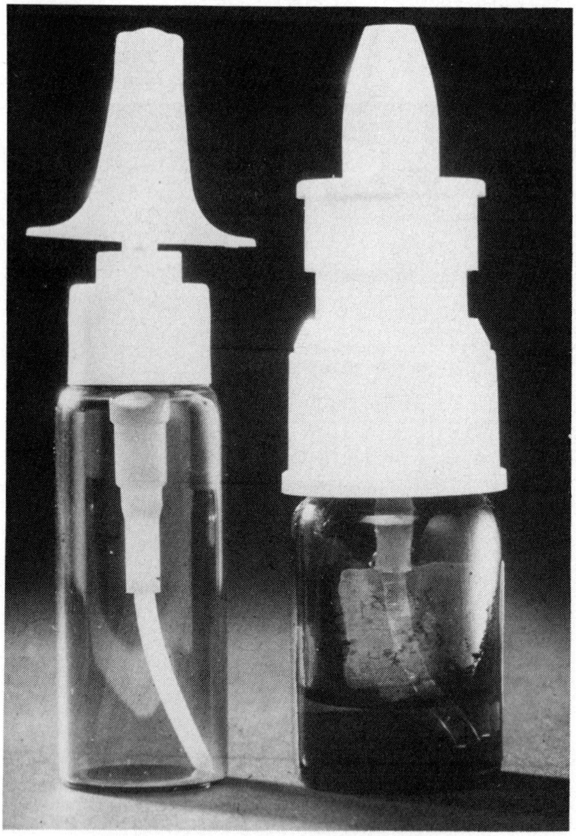

Figure 4: Comparison of an improved metered-dose nebulizer (prototype No. 2, shown on the right), with prototype No. 1 nebulizer. This device was manufactured by precision engineering according to stringent criteria of performance.

This device was engineered on the basis of the following requirements, which are considered to be the essential features of a reliable metered-dose nebulizer:

a) Elimination of tilting

The cross-section of the nebulizer developed for the nasal administration of peptides is illustrated in Figure 5. The fitting surface between the nasal applicator and the pump element has been engineered to make it virtually impossible for these two parts to be tilted against one another.

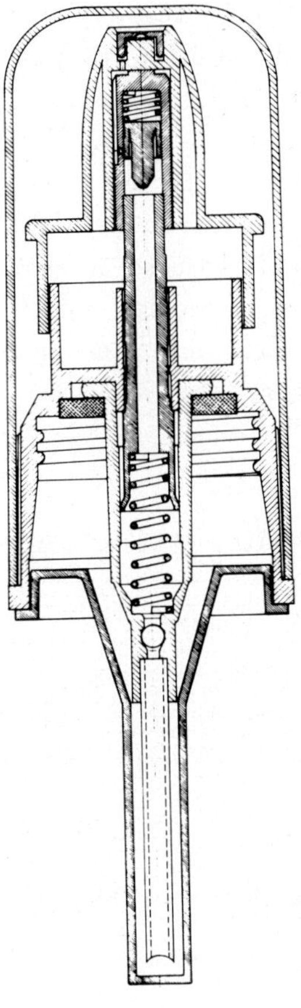

Figure 5: Diagrammatic illustration of the cross-section of the metered-dose nebulizer developed for the intranasal administration of peptides. The device is covered by a protective cap, which has to be removed before each use. The spray head and the nose olive have a close manufacturing tolerance to prevent any tilting during the down-stroke, which opens the spray valve.

b) Protection against microbial contamination

In this design, a spring is installed in the upper part of the nasal applicator, to which a seal is connected; the contents in the pump and in the bottle are thus protected from any outside contamination.

c) Spraying process and droplet size

Using the short-time exposure technique, various stages of the spraying process can be photographed. In the initial stage, a small amount of solution is dispensed in a mushroom-like shape. The "cap" of the mushroom soon breaks off in the form of fairly large droplets and whose "stem" widens out into the shape of a funnel (at 5 ms after the actuation). Fine particles are continuously sheared off from the edge of this funnel during the actual spraying process (at 50 ms after the actuation). After 83 ms, the spraying process is virtually complete. Analysis of the data shows that 90% of the particles have a diameter of close to 50 µm. The large particle diameter obtained with the metered-dose nebulizer, which is clearly different from the small droplets released by a metered-dose aerosol, will prevent the entry of the active ingredient into the bronchial system and lungs (Figure 6). The large particle diameter is favorable for nasal absorption, but not effective by inhalation as shown by the results in the chapter by Sandow and Petri.

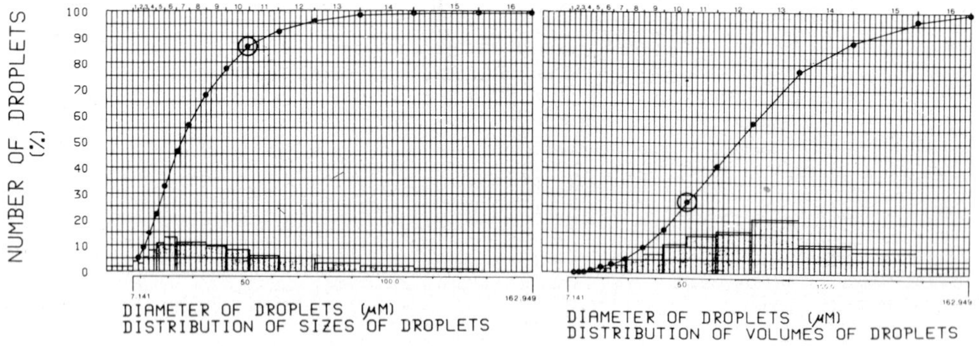

Figure 6: Distribution of the size and the volume of droplets released from the Hoechst metered-dose nebulizer at the time of peak flow from the spray head.

Only the fine particles with a diameter of equal or less than 3 µm will have the chance to enter the lung. The level of these fine particles dispensed from the metered-dose nebulizer was found to be negligible (only 0.014% by the spray weight). This result agrees fairly well with the studies by Fels and Gay (ref. 1) on a mechanically operating "microdose spray". The researchers reported that the probability of occurrence for the droplets with a diameter of less than 5 µm is only 0.12%.

d) Adsorption of active substance on pump components

Individual parts of the pump were incubated for several days with the ^{125}I-labeled active ingredients, or unlabelled peptides, and the extent of adsorption was determined by RIA or by counting of radioactivity. No evidence on the adsorption of the active substance could be established by either methods. When the peptide content in the individual spray doses dispensed after prolonged periods of storage was analyzed by RIA. For pumps with dosage compartments, which had been filled with peptides and left standing at room temperature, no indication of any adsorption of the peptides to the pump surface was obtained.

e) Metering accuracy

The metering accuracy is ensured by the precision engineering of the main section of the dosage compartment, which extends from the ball valve to the seal and from there to the nozzle orifice (Figure 5). The geometrical dimension of various parts of the pump in this area is obviously responsible for the dispensing of a specific quantity of solution for every stroke of the plunger. The dimension and the tolerance of these parts are meticulously controlled during the production of the metered-dose nebulizers.

The spray-to-spray reproducibility of the metered-dose nebulizer is illustrated in Figure 7.

The result confirmed that, beyond the initial priming, the volume of each spray dispensed is highly reproducible; and also showed that the quantity of the solution metered is not dependent upon the amount of solvent remaining in the dosage compartment after different times of application. An exact dosage is obtained at any time. In these two aspects, the metered-dose nebulizer has the advantages over the metered-dose aerosols, i.e., the pressurized products on the market. For comparison, the spraying behavior of a cardiovascular agent, e.g., nitroglycerin, from a metered-dose aerosol was investigated (Figure 8). Apparently, the dosage dispensed by the metered-dose aerosol is dependent upon the volume level of the aerosol remaining in the pressure pack. It was also noticed that the dosage fluctuates greatly once the level of the product in the aerosol container has fallen below a critical mark of 25% of the original volume.

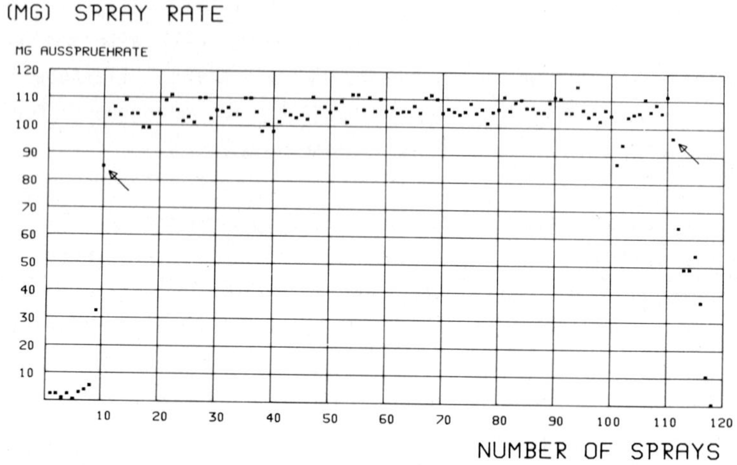

Figure 7: Performance of the metered-dose nebulizer (prototype No. 2) and its spray-to-spray reproducibility, from initial priming (the first 10 spray strokes) until the exhaustion of the peptide solution in the nebulizer.

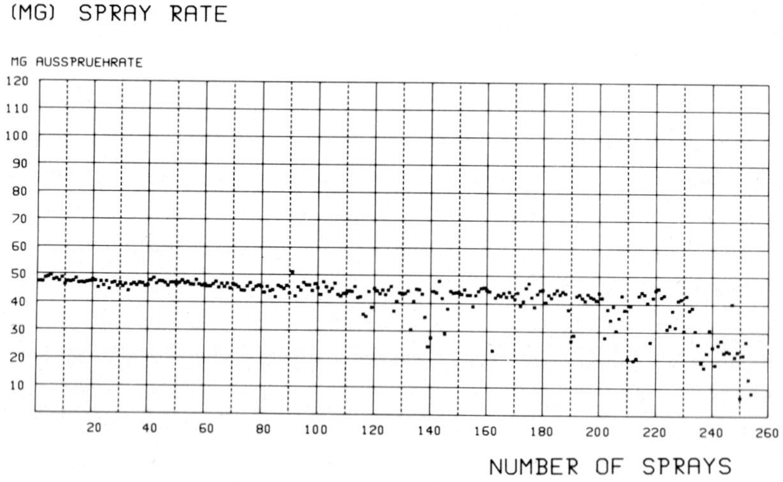

Figure 8: The spray performance of a metered-dose aerosol, which dispenses a cardiovascular preparation containing nitroglycerin, and spray-to-spray reproducibility during a sequential dispensing of 260 spray doses. The performance of this metered-dose aerosol is decreasing with time.

Even though the results suggested that the metered-dose nebulizer, in principle, has a metering accuracy which is slightly superior than the metered-dose aerosol, one should conclude that both systems are equal in their overall performance. The specifications for the testing of a metered-dose aerosol outlined in USP XX and BPC 1973 can also be applied to the metered-dose nebulizers.

f) Pump-to-pump metering accuracy

Because of the dimensional tolerance of the individual plastic parts contained in the metered-dose nebulizer, the spray rate varies somewhat from one pump to another in any given batch. When a group of pumps are tested, a Gaussian-type frequency distribution of the spraying rates is obtained. A typical study is shown in Figure 9, in which 20 metered-dose nebulizers were randomly selected from a batch in accordance with a pre-determined test schedule (see Experimental section A-1) and the total weight lost in each nebulizer after 40 single sprays was determined gravimetrically by reweighing.

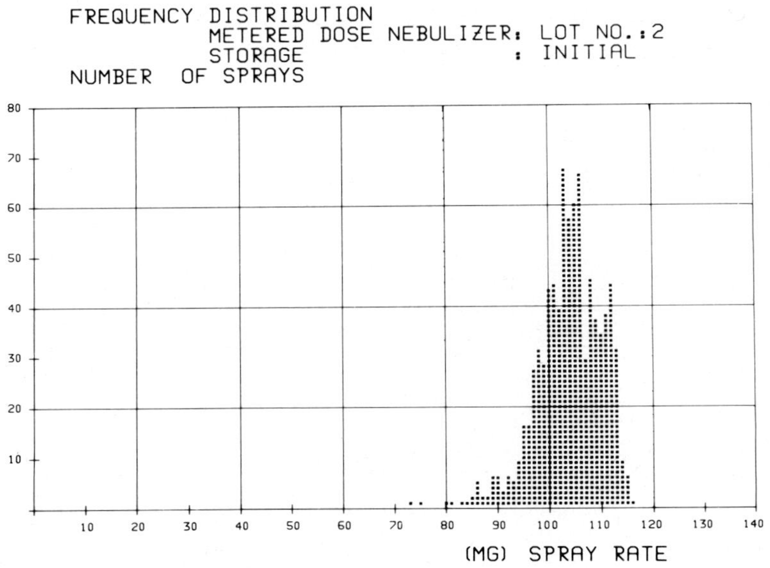

Figure 9: Frequency distribution for a group of 20 metered-dose nebulizers (prototype No. 2). For each pump, the total weight lost following 40 single spray strokes was determined by weighing.

In Figure 9, the individual spray rates for each of the 20 nebulizers were determined following 40 spray strokes, as compared to the results by Yu et al. who reported only the mean values of 8 spray applications per day (ref 2). The pump-to-pump metering accuracy obtained in our measurements agree with data by Fries and Jekle (ref. 3).

g) Sterility

One suitable process for sterilizing the pumps before filling is Gamma-radiation treatment. On the other hand, ethylene oxide is not suitable, because even a small amount of residue could inactivate the peptide in the nebulizer. Pumps are manufactured under the guidelines of strict production hygiene. Random tests for sterility were carried out on more than twenty production batches and the results in each case indicated that the assembled pumps are sterile.

h) Storage Stability

The metering accuracy of three metered-dose nebulizers of different constructions used in the commercial nasal spraying pharmaceutical products in Europe was evaluated. The first type of nebulizer, which is used to deliver a corticoid preparation, yielded a relatively narrow frequency distribution of all 120 spray aliquots dispensed (Figure 10).

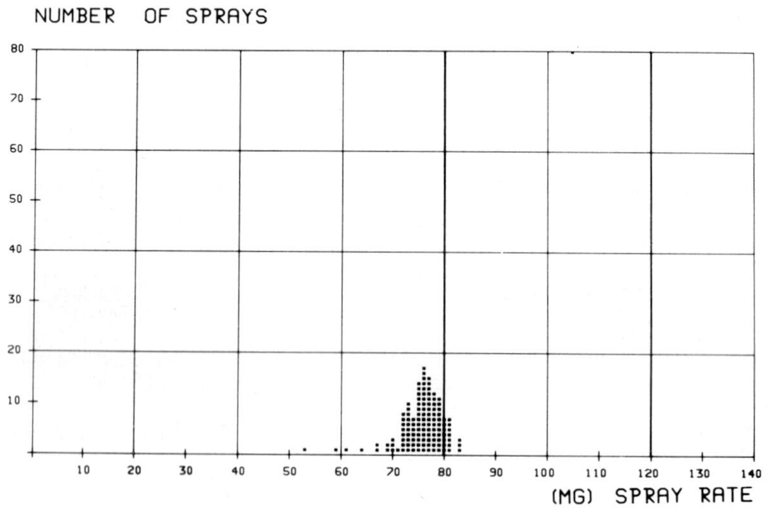

Figure 10: Frequency distribution of a nasal preparation dispensed from a commercial metered-dose nebulizer (Type I).

The second type of nebulizer, which is used to delivery a nasal decongestant, revealed an extremely compact frequency distribution and some signs of breaking up in the frequency pattern with a clear shift towards a smaller spray volume. The lowest value obtained was 0 mg solution, which suggests a complete pump failure in at least one stroke (Figure 11).

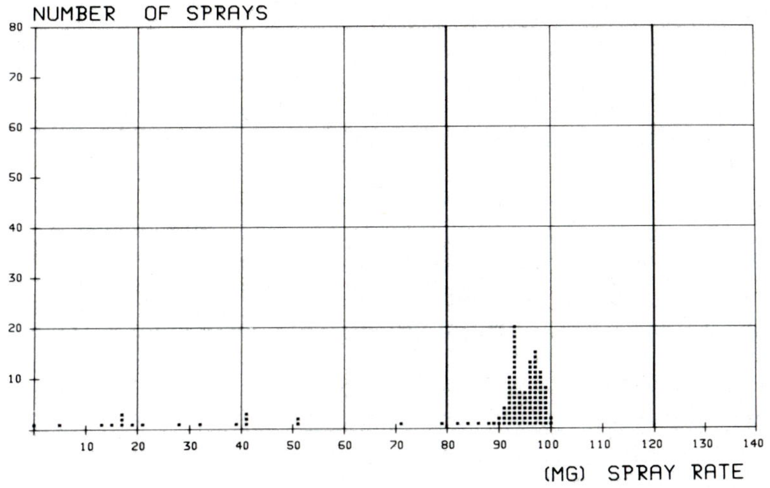

Figure 11: Frequency distribution of a nasal preparation dispensed from a commercial metered-dose nebulizer (Type II). During sequential dispensing, this pump sometimes releases an insufficient volume.

The third type of nebulizer, which is used to deliver another corticoid preparation, exhibited a totally inadequate frequency distribution of the spray aliquots dispensed. A nominal dispensing volume of about 100 mg (or 100 µl) of solution per spray aliquot was obtained with a range between 0 mg and 103 mg (Figure 12).

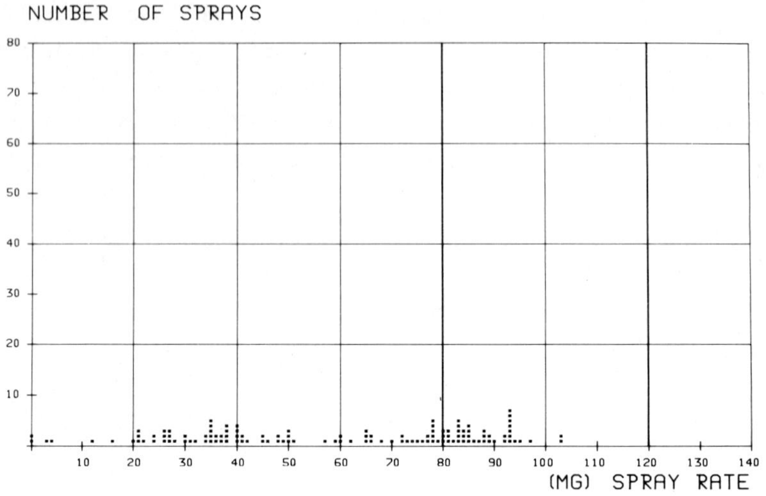

Figure 12: Frequency distribution of a nasal preparation dispensed from a commercial metered-dose nebulizer (Type III). A wide range of spray volumes was obtained during the sequential dispensing.

Storage stability of Hoechst metered-dose nebulizers

It can safely be assumed that for pharmaceutical manufacturers who wish to administer a nasal formulation by means of a metered-dose nebulizer, the decision as to which pump should be used is not the one that can be taken rashly. The particular pump model best suited for the product which has to be dispensed in a precisely predetermined volume and nebulized to the specifications for oral, nasal or bronchial administration is determined in accord with some established internal test criteria. As a rule, these tests have to be carried out within a short time period following the receipt of a prototype pump. Under this condition, a factor that will often be disregarded is the stability of the plastic components in the nebulizer after storage. In the hands of a patient the metered-dose nebulizer and the pharmaceutical solution form a single entity. The metered-dose nebulizer could be stored for an extended period of time before the filling, but once filled and assembled the nebulizer must have a storage stability at least matching that of the pharmaceutical solution to be sprayed. This means that during the storage, even at an elevated temperature, the metered-dose nebulizer must not lose its original metering accuracy, or, if so, only within a narrow allowable range.

It should be pointed out that each metered-dose nebulizer is assembled by fitting together a multitude of individual plastic parts, several of them are made of different polymeric materials. It is not only the size of the dosage compartment that determines the amount of solution applied at each spray; all the individual parts in the pump contribute to the absolute dosage quantity and to the metering accuracy. For instance, the influence of the coil spring could be considerable, though it is simply a component which returns the system to its original position after each dose application (Figure 13).

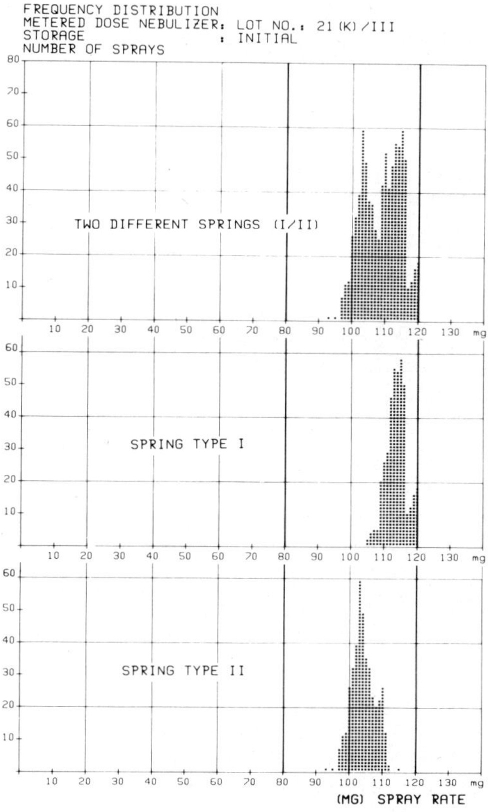

Figure 13: The effect of some technical modifications in the type of coil springs on the spray performance of the Hoechst metered-dose nebulizer. Two different types of coil springs (I and II) were tested for comparison.

Even the coil springs with the same tension, but with a small change in the number of turns, which may already affect the absolute dosage amount per stroke. It is indicated by a widely-dispersed frequency distribution.

The system tested (Figure 13) contained a liquid formulation, which was sprayed under a considerable pressure (up to 5 atm). The leak-tightness of this system was achieved by using a "press fit", or undercuts, and a sealing around the plastics parts. It is possible that in the operational temperature range and, especially under the mechanical stress, some interchange of the molecules and, hence, some dimensional changes in the plastic parts may occur.

The initial spray rates for one of the Hoechst metered-dose nebulizers were compared with the spray rates from the same pump stored at room temperature for six months in Figure 14. The results clearly indicated that the spraying behavior has remained the same after storage under these conditions.

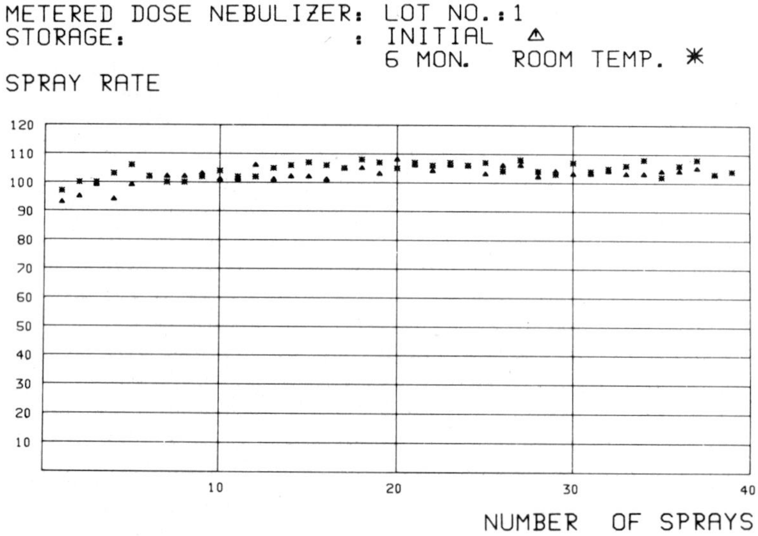

Figure 14: Performance of the metered-dose nebulizer during initial testing and after 6 months of storage at room temperature.

After assembly and filling with LHRH, TRH or buserelin, the Hoechst metered-dose nebulizers were subjected to an intensive stability testing program under various elevated temperature conditions and their performance was found to be satisfactory. Other types of metered-dose nebulizers, which were currently on the market, were observed to exhibit a different thermal stability behavior. One type of the metered-dose nebulizer (by manufacturer

A) lost its initial accuracy, after storage at 40°C for 3 months, but no major change occurred at room temperature for 5 months (Figure 15).

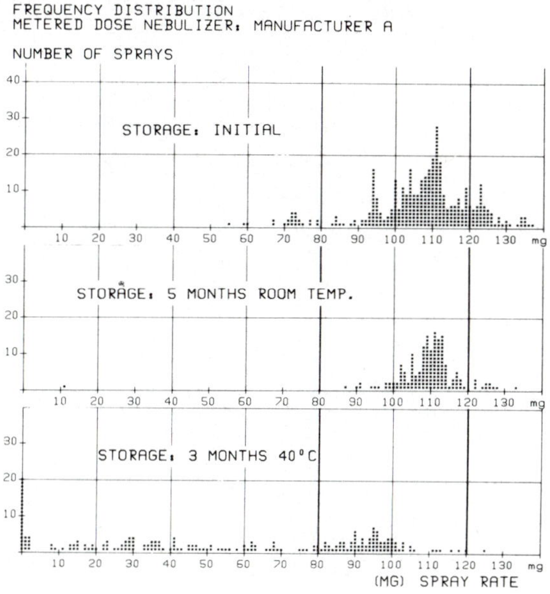

Figure 15: Stability of a commercially available metered-dose nebulizer by manufacturer A, after extended storage at elevated and room temperatures. The performance was substantially reduced after storage at 40°C for 3 months.

Under the same storage conditions, another type of nebulizer, by manufacturer B, has lost its performance at both elevated and room temperatures as demonstrated by the shift of the frequency distribution in the direction of smaller spray volumes (Figure 16).

The frequency distribution for the nebulizer by manufacturer C has become widened and shifted to a smaller spray volume after stored at room temperature for 12 months. At 40°C, the nebulizer has become unusable after 6 months (Figure 17).

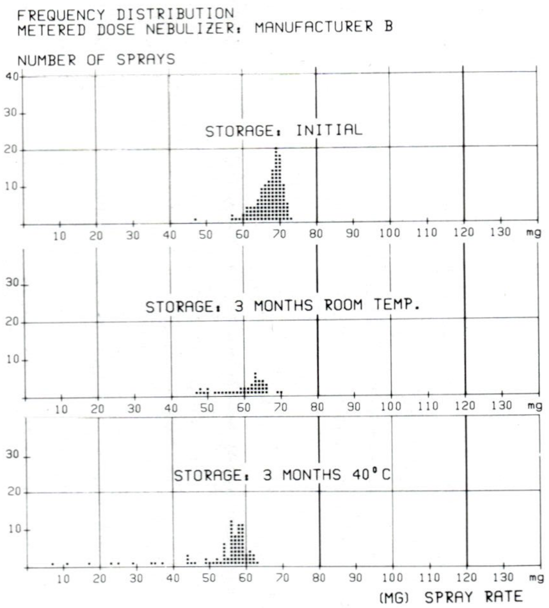

Figure 16: Stabililty of another type of metered-dose nebulizer, the loss of performance was also noted after stored for 3 months at +40°C.

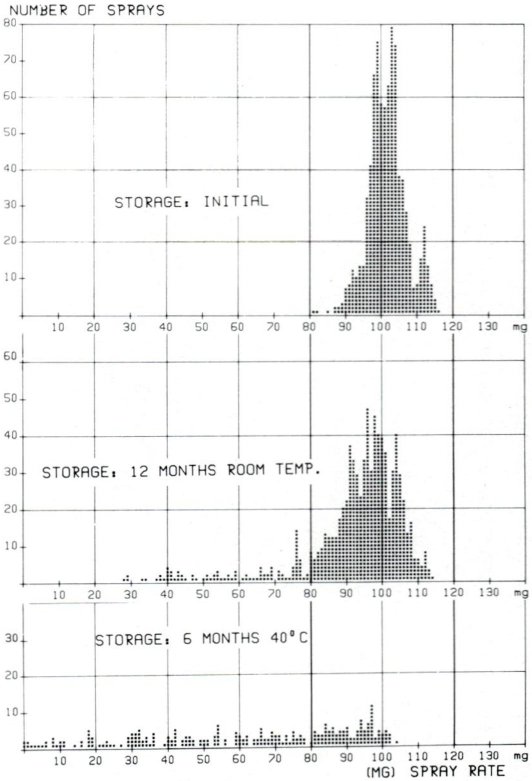

Figure 17: Stability of a third commercially available metered-dose nebulizer. This device became totally unusable after stored at 30°C for 6 months.

On the other hand, the Hoechst nebulizer (ref. 4) showed a rather satisfactory stability behavior even after stored for 20 months at room termperature (Figure 18) and at 30°C (Figure 19). The performance was still acceptable after 8 months at 40°C.

Apparently, the prolonged exposure to the elevated temperatures of 30°C and 40°C has no adverse effect on the spraying performance of the Hoechst nebulizers (Figure 19).

All the data generated so far have demonstrated that this dosage pump is acceptable as a practical application aid and also fulfills the stringent criteria for the intranasal administration of peptides (ref. 5), as a metering device, over the shelf life of the peptides, e.g. TRH, LHRH and LHRH agonist, like buserelin. On the other hand, several types of metered-dose nebulizers, which are currently on the market, exhibit a wide and unpredictable difference in their storage stability and also in their metering accuracy, which are dependent upon storage conditions and duration of storage.

The test results lead to the conclusion that at the present stage of technical development, it is possible to produce a metered-dose nebulizer with a metering accuracy at least equivalent to that of the metered-dose aerosol. The metered-dose nebulizers are the devices which dispense a pharmaceutical by dividing its solution formulation into precisely reproducible aliquots or individual spray doses. Therefore, they must have exactly the same performance over the entire shelf life of the preparation.

ACKNOWLEDGMENT

The authors would like to acknowledge the collaboration and contributions of E. Ebel, W. De Felice, M. von der Ohe, H. Adenauer, W. Zott, J. Klamann and H. Drager for the photomicroscopic analysis of the size and the distribution of droplets, and the assistance of P. Bischoff in the preparation of this manuscript.

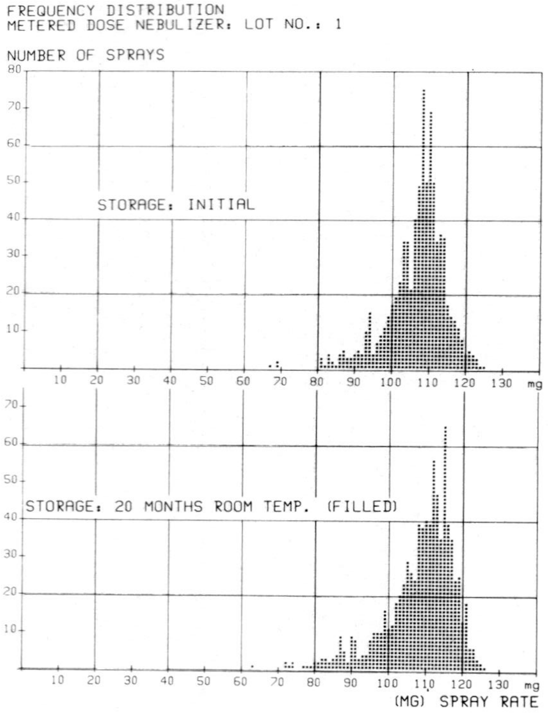

Figure 18: The performance of the Hoechst's metered-dose nebulizer, which contains peptide preparations, after stored for 20 months at room temperature.

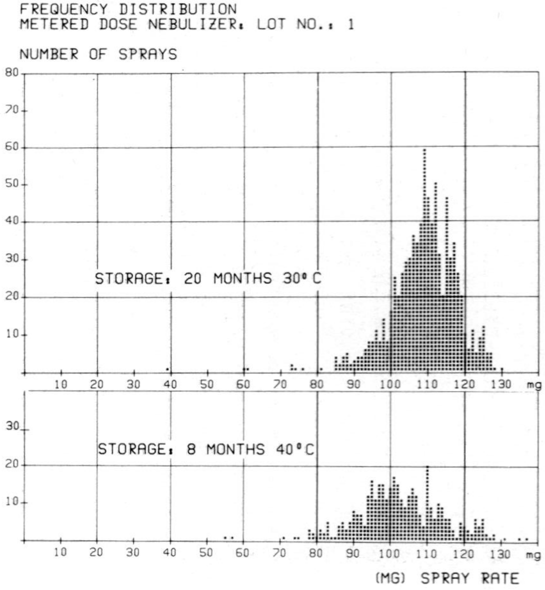

Figure 19: The performance of the Hoechst's metered-dose nebulizer after prolonged storage at elevated temperatures, for 20 months at 30°C or for 8 months at 40°C, the nebulizer still met the predetermined limits of acceptance.

REFERENCES

1) P. Fels and M. Gay; Vergleichende Studie zwischen einem Zerstauberspray and einem Mikrodosierspray bezuglich der freigesetzten Dosen und der Haufigkeitsverteilung der gebildeten Tropfchen, Pharm. Ind., 44 (10a) 958-961 (1982).
2) C. D. Yu, R. Jones, J. Wright, and M. Henesian; Characterization of dose delivery and spray pattern of a metered-dose FLUNISOLIDE nasal spray, Drug Develop. & Indus. Pharm., 9 473-483 (1983).
3) W. Fries and K. Jekle; Untersuchung der Dosiergenauigkeit mechanischer Pumpdosiersprays im Vergleich zu Treibgasaerosolen, Pharm. Ind., 44 189-192 (1982).
4) W. Petri, R. Seidel, and J. Sandow; A pharmaceutical approach to long-term therapy with peptides, Int. Congress of Endocrinology, Satellite Symposium VII on LHRH and Its Analogues, Quebec City, 1984.
5) J. Sandow, G. Jerabek-Sandow, B. Krauss, and M. Schmidt-Gollwitzer; Pharmacokinetics and metabolism of LHRH agonists, clinical aspects. Int. Congress of Endocrinology, Satellite Symposium VII on LHRH and Its Analogues, Quebec City, 1984.

Transnasal Systemic Medications, edited by Y.W. Chien
Elsevier Science Publishers B.V., Amsterdam, 1985 — Printed in The Netherlands

INTRANASAL ADMINISTRATION OF PEPTIDES BIOLOGICAL ACTIVITY AND THERAPEUTIC EFFICACY

J. SANDOW and W. PETRI
Hoechst AG, D-6230 Frankfurt 80, Germany F.R.

SUMMARY

The biological activities of hypothalamic releasing hormones and pituitary hormone analogs were evaluated in the experimental animals. Using the anaesthetized rat, the bioequivalent dose required by intranasal instillation to induce a hormonal effect of similar magnitude to i.v. injection was determined to calculate the nasal bioavailability of various peptides: A nasal absorption of 20% was achieved for thyrotropin-releasing hormone (TRH) by TSH release assay, 1-5% for luteinizing hormone-releasing hormone (LHRH) and several agonist analogs by LH release, ovulation induction and ovarian ascorbic acid depletion assays, 12% for an ACTH analog (heptadecapeptide, alsactide) by corticosterone release assay. The results indicated that monitoring of a hormonal effect is generally the more effective and meaningful approach to the determination of the extent of nasal absorption, since the serum levels of peptides are relatively low and their assay is analytically difficult and time consuming.

The results of the therapeutic efficacy studies for a nasal spray formulation of LHRH indicated that this preparation is suitable for early treatment of cryptorchidism in the children. Studies with buserelin (an LHRH agonist analog) yielded a nasal bioavailability of about 2.5% in humans in the phase I study on gonadotropin release, serum agonist level, and urinary excretion of immunoreactive buserelin. The therapeutic efficacies in female contraception, endometriosis and prostate carcinoma were also evaluated. The hormonal effect of this nasal spray formulation was observed to be reproducible, even with nasal inflammation. After the repeated multiple-dose administrations, pituitary gonadotropin secretion was desensitized and the secretion of gonadal steroids was reduced to the levels equivalent of castration. Under these conditions, the pharmacokinetic analysis of drug levels was found to be useful and appropriate to monitor the nasal absorption of peptides during therapy.

For the therapeutic uses of peptides by self-administration, the convenient method of nasal spray offers a valuable clinical option.

INTRODUCTION

During the last twenty years, peptides have become increasingly important as the new therapeutic agents. This is a consequence of the isolation and structural determination of numerous natural peptides, particularly, the discovery of hypothalamic releasing hormones and pituitary hormones. These peptides have been made available for clinical investigation through chemical synthesis, and the spectrum of their biological activities has been markedly changed and improved by the development of hormone analogs. The advantages of using such peptide hormones and their analogs for medication are attributed to their highly specific activity and excellent biological tolerance, resulting in the absence of side effects frequently observed with other synthetic drugs. One major problem remains, that is: all of these peptides are highly susceptible to metabolism by the gastro-intestinal enzymes, so new methods of drug delivery have to be developed to replace the convenient oral route of administration. If peptides are to be used as the viable therapeutic agents for long-term treatment, two possible approaches are evident, namely to administer the peptide by infusion from a small portable infusion pump or from a sustained-release drug delivery system, and, alternatively, by exploring the possibility of intranasal administration. In this investigation, the biological effect of hypothalamic-releasing hormones and pituitary hormone analogs following the intranasal administration was evaluated in experimental animals, and also in the humans. The results confirm that the use of metered-dose nebulizer for the intranasal administration of peptides is a practical approach to the medication by self-administration.

BIOLOGICAL ACTIVITY OF PEPTIDES BY NASAL ADMINISTRATION

In the course of our studies, the nasal absorption of several peptide hormones in the rat and in the human was investigated. Early examples were the nasal administration of oxytocin to induce uterine contractions (ref. 1) and the accelerated delivery of vasopressin and its analogues (ref. 2-5). Other peptides have also been administered intranasally at a biologically effective dose, e.g. secretin (ref. 6), angiotension analogs (ref. 7), and growth hormone-releasing factor (ref. 8). These early studies have already outlined the important principles for nasal therapy with peptides. The results suggested that the compound selected for development should be sufficiently potent to compensate for the low rate of nasal absorption, which demands a dose higher than that by parenteral route of administration. This usually can be achieved by synthesis of a potent agonist analog.

The first hypothalamic regulatory hormone to be introduced into clinical medicine was the thyrotropin-releasing hormone (TRH), which is used in the diagnosis of thyroid function. There are some indications which suggest that TRH has a role beyond the thyroid function, it is also a peptide neurotransmitter in the brain as well as in the peripheral neural tissue. The nasal absorption of TRH was evaluated in rats (Figure 1).

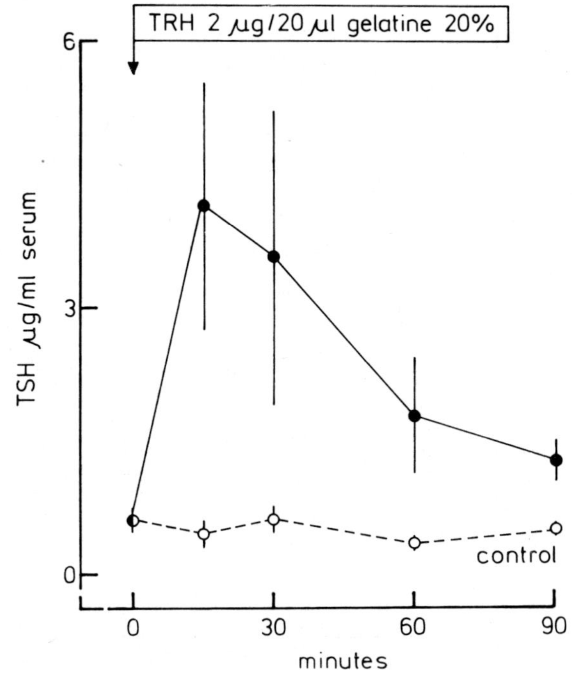

Figure 1: Nasal absorption of TRH in urethane-anaesthetized male rats (200 g) by instillation of 2 μg of TRH through a polyethylene sheated cannula into one nostril. The release of TSH in the serum was measured by RIA. Each data point is the mean value ± standard deviation of 6 rats.

The results indicated a rapid increase in the serum level of TSH with the peak concentration reached at 15 minutes. Calculation of the nasal bioavailability in terms of equieffective dose required for TSH release after i.v. and intranasal administrations indicated that 20% TRH is absorbed through the nasal mucosa. Based on these results, a TRH nasal spray test was developed for clinical diagnosis of thyroid function. While the usual TRH test is performed by the i.v. injection of a dose of 200-400 μg TRH, the intranasal TRH test uses a dose of 2 mg (Figure 2). The intranasal administration of

TRH yields a rapid stimulation of the TSH release with a maximum level reached after 20-30 minutes. The disadvantages of the intravenous TRH test, including the side effects like flushing and hypotensive reactions, are significantly reduced when the nasal spray test is used. To date, however, no therapeutic indications for TRH have been confirmed, although its use has been recommended in the re-animation after brain injury or neurosurgical operations.

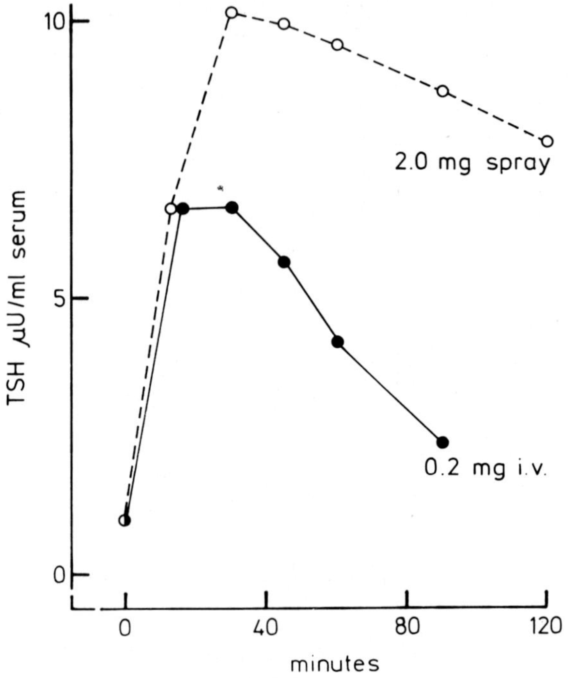

Figure 2: The performance of TRH nasal spray test in humans for thyroid function: comparison in the serum levels of TSH between the i.v. injection of 0.2 mg and nasal administration of 2 mg.

1) Adrenocorticotropic Hormone (ACTH)

There have been numerous attempts to develop preparations of ACTH for nasal application. One particular problem is the selection of an appropriate vehicle, since long-term use of oily suspensions may lead to some unwanted complications of local granuloma formation (ref. 9). The clinical uses of ACTH to reproduce and to reinforce the physiological pattern of cortisol secretion in the humans have several important restrictions on its application at certain times of the day. The injectable ACTH formulations with a prolonged release pattern are not suitable for long-term therapy, because they disrupt the physiological pattern of secretion and they may also induce adrenal atrophy. On the other hand, ACTH substitution by a daily nasal application early in the morning may prevent this complication. Thus, ACTH substitution would not only be envisaged as a form of therapy for substitution after hypophysectomy, but more importantly to support the endogenous daily rhythm of corticol secretion. In our studies, a short-chain analogue of ACTH consisting of 17 amino acids was used. This peptide, /β-Ala^{1},Lys^{17}/ACTH(1-17)heptadecapeptide-4-amino-butylamide (alsactide, Hoe 433), is 5 to 8 times more potent than the natural ACTH or its steroidogenic sequence, ACTH(1-24)tetracosipeptide (tetracosactin, Synacthen^{TM}). In the dexamethasone-blocked rats, a nasal dose of 100 µg ACTH-17 (alsactide, Synchrodyn^{TM}) was found to be equieffective with a s.c. dose of 9 µg on the corticosterone release (Figure 3).

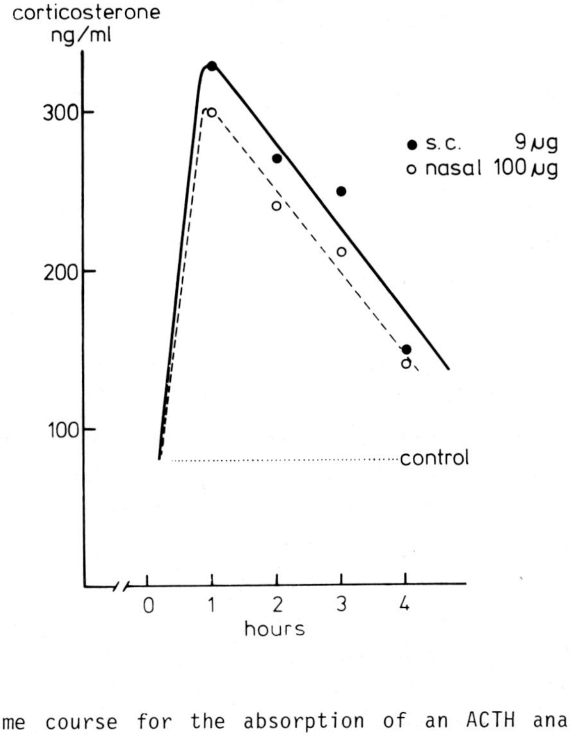

Figure 3: The time course for the absorption of an ACTH analog in rats by nasal and subcutaneous administrations. The analog, alsactide (a heptadecapeptide of ACTH), was instilled into the nasal cavity in a volume of 20 µl/rat. Each data point is the mean value of the corticosterone release in a group of 6 rats.

Based on the effect on the corticosterone release and adrenal ascorbic acid depletion, a nasal bioavailability of 12% was calculated for this heptadecapeptide.

In the dose-titration studies in humans, the nasal spray of a dose of 100 µg was observed to induce a significant increase in the duration of cortisol release, which last for more than 4 hours, whereas the aldosterone secretion was not stimulated at this dose (Figure 4). The pattern of corticosterone secretion after a single dose of nasal spray is similar to the daily endogenous cortisol peak (ref. 10).

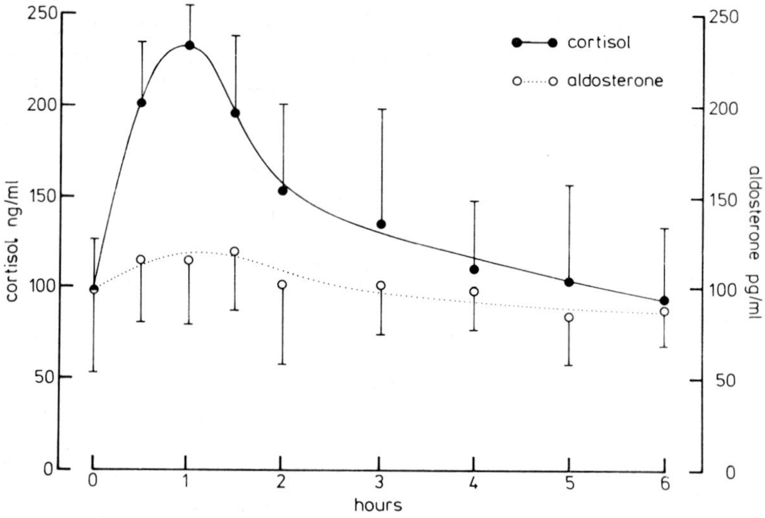

Figure 4: The biological effects following the nasal absorption of ACTH in humans. The ACTH analog (alsactide, a heptadecapeptide) was administered from a metered-dose nebulizer. Each data point is the mean ± SEM of the serum cortisol and aldosterone levels of 10 subjects. At the dose tested, cortisone secretion is stimulated, whereas aldosterone secretion is unaffected (ref. 10).

2) Luteinizing Hormone-releasing Hormone (LHRH)

The structure of LHRH (Gonadorelin) was elucidated in 1971 by the group of Schally. In the initial clinical trials, only the diagnostic use for the stimulation of gonadotropin secretion was confirmed, whereas the practical difficulties in the frequent daily administration of LHRH at regular intervals by injection became apparent. The reason for such a limitation is the requirement for a pulsatile maintenance of pituitary gonadotropin secretion by LHRH, at a relatively constant rate of one LH pulse per 90-120 min. For the treatment of hypothalamic amenorrhea and idiopathic hypogonadotropic hypogonadism in men and women, the use of a pulsatile infusion pump has become mandatory. This technically demanding procedure can, in some instances, be replaced by the more convenient use of an LHRH nasal spray. In early clinical studies, it was found that administration of a dose of 2 mg LHRH by nose drops stimulates LH secretion in a similar manner as the intravenous injection of 50 µg LHRH (ref. 11). On the other hand, a nasal bioavailability of 1% was determined from pharmacokinetic measurements (ref. 12).

A nasal spray formulation was developed at Hoechst AG for the treatment of cryptorchidism in boys (ref. 13). A transient activation of the pituitary-testicular axis is known to be frequently effective in stimulating the descent of the cryptorchid testis (ref. 14). Such treatment is necessary because the prognosis of the fertility in the patients with cryptorchid testes is initially favorable if the treatment is initiated at an early stage, but, subsequently, the efficacy of the treatment progressively declines because of increasing degenerative changes in the cryptorchid tissue. Previously, the transient activation was achieved by the injections of human chorionic gonadotropin (HCG), a procedure which requires injections and is not well tolerated by the infants; and it sometimes leads to some symptoms of androgenic stimulation, which are unwanted in prepubertal children. The intranasal administration of LHRH by nasal spray has been found effective with a multiple daily dose regimen, e.g. 6 times at 200 µg/spray or 3 times at 400 µg/spray, or in a single daily dose of 100 µg/spray (ref. 14, 15). It is surprising to observe that the nasal absorption of LHRH administered by nasal spray is very reliable and is not affected by common colds or intercurrent rhinitis, which may be a consequence of the rapid rate of nasal absorption and the contribution of the lymphatic system to peptide transport towards the anterior pituitary gland (ref. 16). In a study with the LHRH analog, buserelin, experimental rhinitis was induced by histamine and the LH release after the nasal administration of buserelin was compared before and during the experimentally induced nasal inflammation (Figure 5). Results suggested that there is no difference in the LH release induced.

A new application for the LHRH nasal spray is long-term maintenance therapy of spermatogenesis in the hypogonadal men. Once the testicular development and spermatogenesis have been achieved by the pulsatile LHRH therapy, the patients can then be transferred to a maintenance regimen of LHRH by nasal spray administration at the interval of one spray for every 2 hours during the day (ref. 19).

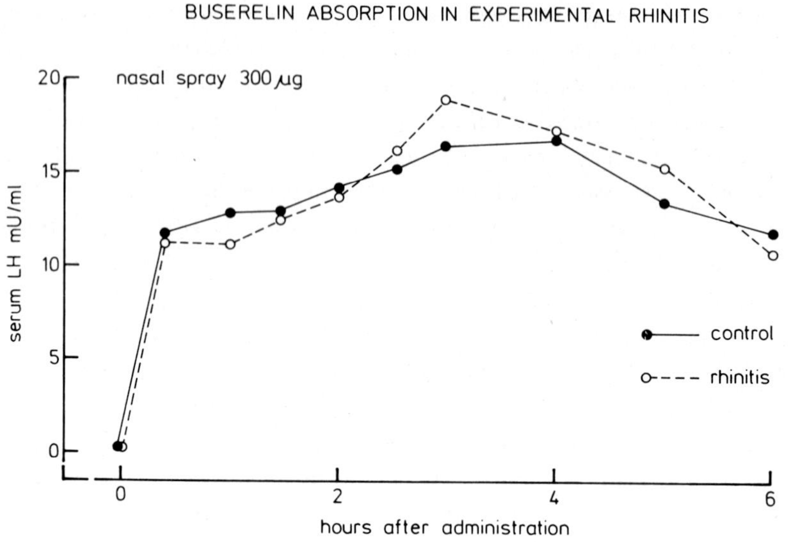

Figure 5: The nasal absorption of an LHRH agonist, buserelin, during an experimental rhinitis induced by histamine. No difference in the LH release was noted, indicating that the process of nasal absorption is rapid and unaffected by the increase in nasal blood flow.

Effect of the routes of administration

In the initial studies, we evaluated the doses required for the induction of ovulation and the depletion of the ovarian ascorbic acid content in rats treated with LHRH and LHRH agonists via various routes of administration. It was found that the nasal route of administration is the most efficient way, requiring a 100-fold multiple of the doses by either subcutaneous or intravenous injection, while the rectal or vaginal administration are 4-6 times less effective and also inconvenient. On the other hand, oral bioavailability of LHRH and its analogues was extremely low, requiring a 3,000- to 10,000-fold higher dose than by injection or 30-100 times more than the nasal dose (Table 1).

TABLE 1 - Effect of administration route on the relative efficacy of LHRH and agonists in the induction of ovulation and depletion of ovarian ascorbic acid in rats.

Route of administration	relative effective dose: ovulation	relative effective dose: ascorbic acid
s.c./i.v.	1	1
nasal	100	100
rectal	400	400
vaginal	600	---
oral	3,000	10,000

The feasibility of repeated vaginal administration was explored in a short-term study with a LHRH analog, D-Leu^6-ethylamide (Leuprolide), in rats by Okada et al. (ref. 18) to achieve pituitary desensitization. The biological effect of nasal administration of LHRH analogue on the termination of pregnancy was also investigated (ref. 19). Oral absorption of LHRH and related analogues was low, requiring a dose which is 3,000 to 10,000-fold higher than by injection.

The buccal absorption was also explored to some extent in response to the clinical finding that buccally administered oxytocin is suitable to induce uterine contractions at the time of parturition. A special film tablet was designed by Prof. Merkle and Mr. Anders at the University of Heidelberg in Germany. This film tablet can be administered to an anesthetized rat and the drug becomes available for buccal absorption by diffusion into the saliva. This buccal therapeutic system was found in close contact, by adhesion, to the buccal mucosa. However, an extremely low rate of absorption across the buccal mucosa was reported, which was also confirmed by the results of human studies. In male subjects, a buccal administration of 5 mg of either LHRH or LHRH analogues, buserelin, failed to raise the serum levels of LH and FSH. Thus, the buccal administration should be ruled out for the clinical uses of hypothalamic regulatory hormones.

3) LHRH analogs

There are two classes of LHRH analogs suitable for therapeutic application by nasal spray: LHRH agonists and LHRH antagonists.

The LHRH agonists are a group of LHRH analogs which act initially to stimulate the release of gonadotropin, followed by the progressive desensitization of gonadotropin secretion and testicular/ovarian down-regulation, resulting in a suppression of the gonadal steroid secretion (ref. 20). The agonists have found their clinical applications in the treatment of endocrine disorders and hormone-dependent tumors (ref. 21, 22).

The second group of LHRH analogs are the LHRH antagonists, which have a highly specific inhibitory action on the stimulating effect of endogenous LHRH, and on the effect of exogenous LHRH. The antagonists are decapeptide analogs of LHRH, with modification of several amino acids in the peptide chain to enhance the resistance to enzyme attack. It is, therefore, not surprising to observe that these antagonists exhibit a rather high level of nasal bioavailability, up to 20%, as demonstrated by biological studies in monkeys.

In our studies with several agonists of LHRH (1-9) nonapeptide-ethylamide type, such as D-Leu^{6}-ethylamide, D-Trp^{6}-ethylamide and D-Ser(But)^{6}-ethylamide (buserelin, Hoe 766), it was found that the bioavailabilities of these peptides by nasal administration in the rats, either by single dose administration or by repeated daily administration over 14 days, are quite similar in the order of magnitude, despite some small differences in their biological potencies. In the rat, the long-term daily treatment by nasal instillation is possible in the adult animal with a body weight of 150-200 g, under a light ether anaesthesia, for a time period of 14-28 days. A special cannula, which contains a protective polyethylene sheating attached to a Hamilton syringe, was found suitable for accurate dosing by nasal instillation.

THERAPEUTIC EFFICACY OF PEPTIDES BY NASAL ADMINISTRATION

These studies were all performed with a specially-designed metered-dose nebulizer outlined in the chapter by Petri et al. Two different peptide formulations were investigated, one contained buserelin at a concentration of 100 µg per 100 µl (the dispensing volume of the metered-dose nebulizer), with benzyl alcohol as the preservative; and the second formulation contained buserelin at a concentration of 150 µg per 100 µl, with benzalkonium chloride as the preservative. In phase I studies, the biological activities of this nasal spray were evaluated by measuring the gonadotropin release, in comparison with s.c. or i.v. injection. A nasal bioavailability of 2.5% was found in one study. Interestingly, the time course for LH release after nasal administration resembled the pattern following a subcutaneous injection, which is characterized by a gradual increase to peak levels after about 30-60 min.. This pattern is rather different from the rapid increase to high levels observed 5-10 min. after an intravenous injection.

Pharmacokinetic methods were developed to analyze buserelin absorption following the nasal spray administration (ref. 23). After a nasal dose of 400 µg buserelin, plasma LH level increased rapidly within 30 minutes to a peak level and remained at the elevated concentration for more than 6 hours (Figure 6), while the plasma concentration of buserelin increased rapidly, remained at the peak level only for a relatively short period of time, and then declined to the non-detectable level within 2 hours. The plasma buserelin profile observed was similar to that seen after an s.c. injection.

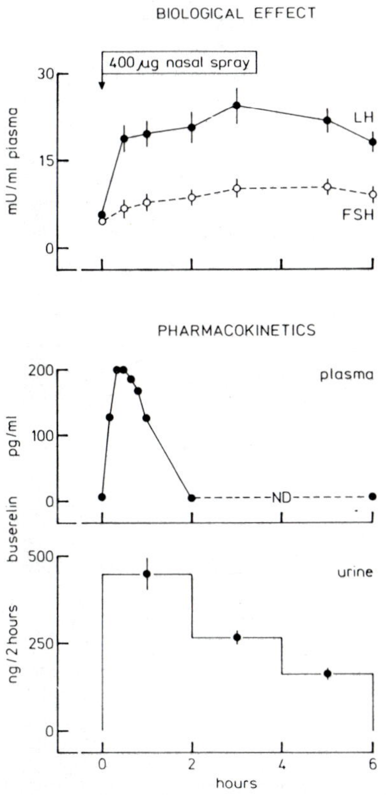

Figure 6: Biological activities, plasma and urine levels of buserelin in 6 male volunteeers after the nasal administration of buserelin at a dose of 400 µg. Note that the release of LH and FSH persists for 6 hours, whereas the plasma level of buserelin decreases rather rapidly. Urinary excretion of immunoreactive buserelin was used to monitor peptide absorption.

The discrepancy observed between the drug level and the induced biological activities is apparently a result of high affinity of the pituitary LHRH receptors for the LHRH agonists, like buserelin, and the long retention of buserelin at the pituitary receptor site is due to its resistance to enzyme inactivation. In the dose-titration studies with the nasal spray formulations, the urinary excretion profiles of buserelin were found to be dose- and time-dependent (Figure 7). A nasal bioavailability of about 1% was calculated from the pharmacokinetic analysis, using a s.c. dose of 5 µg as the reference, while the result of LH-release studies indicated a nasal bioavailability of 2.5%. For another agonist, /D-Nal(2)^{6}/LHRH (nafarelin), a nasal bioavailability of about 2% was reported (ref. 24).

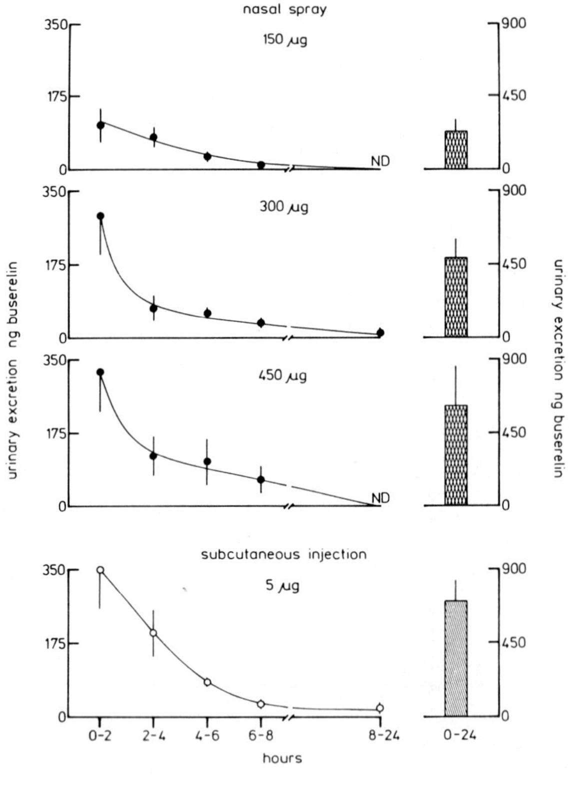

Figure 7: Urinary excretion profiles of buserelin following nasal administration in the male human volunteers. Nasal spray doses of 150-450 µg were compared with the subcutaneous injection of 5 µg. Note the time-dependent excretion of immunoreactive buserelin in the urine. Columns indicate the total urinary excretion within 24 hours after treatment.

In the studies on therapeutic efficacy, the absorption of peptide from the nasal administration site is conveniently monitored by measuring the urinary excretion of immunoreactive buserelin (ref. 23). This can be performed on either a 24-hour urine sample, or in the urine sample collected over a certain time period after nasal administration. For example, in the low dose studies with buserelin in the female contraception (ref. 25), urine was collected for 2 hours before administration of a nasal dose of 400 µg and then at 2-hour intervals for up to 6 hours after treatment, because the urinary excretion of buserelin is time-dependent. In the contraceptive study, the effect of different modes of administration, i.e., the nasal spray administered into the nasal cavity as prescribed, inhaled through the nose during forced inhalation, or sprayed into the oral cavity during forced inhalation, were compared. In two of the subjects, the nasal spray administration resulted in a time-dependent urinary excretion of buserelin with a total excretion of 3.39 and 1.61 µg/6 hours, respectively (Table 2). Results also indicated that the oral inhalation is much less effective for the LHRH analogs, like buserelin, which are not absorbed effectively from the bronchial epithelium.

TABLE 2 - Contraceptive use of buserelin in human subjects (n=2): pharmacokinetic monitoring of the absorption following different modes of administration.

dose (400 µg)	period (hours)	urinary excretion (ng/2 hours): nasal spray	nasal inhalation	oral inhalation
Subject #1				
pre-treatment	4 hours	0	0	0
post-treatment	0-2	1894	660	237
	2-4	1076	302	115
	4-6	421	no sample	59
total excretion		3391	962	411
Subject #2				
pre-treatment	4 hours	0	0	0
post-treatment	0-2	1058	780	57
	2-4	394	376	27
	4-6	189	154	0
total excretion		1614	1310	84

In comparison with the lack of absorption by the buccal route, inhalation of buserelin through the mouth was at least marginally effective, though it was insufficient for any clinical effects.

In the therapeutic efficacy studies, the nasal buserelin spray is generally administered as a maintenance therapy, 3 times or more a day. Initial suppression is achieved by high-dose injections or long-term infusion over several days (ref. 26). The maintenance therapy with nasal buserelin spray has the advantage of being easily adjustable by administering multiples of the single spray dose. In the children with precocious puberty, frequent administration (8 times daily) was found to be effective to suppress the secretion of gonadal steroids, even without an initial injection period. However, the daily total dose which can be given by nasal spray is limited, and, in the case of insufficient suppression or escape from previous suppression, the regimen should be changed to the injection method for a duration at least until a full suppression has been achieved again.

The treatments currently under investigation with the nasal spray formulation of buserelin are endometriosis (ref. 27, 28), precocious puberty and hormone-dependent tumors, e.g. prostate and mammary carcinoma (ref. 26, 29-31). The reversible suppression of pituitary-ovarian function is also investigated as a new approach to female contraception, based on the sequential administration of a nasal peptide spray to inhibit ovulation (ref. 32), and a progestagen to achieve secretory transformation of the endometrium and thus a regular, predictable bleeding pattern (ref. 25).

CONCLUSIONS

Experimental and clinical evidences confirm that the nasal administration is a practical approach to therapy with many drugs, with the advantages of rapid absorption, which is relatively similar to a subcutaneous injection, ease of administration and good local tolerance. One example is the development of nasal spray formulations for peptides, particularly, the hypothalamic regulatory hormones and their analogs (Table 3). The nasal administration has a bioavailability generally between 1 and 20%, depending upon the molecular weight and physicochemical properties of the peptide as well as its enzyme resistance and other factors. The nasal absorption of GRF, a peptide with 44 amino acids, is encouraging (ref. 8) There are many practical benefits realized in the therapy by nasal administration, because the patients can administer the medication themselves without the use of a biomedical device, or a sustained release formulation. The time of the day can be selected at will, endogenous biological rhythms can be preserved and reinforced as in the case of ACTH.

TABLE 3 - Peptides active by nasal administration: Relationship between nasal bioavailability and molecular weight

peptides	absorption %	no. amino acids
thyrotropin-releasing hormone (TRH)	20	3
vasopressin analogs	6-12	9
LHRH, agonists and antagonists	1-10	9-10
ACTH analogs	12	17-18
growth hormone-releasing factor (GRF)	1- 2	40-44

Nasal spray formulations also facilitate the diagnostic applications of peptides, by reducing the side-effects commonly observed in the intravenous testing, and the long-term therapeutic uses. There are several obvious benefits in treatment of infants and children, where the injections often cause a psychological trauma. The limitations of nasal peptide spray therapy are imposed by the low level of bioavailability and the need for a good patient compliance, if multiple daily doses should be required. The peptide to be administered nasally should be readily soluble in a well-tolerated vehicle and absorbed to a sufficiently high extent to make this mode of administration economical. Nasal spray administration is one of the important options when long-term treatment with peptides is envisaged.

ACKNOWLEDGMENTS

The authors would like to express their appreciation to NIH and NIADDK, National Hormone and Pituitary Program, and G. D. Niswender and A. F. Parlow for the generous supply of RIA reagents for preclinical animal studies, to Professors H. Croxatto, A. Angeli and Saitoh for their contributions in the clinical studies, M. Hahn, S. Kille, W. Stoll and G. Klante for their technical assistance, as well as the skillful secretarial assistance in preparation of the manuscript by P. Bischoff.

REFERENCES

1) N. E. Borglin, Intranasales Oxytocin als wehenstimulierendes Mittel, Zentralblatt fur Gynakologie 85 1-7 (1963).
2) D. R. Brown and D. L. Uden, The use of 1-desamino-8-D-arginine vasopressin (DDAVP) in the management of neurogenic diabetes insipidus, Minnesota Mecidine 62 427-432 (1979).
3) W. E. Cobb, S. Spare and S. Reichlin, Neurogenic diabetes insipidus: management with DDAVP (1-desamino-8-D-arginine vasopressin), Annals Int. Med., 88 183-188 (1978)
4) W.N.P. Lee, B. M. Lippe, S. H. La Franchi and S. A. Kaplan, Vasopressin analog DDAVP in the treatment of diabetes insipidus., Am. J. Dis. Child., 130 166-169 (1976).
5) F. Ziai, R. Walter and I. M. Rosenthal, Treatment of central diabetes insipidus in adults and children with desmopressin, Arch. Int. Med., 138 1382-1385 (1978).
6) P. B'Hend, B. Haldemann, B. Hadorn, M. Kleeb and H. Luthi, Stimulation of pancreatic secretion in man by secretin snuff, Lancet, I 509-510 (1973).
7) B. A. Scholkens, R. Lux and R. Steinbach, Hypotensive action of an intra-nasally applied angiotension II-antagonist, Archives internationales de Pharmacodynamie et de Therapie, 229 244-250 (1977).
8) W. S. Evans, J. L. C. Borges, D. L. Kaiser, M. L. Vance, R. P. Sellers, R. M. MacLeod, W. Vale, J. Rivier and M. O. Thorner, Intranasal administration of human pancreatic tumor GH-releasing factor-40 stimulates GH release in normal men, J. Clin. Endocr. Metab., 57 1081-1083 (1983).
9) G. Baumann, A. Walser, P. A. Desaulles, F. J. A. Paesi and L. Geller, Corticotropic action of an intra-nasally applied synthetic ACTH derivative, J. Clin. Endocrin., 42 60-63 (1976).
10) A. Angeli, F. Orlandi, P. Paccotti, A. Caveggia and F. Ceresa, Studio della risposta glico- e mineralocorticoide alla somministrazione acuta di un nuovo derivato sintetico dell'ACTH: /β -ALA^1, LIS^{17}/ ACTH$^{1-17}$-4-amino-n-butilamide, J. Endocrinol. Invest., 4 267-270 (1981).
11) H. G. Solbach and W. Wiegelmann, Intranasal application of luteinizing-hormone-releasing hormone, Lancet, I 1259 (1973).
12) J. P. Bourguignon, H. G. Burger and P. Franchimont, Radioimmunoassay of serum luteinizing-hormone-releasing hormone (LHRH) after intra-nasal administration and evaluation of the pituitary gonadotrophic response, Clinical Endocrinology, 3 437-440 (1974).
13) W. Petri, R. Seidel and J. Sandow, A pharmaceutical approach to long-term therapy with peptides. In LHRH and Its Analogues - Satellite Symposium VII. Int. Congress of Endocrinology, Quebec City, 1984, in press.
14) F. Hadziselimovic, J. Girard, B. Herzog and G. Stalder, Hormonal treatment of cryptorchidism, Horm. Res., 16 188-192 (1982).
15) R. Illig, T. Torresani, H. Bucher, M. Zachmann and A. Prader, Effect of intranasal LHRH therapy on plasma LH, FSH and testosterone, and relation to clinical results in prepubertal boys with cryptorchidism, Clinical Endocrinology 12 91-97 (1980).
16) P. G. Gopinath, G. Gopinath and T. C. Anand Kumar, Target site of intranasally sprayed substances and their transport across the nasal mucosa: a new insight into the intranasal route of drug delivery, Current Therapeutic Research, 23 596-607 (1978).
17) D. Klingmuller, M. Meschi and H. U. Schweikert, Successful intranasal administration of LHRH in men with hypogonadotropic hypogonadism, Journal of steroid biochemistry, 20 A62 (1984).
18) H. Okada, I. Yamazaki, Y. Sakura, T. Yashiki, T. Shimamoto, and H. Mima, Desensitization of gonadotropin-releasing response following vaginal consecutive administration of leuprolide in rats, J. Pharm. Dyn., 6 512-522 (1983).

19) I. Yamazaki, Differences in the pregnancy-terminating effectiveness of an LHRH analogue by subcutaneous, vaginal, rectal, and nasal routes in rats, Endocrinol. Japan, 29 415-421 (1982).
20) J. Sandow, Inhibition of pituitary and testicular function by LHRH analogues. In Progress towards a male contraceptive (S. L. Jeffcoate and M. Sandler, Eds.), John Wiley & Sons Ltd., London (1982) pp. 19-39.
21) J. Sandow, Clinical applications of LHRH and its analogues, Clin. Endocr., 18 571-592 (1983).
22) J. Sandow, Therapeutic use of LHRH analogs in reproductive disorders. In Andrology: Infertility and sterility, (1984), in press.
23) J. Sandow G. Jerabek-Sandow, B. Krauss and M. Schmidt-Gollwitzer, Pharmacokinetics and metabolism of LHRH agonists, clinical aspects. In LHRH and Its Analogues - Satellite Symposium VII. Int. Congress of Endocrinology, Quebec City (1984), in press.
24) S. T. Anik, G. McRae, C. Nerenberg, A. Worden, J. Foreman, J. Y. Hwang, S. Kushinsky, R. E. Jones and B. Vickery, Nasal absorption of Nafarelin acetate, the decapeptide /D-Nal(2)^6/LHRH, in rhesus monkeys I., Journal of Pharmaceutical Sciences, 73 684-685 (1983).
25) M. Schmidt-Gollwitzer, W. Hardt, K. Schmidt-Gollwitzer and M. von der Ohe, The contraceptive use of buserelin, a potent LHRH agonist: clinical and hormonal findings. In LHRH Peptides as Female and Male Contraceptives (G. I. Zatuchni, J. D. Shelton & J. J. Sciarra, Eds.), Harper & Row, Philadelphia, (1982) pp. 199-215.
26) V. Borgmann, W. Hardt, M. Schmidt-Gollwitzer, H. Adenauer and R. Nagel, Sustained suppression of testosterone production by the luteinising-hormone releasing-hormone agonist buserelin in patients with advanced prostate carcinoma, Lancet, II 1097-1098 (1982).
27) A. Lemay and G. Quesnel, Potential new treatment of endometriosis - reversible inhibition of pituitary-ovarian function by chronic intranasal administration of a LHRH agonist, Fertil. Steril., 38 376-377 (1982).
28) R. W. Shaw, H. M. Fraser and H. Boyle, Intranasal treatment with luteinizing-hormone-releasing hormone agonist in women with endometriosis, Br. Med. J., 287 1667 (1983).
29) N. Faure, A. Lemay, A. Belanger and F. Labrie, Inhibition of androgen biosynthesis in the human male by chronic administration of /D-Ser(TBU)^6-des-Gly-NH_2^{10}/LHRH ethylamide (buserelin). In LHRH Peptides as Female and Male Contraceptives (G. I. Zatuchni, J. D. Shelton and J. J. Sciarra, Eds.), Harper & Row, Philadelphia, (1982) pp. 307-320.
30) N. Faure, F. Labrie, A. Lemay, A. Belanger, Y. Gourdeau, B. Larouche and G. Robert, Inhibition of serum androgen levels by chronic intranasal and subcutaneous hormone (LHRH) agonist in adult men, Fertil. Steril., 37 416-424 (1982).
31) J. G. M. Klijn, and F. H. deJong, Treatment with a luteinizing-hormone releasing-hormone analogue (buserelin) in premenopausal patients with metastatic breast cancer, Lancet, II 1213-1216 (1982).
32) W. Hardt and M. Schmidt-Gollwitzer, Sustained gonadal suppression in fertile women with the LHRH agonist buserelin, Clin. Endocrinol., 19 613 (1983).
33) C. Bergquist, S. J. Nillius and L. Wide, Intranasal LHRH agonist treatment for inhibition of ovulation in women: clinical aspects, Clin. Endocr., 17 91-98 (1982).

Transnasal Systemic Medications, edited by Y.W. Chien
Elsevier Science Publishers B.V., Amsterdam, 1985 – Printed in The Netherlands

INTRANASAL ADMINISTRATION OF NAFARELIN ACETATE CONTRACEPTION AND THERAPEUTIC APPLICATIONS

B. H. VICKERY, S. ANIK, M. CHAPLIN and M. HENZL
Syntex Research
Palo Alto, California 94304

INTRODUCTION

Luteinizing hormone-releasing hormone (LHRH), in common with a number of other peptide hormones, must be secreted in a pulsatile fashion in order to trigger and maintain the release of gonadotropin and, thus, ensure the correct functioning of the reproductive cascade, which results in gametogenesis and gonadal steroidogenesis (ref. 1, 2). Continuous administration of LHRH was reported to result in a down-regulation of the homologous pituitary receptors and interruption of the normal release patterns of gonadotropins (ref. 3, 4).

Some highly potent agonistic analogs of LHRH have been synthesized. Unfortunately, their increased potency is the result of the increase in receptor binding affinity and/or the protection from metabolism, both of which favor a sustained occupancy of the receptor and thus a down-regulation of receptors. It, therefore, is unlikely that the highly potent LHRH agonistic analogs will be useful for the treatment of infertility. They are, however, under intensive investigation for possible antifertility activities and for the treatment of gonadal hormone-dependent syndromes and neoplasias.

LHRH and its analogs have a relatively short circulatory half-life and require administration of one or more times daily to achieve a desired effect. In addition, due to enzymatic degradation and/or their extremely poor absorption from the gastrointestinal tract, a very large and economically unacceptable dose (1000 to 10,000 times of the parenteral dose) is required to be therapeutically effective by oral administration, while frequent administration by parenteral route is not desirable. Although parenteral administration may be tolerable, with reasonable compliance, in the treatment of life threatening disease, such as prostatic carcinoma, or even for precocious puberty, these points become arguable in endometriosis therapy and for contraception. For these reasons, alternative drug delivery via transmucosal, and, in particular, the intranasal route has been explored.

Since these peptides have a reasonably low molecular weight and are lipophilic in nature, they should be absorbed by these transmucosal routes; even though the bioavailability is expected to be only a low fraction of that resulting from injection.

It, therefore, becomes important to select a highly potent, lipophilic long-acting LHRH analog to maximize the efficacy by intranasal administration. Nafarelin acetate ([6-D-(2-naphthyl)alanine]LHRH; [D-Nal(2)^6]LHRH; RS-94991), whose structure is shown in Fig. 1, has been identified to be such an analog.

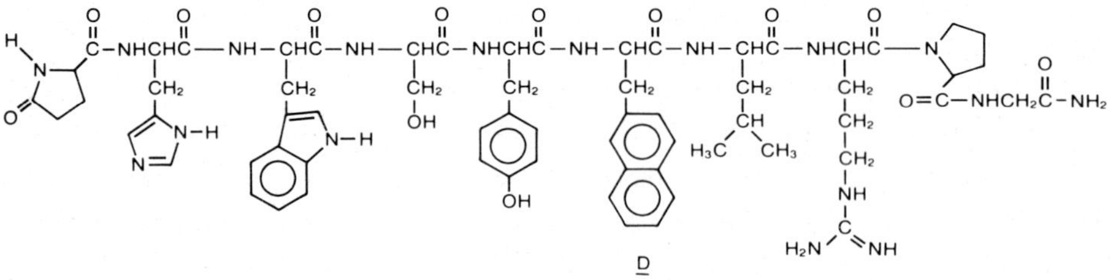

[D-Nal(2)^6]LHRH
Nafarelin

Figure 1. The chemical structure of nafarelin.

Pharmacological Studies of Nafarelin Acetate:

Nafarelin acetate is a classical agonistic analog of LHRH in that it binds to rat pituitary cell receptors with a K_A of 2.1 x 10^{10} (ref. 5), in an assay based on the displacement of [^{125}I-D-Ser(tBu)^6, Pro^9-NHEt]LHRH under *in vitro* conditions (ref. 6). This value is similar in magnitude to that of another well-described analog, [D-Trp^6, Pro^9-NHEt]LHRH (4.1 x 10^{10}). The binding to pituitary cell receptors results in the release of LH; and, in the *in vitro* dispersed rat pituitary cell system, nafarelin acetate again was found to be equivalent in potency to [D-Trp^6, Pro^9-NHEt]LHRH and was 100 folds more potent than LHRH itself (Fig. 2). The documented extrapituitary effects of LHRH analogs in rats (ref. 7) were also exhibited by nafarelin. In an *in vitro* system, which used granulosa cells obtained from immature, hypophysectomized, diethylstilbestrol - treated female rats, nafarelin was found to suppress the FSH-stimulated production of estradiol (ref. 8).

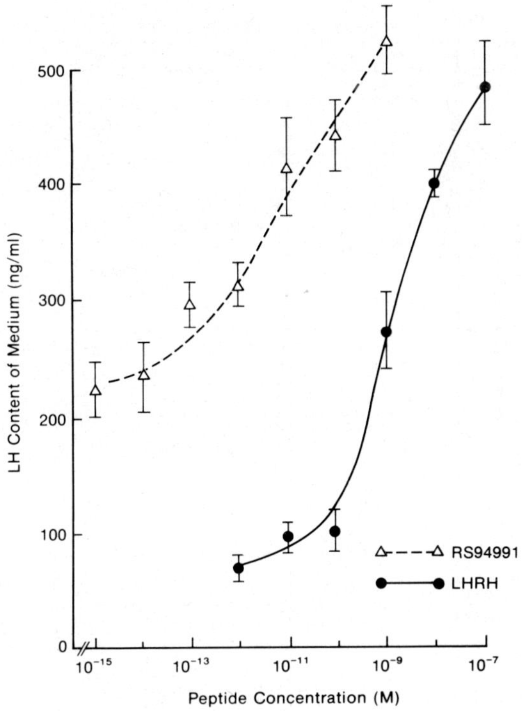

Figure 2. In vitro release of LH from the dispersed rat pituitary cells.

Administration of nafarelin, once or twice daily, to female rats was observed to suppress estrous cyclicity. Direct comparison in this assay with [D-Trp^6, Pro^9-NHEt]LHRH indicated that nafarelin is twice as potent (ref. 9). Comparison with LHRH suggested that nafarelin is 190-230 times more potent than LHRH. Thus, nafarelin is relatively more potent by in vivo evaluation than by in vitro testing.

Pharmacokinetic Studies of Nafarelin Acetate:

In metabolic and dispositional studies, [^{14}C] nafarelin and [^{3}H]LHRH were administered intravenously to female rats at approximately equimolar doses. The results showed that the plasma $t_{1/2}$ is 34 minutes for nafarelin and 7 minutes for LHRH (Fig. 3). The rates of clearance were 2.3 and 11.0 ml/minute for nafarelin and LHRH, repectively. These differences would account for the increased potency observed in in vivo relative to that observed in in vitro.

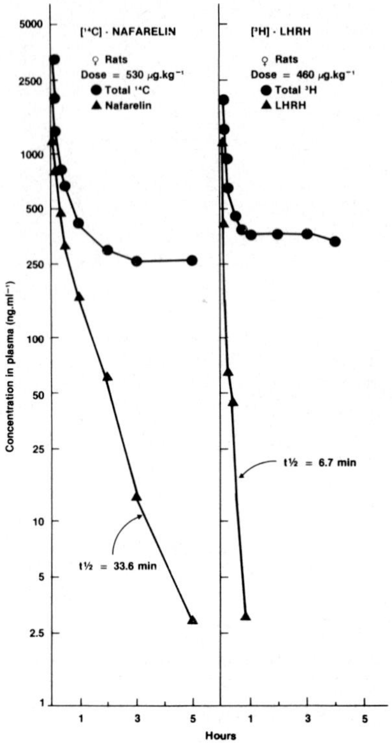

Figure 3. Comparison of the circulating $t_{1/2}$ of nafarelin and LHRH in rats following the bolus intravenous injection of equimolar quantities.

Subcutaneous administration of 10 μg/kg of nafarelin to male dogs was noted to cause an immediate elevation of plasma levels of LH and testosterone. As these doses were repeated on a daily basis, the pre-injection levels of LH and testosterone were lowered and the stimulatory response was progressively decreased (ref. 10). Castrate levels of testosterone were reached after about 1 week, which resulted in a suppressed function of the accessory organs. Ejaculation ceased and a marked decline was observed in the size of even the hyperplastic prostate in geriatric dogs (ref. 11). Similar loss in the responsivity of FSH was also noted. The combined lowering of LH, FSH and testosterone resulted in aspermatogenesis. A supplementation of the circulating levels of testosterone was reported to reverse the hypoandrogenicity of the accessory organs, but did not affect the testicular regression. Besides the potential for male contraception suggested by these effects, there has been some interest in the possibility of gonadoprotective effects against cancer chemotherapeutic agents (ref. 12, 13). It has recently been shown that some chemotherapeutic agents also exert similar effects on testicular function in dogs as in men (ref. 14, 15); and the hypothesis that induction of a temporary pseudo-prepubertal state with LHRH analogs during chemotherapy will prevent sterilization, is presently undergoing evaluation.

The female rhesus monkey is a convenient animal model for predicting the effects of LHRH agonists in women. Daily administration of nafarelin was observed to cause a dose-dependent inhibition of ovulation (Table 1), with a complete inhibition of ovulation at a dose of 5 µg per day by intramuscular injection.

TABLE 1. EFFECT OF DAILY INTRAMUSCULAR INJECTION OF NAFARELIN ACETATE ON OVULATION IN RHESUS MONKEYS

Dose (µg/Day)	Number of Animals	Ovulatory Cycles / Treated Cycles
-	5	15/15
0.31	3	6/9
1.25	3	1/9
5.0	3	0/9
20.0	2	0/6

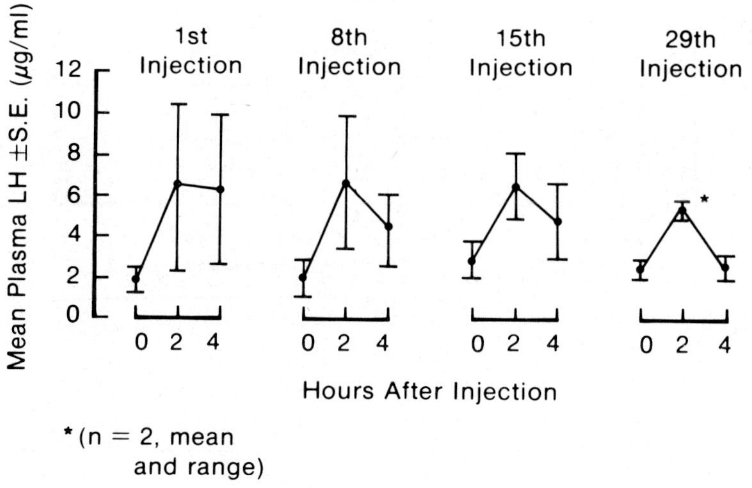

Figure 4. Plasma LH levels in the female rhesus monkeys at various times after the consecutive daily intramuscular injection of 5 µg of nafarelin for 29 days.

As this dose continued, the pituitary responsivity to each injection, though progressively declining, was still noticeable, (Fig. 4); but the preovulatory estrogen and LH surges failed to occur (Fig. 5). After termination of long-term administration, a rapid resumption of normal ovulatory ovarian function was observed (Fig. 6).

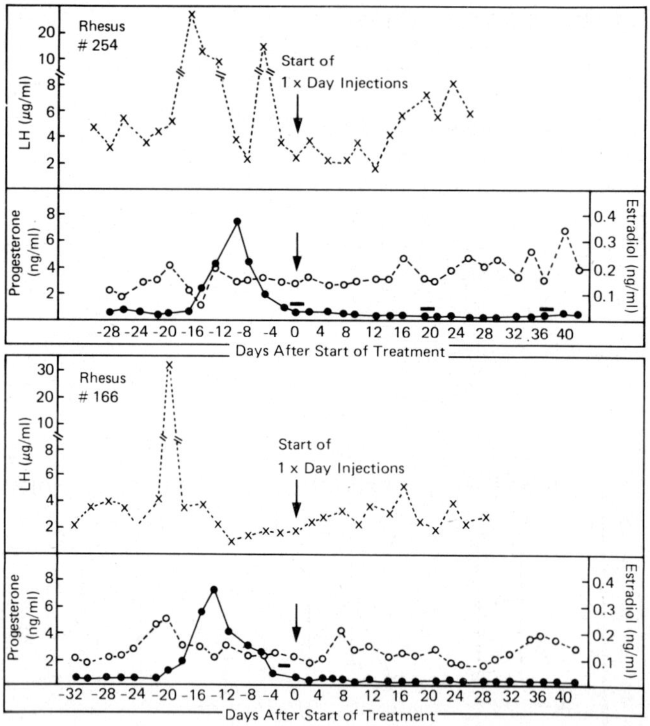

Figure 5. Plasma levels of LH(x), estradiol (o) and progesterone (•) in two female rhesus monkeys before and during the treatment with 5 μg per day of nafarelin by intramuscular injection.

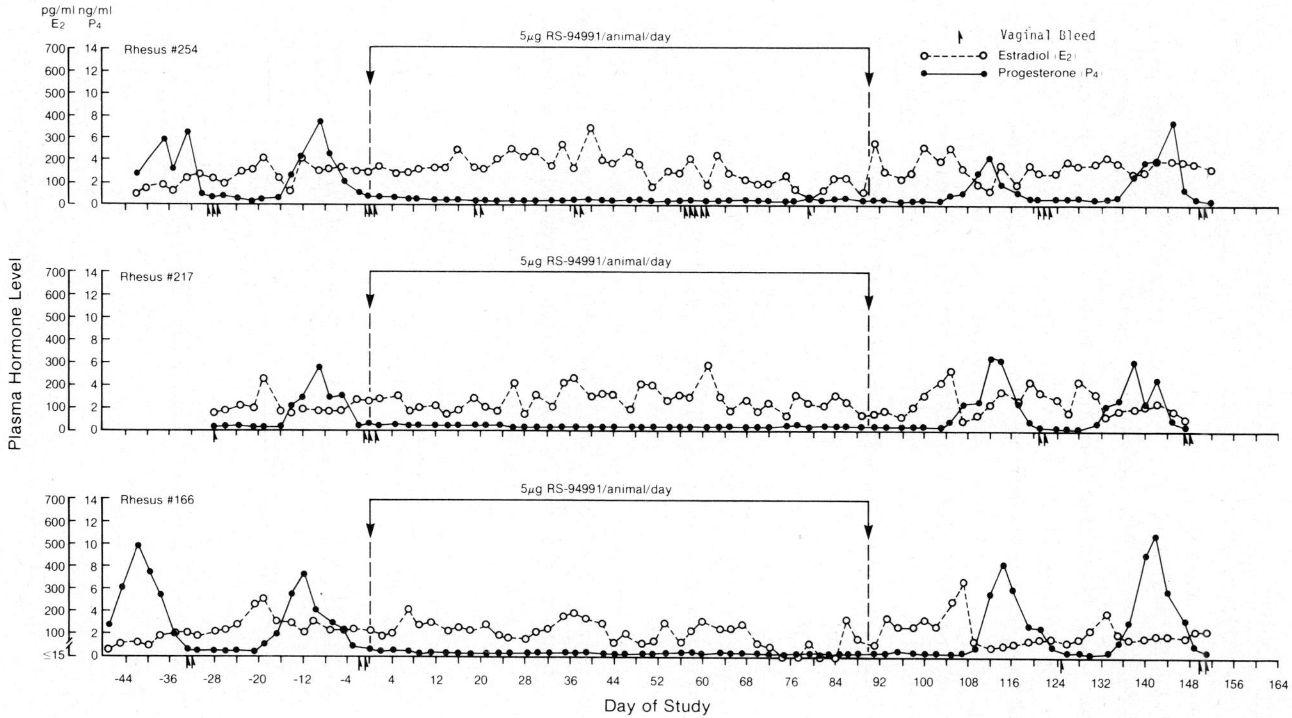

Figure 6: Plasma levels of estradiol and progesterone and menstrual flow pattern in three female rhesus monkeys before, during and after 90 consecutive days of treatment with 5 μg of nafarelin.

The high potency of nafarelin in the monkey was addressed through metabolism and dispositional studies. The plasma $t_{\frac{1}{2}}$ of nafarelin and LHRH after intravenous administration were found to be 120 and 33 minutes, respectively. In addition, the rate of systemic clearance of nafarelin was 12 times slower than that of LHRH, while the volume of distribution of nafarelin was 3.5 times smaller than that of LHRH. In summary, nafarelin remained in the plasma at higher concentrations for a longer period of time than did LHRH. Some explanations for these observations were provided by the findings that: a) the enzymes present in the plasma of rhesus monkeys rapidly metabolize LHRH, but not nafarelin; and b) nafarelin is highly bound to plasma proteins (80%) in contrast to LHRH (25%), which could act as a circulatory depot of nafarelin and slow down its metabolism.

Nasal Administration in Monkeys

Having established the biological effects of nafarelin in animal models, the feasibility and the potential of intranasal administration of nafarelin by various formulations were evaluated. As by injection, a dose-dependent inhibition of ovulation was observed following daily administration of nafarelin in the dose range of 62-250 µg, which was administered as a 100 µl-spray from a metered-dose pump. The 250 µg/day was determined to be the completely effective dose (Fig. 7), which produced a biological activity equivalent to 5 µg/day by injection, indicating a relative bioefficacy of ~2%.

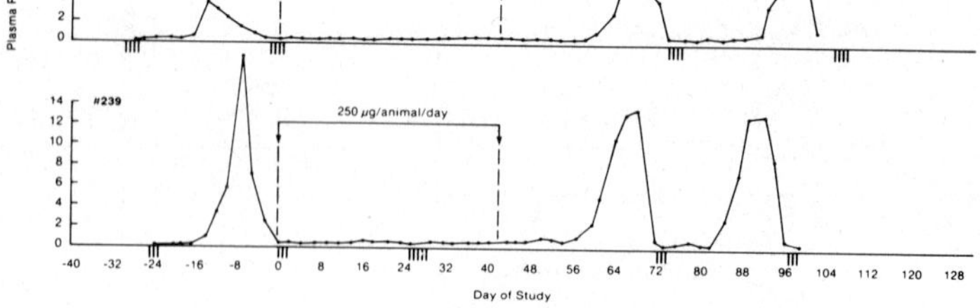

Figure 7. Plasma levels of progesterone and menstrual flow pattern in three female rhesus monkeys before, during and after 42 days of the consecutive daily intranasal administrations of 250 µg of nafarelin.

While evaluation of ovulation-inhibiting activity is a valid demonstration of the absorption of nafarelin, such an assay, however, lacks the precision required for quantitative measurement of absorption. For further work on the optimization of nasal absorption, a highly sensitive and specific radioimmunoassay method was developed (ref. 16). When this assay method was used to quantitate the actual circulating levels of nafarelin in the plasma of rhesus monkeys following various nasal doses, a non-linear profile was obtained (Fig. 8). The administered dose was varied by administering a constant volume of the drug solution with different concentrations. However, the data in Figure 8 suggested that a proportionality exists between absorption and concentration.

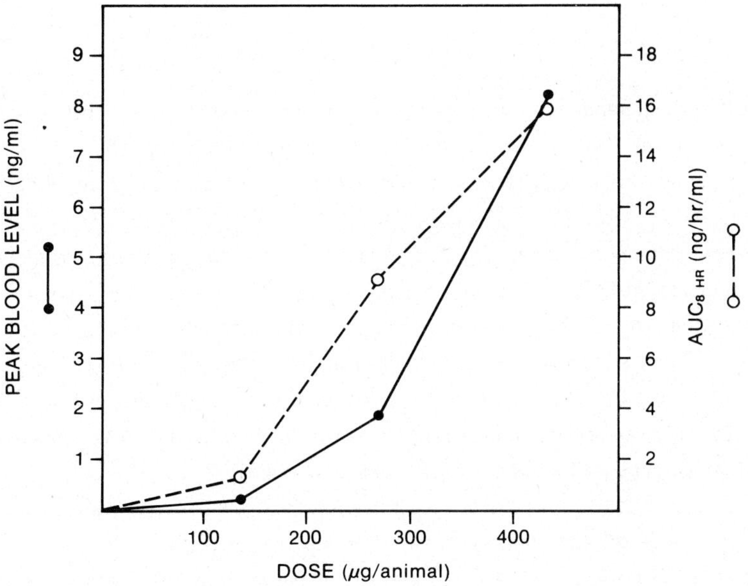

Figure 8. Effect of dose on the peak blood levels and the area under the curve (AUC), measured over an 8-hour period, following the intranasal administration of nafarelin in monkeys.

In fact, when the blood levels were normalized to the concentration of nafarelin in the solution administered (Fig. 9), it became clear that there is a linear correlation between absorption and concentration.

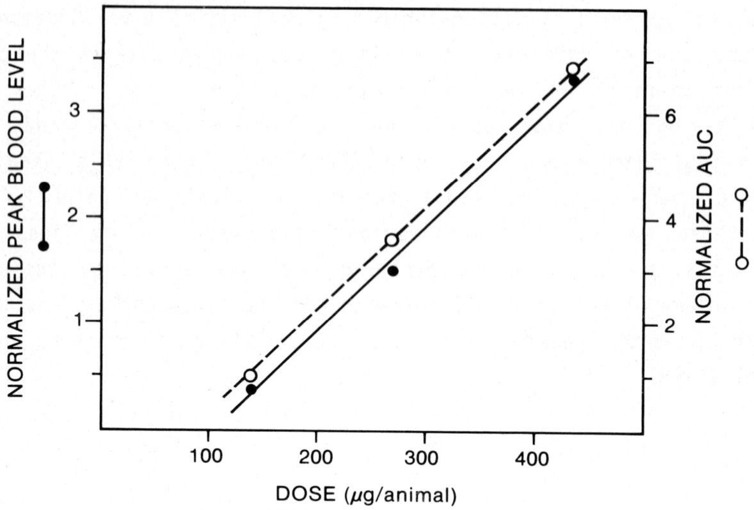

Figure 9. Linear dependency of the peak blood levels and the area under the curve (AUC), which have been normalized by the concentration of nafarelin, on the doses administered intranasally to monkeys.

Therefore, the results suggested that, at least in these monkeys, the intranasal bioavailability can be enhanced and maximized by administration of a concentrated solution. The reasons for this correlation are not known, although it is conceivable that saturation of the degradative enzymes in the nasal mucosa could play some role. In practice, the upper limit of this correlation is restricted by the solubility of nafarelin in the appropriately buffered and preserved solutions, i.e., 2.5-3.0 mg/ml.

Clinical Evaluations of Intranasal Nafarelin Administration

Extensive evaluations of the clinical pharmacology of nafarelin in both men (ref. 17) and women (ref. 18) by injection had confirmed the intrinsic potency of this analog in the clinical setting. Determination of the blood levels of nafarelin following intranasal administration in men and women confirmed the relevance of the results generated in monkeys. Again, increase of drug concentration in the dosage administered was observed to enhance the nasal bioavailability. The circulatory $t_{1/2}$ of the compound administered nasally was found to be rather similar to that by subcutaneous injection (Fig. 10).

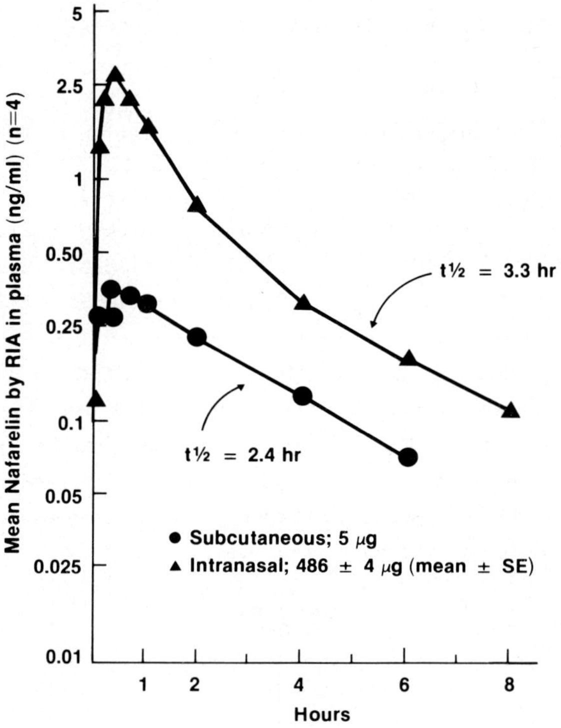

Figure 10. Plasma disappearance curves in the women following the subcutaneous injection of 5 μg or the intranasal administration of 486 (±4) μg of nafarelin.

Plasma protein binding of nafarelin, acting as an effective depot for the drug, was again observed. The combination of relatively high bioavailability (5%) and prolonged plasma $t_{\frac{1}{2}}$ and extensive plasma protein binding would be expected to yield a high efficacy for intranasal administration. This was demonstrated by the studies in which the biological efficacy was assayed by the inhibition of ovulation and by the time to the suppression of ovarian steroidogenesis (Table 2).

TABLE 2. INHIBITION OF OVULATION AND SUPPRESSION OF OVARIAN HORMONAL FUNCTION BY NAFARELIN ACETATE FOLLOWING INTRANASAL SPRAY

Dose (μg/day)	No. of Subjects	Ovulation Not Suppressed	Luteinization	Anovulation	E_2 <30 40 Days	pg/ml in 20 Days
125	6	3(50%)	2(33%)	1(17%)	-	-
250	5	0(0%)	2(40%)	3(60%)	1(20%)	0(0%)
500	2	0(0%)	0(0%)	2(100%)	2(100%)	0(0%)
1000	6	0(0%)	0(0%)	6(100%)	2(33%)	4(67%)

In fact, the relative bioavailability determined by biological effect increased to 10% when judged by the time needed for the achievement of postmenopausal estrogen levels. This finding was applied to the treatment of endometriosis, and the results indicated that the intranasally administered nafarelin is extremely therapeutic, whether judged by regression of the lesions (ref. 19), or by relief of the pain (Fig. 11).

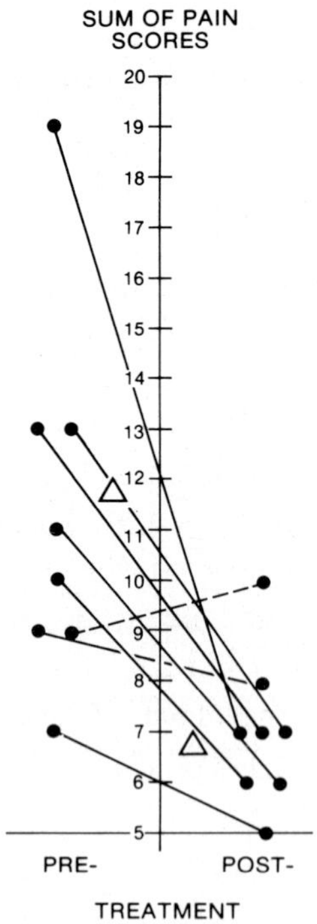

Figure 11. Pain scores in women with endometriosis prior to and after the 6 months of daily intranasal treatment with 500 μg of nafarelin keys: (●) individual patients; (△) average of all values.

The efficacy noted in the treatment of endometriosis by intranasal nafarelin administration has encouraged us to pursue this route of administration also for other indications. Ongoing trials include idiopathic true precocious puberty and prostatic carcinoma. Literature reports on other agonists have indicated a poor response to the nasal medication alone, although intranasal administration instituted following a course of injectable therapy seems to be efficacious (ref. 20, 21). Preliminary results with nafarelin suggest that nasal treatment alone will be adequate in these syndromes.

In addition, the results of an ongoing contraceptive trial, involving the intranasal administration of nafarelin to women, indicated that even the lowest daily dose tested (125 μg) has resulted in complete anovulation and a high percentage of cases of amenorrhea and hot flashes (ref. 22). The data clearly suggested that once-a-day intranasal administration will be a convenient and sufficient modality for female contraception.

At present, it appears that the only potential utility of LHRH agonists which may not be achieved by intranasal administration is the control of male fertility. In fact, the attainment of azoospermia in men has proven remarkably elusive even by injectable therapy (ref. 23, 24). There is some suggestion that a continuously circulating blood level of LHRH agonists is required (ref. 25, 26). Whether this is simulated by the "megadose"-type injectable therapy with leuprolide, a potent LHRH analog, in prostatic carcinoma patients (ref. 27) or whether the noted absence of spermatogenesis in such cases is more a reflection of the debilitating effects of the disease (ref. 28) is not known. However, the use of absorption enhancing agents has recently been reported to increase the transmucosal bioavailability of other LHRH analogs by 4-6 folds in animal models (ref. 29). If the resistance of the male to the treatment is merely a question of dose, then perhaps the addition of these or other enhancers to the formulation, particularly in combination with the LHRH analogs as highly potent as nafarelin, may allow even this indication to respond to intranasal administration.

REFERENCES

1) P. E. Belchetz, T. M. Plant, Y. Nakai, E. J. Keogh, and E. Knobil, Hypophysial response to continuous and intermittent delivery of hypothalamic gonadotropin-releasing hormone, Science, 202 631 (1978).
2) T. F. Davies, A. Gomez-Pan, M. J. Watson, C. A. Mountjoy, J. P. Hanker, G. M. Besser, and R. Hall, Reduced "gonadotropin response to releasing hormone" after chronic administration to impotent men, Clin. Endocrinol. (Oxf), 6 213 (1977).
3) C. Bergquist, S. J. Nillius, G. Skarin, and L. Wide, Inhibitory effects on gonadotrophin secretion and gonadal function in men during chronic treatment with a potent stimulatory luteinizing hormone-releasing hormone analogue, Acta Endocrinol. (Copenh), 91 601 (1979).
4) J. DeKonig, J. A. M. J. Van Dieten, and G. P. Van Rees, Refractoriness of the pituitary gland after continuous exposure to luteinizing hormone releasing hormone, J. Endocrinol., 79 311 (1978).
5) R. N. Clayton, unpublished data.
6) R. N. Clayton, and K. J. Catt, Receptor-binding affinity of gonadotrophin-releasing hormone analogs: analysis by radioligandreceptor assay, Endocrinology, 160 1154 (1980).
7) A. J. W. Hsueh, and G. F. Erickson, Extrapituitary action of gonadotropin-releasing hormone: direct inhibition of ovarian steroidogenesis, Science, 204 854 (1979).
8) A. J. W. Hsueh, unpublished data.
9) J. J. Nestor, Jr., T. L. Ho, R. A. Simpson, B. L. Horner, G. H. Jones, G. I. McRae, and B. H. Vickery, The synthesis and biological activity of some very hydrophobic analogs of luteinizing hormone releasing hormone, J. Med. Chem., 25 795 (1982).
10) B. H. Vickery, G. I. McRae, W. Briones, A. Worden, R. Seidenberg, B. D. Schanbacher, and R. Falvo, Effects of an LHRH agonist analog upon sexual function in male dogs: suppression, reversibility and effect of testosterone replacement, J. Androl., 5 28 (1984).
11) B. H. Vickery, G. I. McRae, and H. Bonasch, Effect of chronic administration of a highly potent LHRH agonist upon prostatic size and function in geriatic dogs, The Prostate, 3 123 (1982).
12) L. M. Glode, J. Robinson, and S. F. Gould, Protection from cyclophosphamide-induced testicular damage with an analogue of gondotropin-releasing hormone, Lancet, May 2 1132 (1981).
13) L. M. Glode, J. Robinson, S. F. Gould, T. M. Nett, and D. Mervill, Protection of spermatogenis during chemotherapy, Drug Exptl. Clin. Res., 8 367 (1982).
14) D. V. Link, D. P. Waller, J. C. Goodpasture, L. J. D. Zaneveld, and B. H. Vickery, Effects of combined cyclophosphamide-doxorubicin on male reproductive function in dogs, The Pharmacologist, 25 229 (1983).
15) J. Goodpasture, E. Bostwick, K. Bergstrom, and B. H. Vickery, Dog reproductive parameters during and after long term cyclophosphamide administration, J. Androl., 5 16 (1984) (abstract).
16) C. Nerenberg, J. Foreman, N. Chu, M. D. Chaplin, and S. Kushinsky, Radioimmunoassay of nafarelin ([6-(3-(2-naphthyl)D-alanine)]LHRH) in plasma or serum. Anal. Biochem., (1984) in press.
17) D. Heber, R. S. Swerdloff, and M. Henzl, Effects of nafarelin acetate in men. In: LHRH and Its Analogs: Contraceptive and Therapeutic Applications, (B. H. Vickery, J. J. Nestor, Jr., E. S. E. Hafez, Eds.), MTP Press, Lancaster, (1984) p. 257.
18) S. E. Monroe, M. R. Henzl, M. C. Martin, E. Schriock, V. Lewis, S. Kushinsky, C. Nerenberg, and R. B. Jaffe, Ablation of folliculogenesis in women by a single dose of gonadotropin releasing hormone agonist: significance of time in cycle, Fertil. Steril. (1984) in press.

19) E. Schriock, S. E. Monroe, M. R. Henzl, and R. B. Jaffe, Treatment of endometriosis with nafarelin acetate, a potent GnRH agonist, New Engl. J. Med., (1984) in press.
20) A. S. Lider, F. J. Holland, D. C. Costigan, M. R. Jenner, G. Wielgosz, and A. T. A. Fazekas, Intranasal and subcutaneous treatment of central precocious puberty in both sexes with a long acting analog of luteinizing hormone-releasing hormone, J. Clin. Endocrinol. Metab., 58 966 (1984).
21) N. Faure, A. Lemay, G. Tolis, F. Labrie, A. Belanger, and A. T. A. Fazekas, Buserelin therapy for prostatic carcinoma. In: LHRH and Its Analogs: Contraceptive and Therapeutic Applications, (B. H. Vickery, J. J. Nestor, Jr., E. S. E. Hafez, Eds.) MTP Press, Lancaster, (1984) p. 337.
22) S. J. Nillius, C. Bergquist, J. Gudmundsson, and L. Wide, Superagonists of LHRH for contraception in women, J. Steroid Biochem., 20 1373 (1984) (abstract).
23) C. Bergquist, S. J. Nillius, T. Berg, G. Skarin, and L. Wide, Inhibitory effects on gonadotropin secretion and gonadal function in men during chronic treatment with a potent stimulatory luteinizing hormone-releasing hormone analogue, Acta Endocrinol (Copenh), 91 601 (1979).
24) G. Doelle, R. M. Evans, A. N. Alexander, and D. Rabin, Antifertility effects of an LHRH agonist in men. In: LHRH and Its Analogs: Contraceptive and Therapeutic Applications, (B. H. Vickery, J. J. Nestor, Jr., E. S. E. Hafez, Eds.) MTP Press, Lancaster, (1984) p. 271.
25) F. Bint Akhtar, G. R. Marshall, E. J. Wickings, and E. Nieschlag, Reversible induction of azoospermia in rhesus monkeys by constant infusion of a GnRH agonist using osmotic minipumps, J. Clin. Endocrinol. Metabl., 56 534 (1983).
26) F. Bint Akhtar, G. F. Weinbauer, G. H. Vickery, L. M. Sanders, and E. Nieschlag, Pituitary and testicular function in rhesus monkeys under long term sustained release of [D-Nal(2)^6] LHRH in Abstract of 3rd Joint Meeting, British Endocrine Societies, Edinburgh, Scotland, (1984).
27) R. J. Santen, B. Warner, L. M. Demers, M. Dufau, and J. A. Smith, Jr., Leuprolide therapy for prostatic carcinoma. In: LHRH and Its Analogs: Contraceptive and Therapeutic Applications (B. H. Vickery, J. J. Nestor, Jr., E. S. E. Hafez, Eds.). MTP Press, Lancaster, (1984) p. 351.
28) J. Rajfer, R. S. Swerdloff, and D. Heber, Human testicular morphologic characteristics after chronic GnRH analog therapy, Fertil. Steril., 39 440 (1983) (abstract).
29) H. Okada, I. Yamazaki, T. Yashiki, T. Shimamoto, and H. Mima, Vaginal absorption of a potent luteinizing hormone-releasing hormone analogue (leuprolide) in rats. IV: Evaluation of the vaginal absorption and gonadotropin responses by radioimmunoassay, J. Pharm. Sci., 73 298 (1984).

Transnasal Systemic Medications, edited by Y.W. Chien
Elsevier Science Publishers B.V., Amsterdam, 1985 – Printed in The Netherlands

INTRANASAL ADMINISTRATION OF INSULIN EFFICACY AND MECHANISM

J. S. Flier, A. C. Moses, G. S. Gordon, and R. S. Silver
Department of Medicine, Beth Israel Hospital
M. C. Carey
Department of Medicine, Brigham and Women's Hospital
Boston, Massachusetts

ABSTRACT

Studies were conducted to assess the feasibility of administering insulin to man by a nasal spray. Effective administration requires the incorporation of an adjuvant molecule, such as a bile salt (i.e. sodium deoxycholate). In this chapter, the characteristics of insulin administered nasally as a spray with bile salt in normal and diabetic humans will be described. In addition, some recent insights into the structural basis for bile salt activity and possible mechanisms of adjuvant activity will be discussed. Finally, the potential utility of nasally administered insulin in the treatment of diabetes will be outlined.

INTRODUCTION

The treatment of diabetic patients with insulin currently requires that they receive daily parenteral injections. These injections are certainly lifesaving in patients with Type I diabetes, and they are often necessary for metabolic control in patients with Type II diabetes. Nonetheless, hypodermic injection is not an ideal means for insulin delivery. The local discomfort and the perceived lifestyle disruption caused by daily injections deter many patients with Type I diabetes from accepting intensive insulin treatment regimens. In addition, many patients with Type II diabetes refuse to accept insulin therapy entirely. For these reasons, many investigators have attempted to develop alternate, nonparenteral routes of insulin administration, such as enterally, with and without liposome encapsulation (ref. 1, 2), rectally (ref. 3), vaginally (ref. 4), and through the respiratory epithelium (ref. 5). Unfortunately, these attempts have generally met with minimal enthusiasm due to limited and variable absorption of insulin.

Another possible and as yet poorly explored means of insulin delivery is via application to the nasal mucosa. It is already known that certain small peptides can be absorbed through the nasal mucosa as a snuff or directly from aqueous solution (ref. 6-8). However, absorption has typically been low and variable, and many therapeutically important peptides with a larger molecular size, including insulin, are not absorbed to any significant degree. Recent work demonstrating that certain adjuvant molecules can enhance insulin absorption across the nasal mucosa (ref. 9-11) has increased the interest in the potential utility of intranasally administered insulin.

Published reports on attempts to administer insulin by the transnasal route date back to the early 1930's (ref. 12). More recently, Hirai et al. (ref. 9) and Pontiroli et al. (ref. 10) have demonstrated that mixtures of insulin and the solutions of bile salts (glycocholate) or other surface-active agents cause an increase in serum insulin levels sufficient to lower the blood glucose concentration. However, these reports failed to answer the questions regarding the kinetics, reproducibility, and efficacy of this route of insulin administration. As a result, little attention has been focused on these reports. Very recently, this issue has been readdressed and data have been presented that when insulin is mixed with an appropriate bile salt, it can be delivered to the bloodstream by the nasal route with reproducible kinetics and acceptable efficiency (ref. 11).

This chapter will primarily focus on recent work related to the intranasal delivery of insulin aided by adjuvant molecules.

NASAL INSULIN DELIVERY IN NORMAL SUBJECTS

The initial studies involved the administration of insulin-bile salt sprays to 25 control subjects and a limited number of patients with Type I and Type II diabetes in the fasting state (ref. 11). The commercially available regular porcine insulin (U-500) and highly purified Na deoxycholate were used and delivered by a commercial pump spray device at a volume of approximately 80 µl/spray. The results indicated that in the presence of 1% Na deoxycholate, the insulin level in the blood varied linearly with the concentration of insulin in the spray administered (Figure 1).

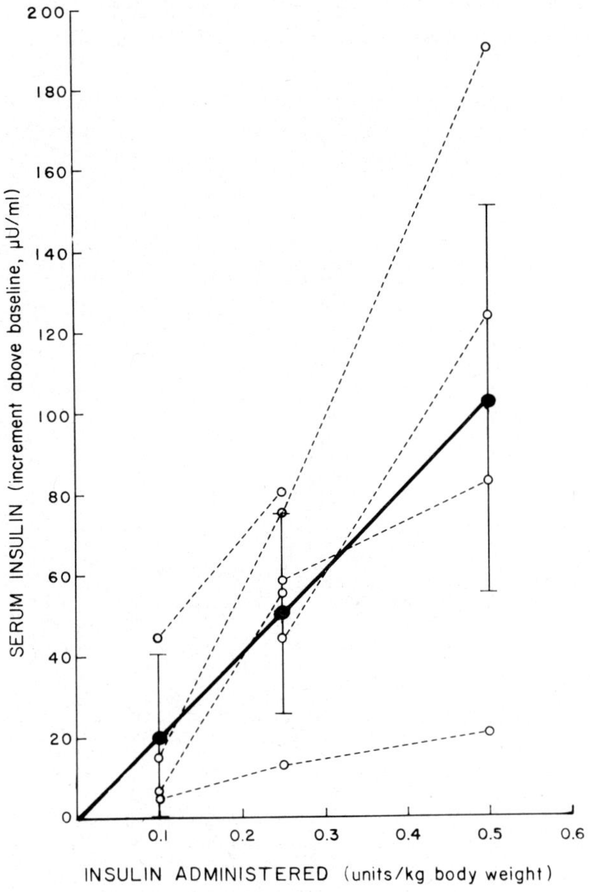

Figure 1: Insulin absorption following graded doses of insulin delivery. Six normal volunteers were administered graded doses of insulin (range: 0.1-0.5 U/kg) in 1% (w/v) Na deoxycholate. Individual responses are shown by the open symbols and dashed line for each subject. The solid symbols and solid line represent the mean peak serum insulin concentration above baseline (for all subjects achieved at each insulin dose). The numbers of subjects studied at each dose were: 0.1 U/kg, N=4; 0.25 U/kg, N=6; 0.5 U/kg, N=5.

When 0.5 U of insulin/kg body weight were administered to a group of subjects, a mean peak plasma insulin level of 110 μU/ml was achieved (Figure 2).

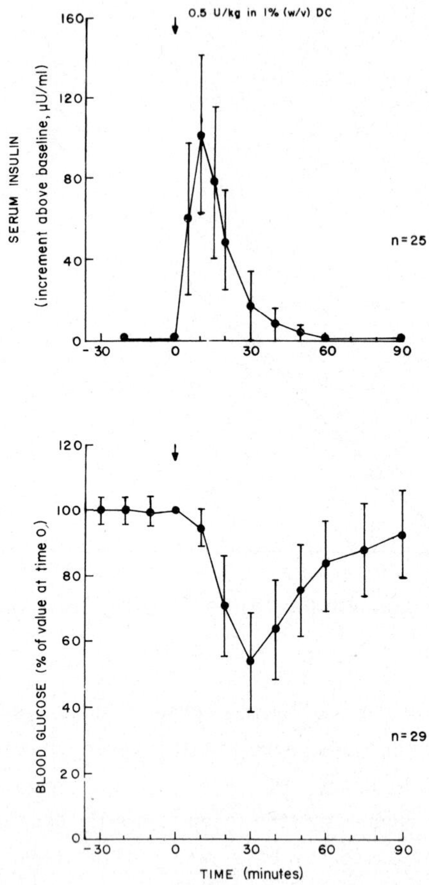

Figure 2: Upper panel: Serum insulin levels (mean ± 1 SD) for 25 normal subjects who received a nasal spray of 0.5 U insulin/kg in 1% (w/v) deoxycholate at time 0. Lower panel: Blood glucose as percentage of the value at time 0 (mean ± 1 SD) versus time for 29 normal subjects who received 0.5 U insulin/kg-1% (w/v) deoxycholate nasal spray at time 0.

The kinetic pattern of nasal insulin absorption with this approach was highly reproducible, with the peak insulin level seen between 10 to 15 minutes after administration. Following the peak level, the plasma insulin concentration fell rapidly with a half-life of approximately 6 minutes. In any one individual given the same dose of insulin, plasma insulin concentrations varied relatively little on multiple administrations. The plasma glucose level was observed to fall in a predictable manner in response to intranasal insulin delivery in normal individuals (Figure 2). In essentially all cases, 0.5 U insulin given intranasally resulted in a 40-60% reduction in the blood glucose level by 30 minutes, followed by a spontaneous rebound of the blood glucose concentration secondary to the expected counterregulatory hormone responses.

Through the comparisons with intravenous administration, it was estimated that between 10 and 20% of nasally administered insulin reaches the bloodstream (Figure 3).

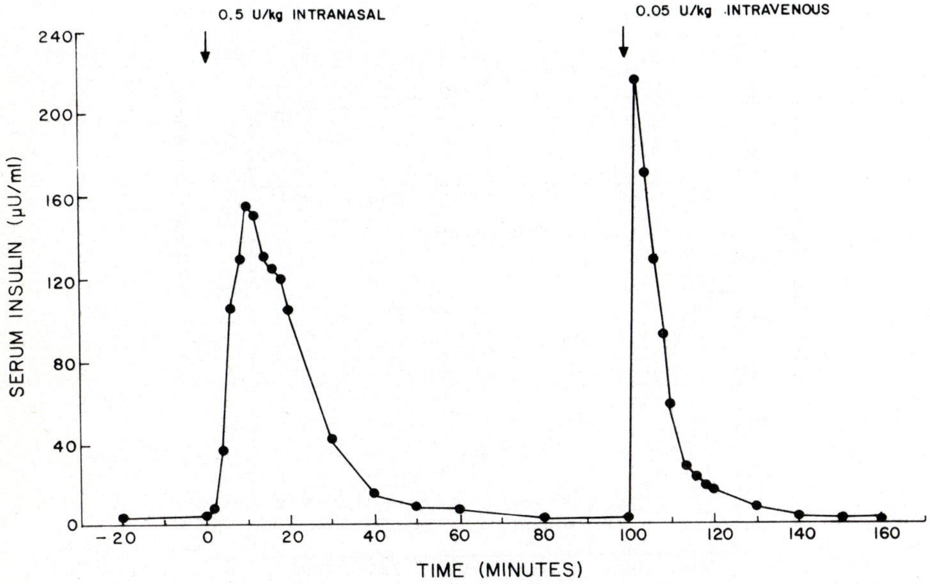

Figure 3: Serum insulin levels in a volunteer who received intranasal administration of 0.5 U/kg in 1% (w/v) deoxycholate as a nasal spray, followed by intravenous injection of 0.05 U/kg. Insulin was administered at the time indicated by the arrows.

NASAL INSULIN DELIVERY IN PATIENTS WITH DIABETES

1) Fasting state:

When insulin is delivered nasally with sodium deoxycholate, the peak plasma insulin levels in the diabetic patients are very similar to those seen in the normal subjects. This is true with respect to both the kinetics and the peak serum insulin levels attained. The pattern of blood glucose responses is somewhat different in diabetics, however. In these individuals, with both Type I and Type II diabetes, the plasma glucose concentrations were observed to fall steeply for the first hour after the insulin nasal spray to a level which is approximately 30-40% below the baseline. In most cases, the plasma glucose concentrations remained at this lower level for the next 3-5 hour (Figure 4).

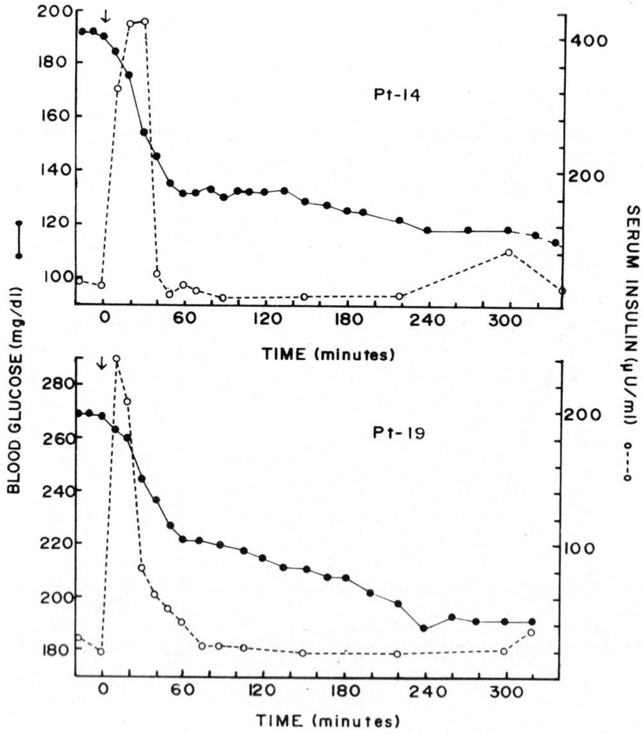

Figure 4: Upper panel: Serum insulin (o---o) and blood glucose (●---●) levels in 2 patients with Type II diabetes following intranasal aerosol administration of 0.5 U insulin/kg with 1% (w/v) deoxycholate (arrow).

In a few individuals, in whom the counterregulatory responses to hypoglycemia is developed, the blood glucose level gradually restored itself despite the continued fasting over the next several hours.

2) Fed State:

More recent studies have demonstrated that when insulin is delivered nasally at mealtime, it serves as an effective buffer against the meal-related rises in the blood glucose level (ref. 13). In these studies, insulin was administered, as a nasal spray, within the first 15-30 minutes after the beginning of the test meal. The results were equivalent among the Type I diabetic patients, who usually take ultralente or NPH insulin, the Type II diabetic patients, who normally receive NPH or Lente insulin, and the Type II diabetic patients, who have never before been treated with insulin. In each case, the nasally administered insulin was found to be extremely effective at reducing or ablating the meal-related hyperglycemia. Moreover, the risk of postprandial hypoglycemia associated with this therapy appeared to be very low.

MECHANISM OF ADJUVANT ACTION

Within the gastrointestinal tract, bile salts are well known to promote the transmembrane movement of endogenous and exogenous lipids (ref. 14) as well as the transmembrane and/or paracellular movement of such small polar molecules as water, electrolytes, aspirin, and oxalate (ref. 15). Because of these functions as well as their surface-active properties on the biomembranes (ref. 16), bile salts have been viewed as potential adjuvants for the transmucosal delivery of drugs, and they have been widely explored for this purpose. Although the micellar properties of bile salt molecules and the details of their interactions with membranes and exogenous lipids have been extensively studied by physical techniques, little is known about the mechanisms by which these molecules enhance the transmucosal absorption of drugs.

As demonstrated experimentally, bile salts were reported to promote the nasal absorption of insulin in man as well as in the laboratory animals. Nevertheless, some previous studies in rats employing a range of bile salt species failed to define any useful structure-activity relationships (ref. 17). Extensive structure-activity studies were recently carried out on a series of purified naturally-occurring bile salts to evaluate their ability to enhance insulin absorption across the human nasal mucosa, when administered as an insulin-bile salt nasal spray. A dramatic difference was noted between bile salt species with closely related structures in their capacity to promote insulin absorption (Figure 5).

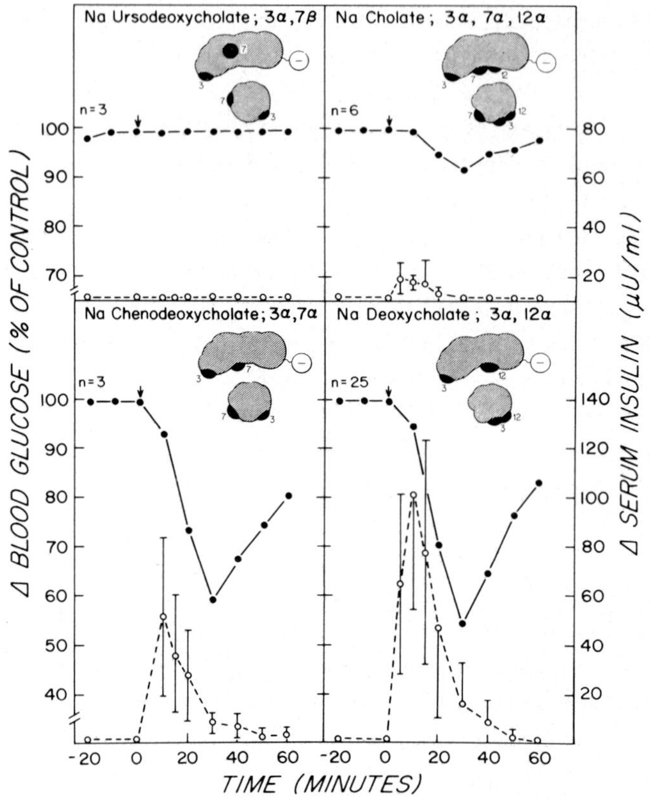

Figure 5: Four different bile salts were administered by spray to normal volunteers as 1% solution with insulin (0.5 U/kg). Blood glucose levels (•), are indicated by per cent of the control (=100%), and plasma insulin levels (o), are indicated by the change over baseline. The arrows indicate the time when insulin-bile salt solution spray was given. The inserts show the schematic representations, in two projections, of bile salt structures.

The efficacy of the bile salts tested was found to be determined by the hydrophobic-hydrophilic balance of the hydroxyl-substituted steroidal nucleus and not by the overall molecule, since the conjugation with polar side groups only reduced the net hydrophobicity, but did not decrease the adjuvant potency of bile salts (ref. 18). This information suggests the strategies for the future development of a safe and effective adjuvant agent.

One of the major objectives in our attempts to develop an adjuvant for the transmucosal administration of insulin or other polypeptides is to identify an effective compound that would not cause local or systemic toxicity. Each of the unconjugated bile salts tested so far was noted to produce some local nasal irritation, as indicated by a brief (3-5 minute) burning sensation in the nose. However, this irritation did not correlate with the adjuvant activity of the bile salt in the structure-activity studies. It was observed that some subtle alterations in the bile salt structure have yielded profoundly different effects on the adjuvant activity and the nasal irritation potential. It also was discovered that the adjuvant activity can be predicted from the physical chemistry of the monomers. These observations raise the possibility that bile salts or related molecules can be structurally engineered to retain the adjuvant activity in promoting the transmucosal drug absorption without retaining the components which potentially produce the toxic side effects.

FUTURE DEVELOPMENTS

We believe that the preliminary data generated so far suggest the potential application of the nasal route for the effective delivery of insulin. The kinetics of transnasal insulin delivery aided by adjuvants would potentially make it suitable for the mealtime administration with the goal of blunting the meal-related hyperglycemia. For this purpose, nasal insulin may be superior to other routes of administration currently available for this treatment. Because of its ease of administration and expected patient acceptability, intensification of the insulin treatment regimes with the aid of intranasal administration could potentially lead to a widespread improvement in glycemic control in both Type I and Type II diabetics. The possibility that in some patients with mild Type II diabetes, in which the transnasal insulin alone might suffice as a therapy, needs further exploration. Further studies of adjuvant molecules aimed at improving their efficacy and reducing their potential of mucosal irritation is certainly necessary and is ongoing.

REFERENCES

1) G. A. Harrison; Insulin in alcoholic solution by mouth, Br. Med. J., 1204-1205 (1923).
2) M. Shichiri, R. Kawamori, Y. I. Goriya, M. Kikuchi, Y. Yamasaki, Y. Shigeta, and H. Abe; Increased intestinal absorption of insulin in a micellar solution: water-in-oil-in-water insulin micelles, Acta. Diabetol. Lat., 15 175-183 (1978).
3) Y. Yamaski, M. Shichiri, R. Kawamori, M. Kikuchi, T. Yaki, S. Arai, R. Tohdo, N. Hakui, N. Oji, and H. Abe; The effectiveness of rectal administration of insulin suppository in normal and diabetic subjects, Diabetes Care, 4 454-458 (1981).
4) N. F. Fisher; The absorption of insulin from the intestine, vagina and scrotal sac., Am. J. Physiol., 67 65-71 (1923).

5) F. M. Wigley, O. H. J. London, S. H. Wood, J. C. Shipp, and R. H. Waldman; Insulin across respiratory mucosa by aerosol delivery, Diabetes, 20 552-556 (1971).
6) A. M. Dashe, C. R. Kleeman, J. W. Czarczkes, H. Rubinoff, and I. Spears; Synthetic vasopressin nasal spray in the treatment of diabetes insipidus, JAMA, 190 113-115 (1964).
7) H. G. Solbach and W. Wiegelmann; Intranasal application of luteinizing-hormone releasing hormone, Lancet, 1 1259 (1973).
8) G. Baumann, A. Walser, P. A. Desaulles, F. J. A. Paesi, and L. Geller; Corticotropic action of an intranasally applied synthetic ACTH derivative, J. Clin. Endocrinol. Metab., 42 60-63 (1975).
9) S. Hirai, T. Ikenaga, and T. Matsuzawa; Nasal absorption of insulin in dogs, Diabetes, 27 296-299 (1978).
10) A. E. Pontiroli, M. Alberetto, A. Secchi, G. Dossi, I. Bosi, and G. Pozza; Insulin given intranasally induces hypoglycemia in normal and diabetic subjects, Br. Med. J., 294 303-306 (1982).
11) A. C. Moses, G. S. Gordon, M. C. Carey and J. S. Flier; Insulin administered as an insulin-bile salt aerosol, Diabetes, 32 1040-1047 (1983).
12) W. S. Collens and M. A. Goldzeiher; Absorption of insulin by nasal mucous membrane, Proc. Exp. Biol. and Med., 29 756 (1932).
13) R. D. Silver, A. C. Moses, M. C. Carey, and J. S. Flier; Insulin-bile salt nasal aerosol markedly reduces postprandial glycemic excursion in diabetics, Diabetes, 33 75A (Abst. No. 299)(1984).
14) M. C. Carey; In The Liver, Biology and Pathobiology (I. M. Arias, H. Popper, D. Schacter and D. Shafritz, Eds.) Raven Press, New York (1982) pp. 429-465.
15) E. L. Forker; Mechanisms of hepatic bile formation, Ann. Rev. Physiol., 39 323 (1977)
16) M. C. Carey; In Bile Acids in Gastroenterology (E. Roda and L. Barbara, Eds.) MTP Press, Boston (1983) pp. 19-56.
17) S. Hirai, T. Yashiki, and H. Mima; Effect of surfactants on the nasal absorption of insulin in rats, Internat. J. Pharmaceut., 9 165 (1981).
18) A. C. Moses, J. S. Flier, G. S. Gordon, R. D. Silver, and M. C. Carey; Transnasal insulin delivery: structure-function studies of absorption enhancing adjuvants, Clinical Research, 32 245A (1984).